D1597714

Human Hybridomas and Monoclonal Antibodies

Human Hybridomas and Monoclonal Antibodies

Edited by

Edgar G. Engleman and
Steven K. H. Foung

Stanford University Medical Center
Stanford, California

James Larrick and
Andrew Raubitschek

Cetus Immune Research Laboratories
Palo Alto, California

Plenum Press • New York and London

Library of Congress Cataloging in Publication Data

Main entry under title:

Human hybridomas and monoclonal antibodies.

Includes bibliographies and index.
  1. Antibodies, Monoclonal. 2. Hybridomas. I. Engleman, Edgar C. [DNLM: 1. Antibodies, Monoclonal. 2. Hybridomas. 3. Immunologic Technics. QW 575 H918]
QR186.85.H86   1985   616.99′4079   85-12401
ISBN 0-306-41982-3

©1985 Plenum Press, New York
A Division of Plenum Publishing Corporation
233 Spring Street, New York, N.Y. 10013

Printed in the United States of America

Contributors

JULIAN L. AMBRUS, JR., Laboratory of Immunoregulation, National Institute of Allergy and Infectious Disease, National Institutes of Health, Bethesda, Maryland 20205

ANN ARVIN, Department of Pediatrics, Stanford University School of Medicine, Stanford University Medical Center, Stanford, California 94305

MAKOTO ASADA, Division of Chemical Toxicology and Immunochemistry, Faculty of Pharmaceutical Sciences, University of Tokyo, Tokyo 113, Japan

TSEHAY ATLAW, Department of Microbiology and Immunology, Queen's University, Kingston, Ontario, Canada K7L 3N6

CLAUDIA J. BENIKE, Department of Pathology, Stanford University School of Medicine, Stanford University Medical Center, Stanford, California 94305

MARCIA BIEBER, Cancer Biology Research Laboratory, Department of Radiology, Stanford University School of Medicine, Stanford, California 94305

WARREN C. BOGARD, JR., Centocor, Malvern, Pennsylvania 19355

S. J. L. BOL, Rotterdam Radiotherapeutic Institute, Rotterdam, The Netherlands.

R. L. H. BOLHUIS, Rotterdam Radiotherapeutic Institute, Rotterdam, The Netherlands

PETER BRAMS, Cancer Biology Laboratory, State University Hospital (Rigshospitalet), DK-2100 Copenhagen, Denmark

KAREN G. BURNETT, Hybritech, San Diego, California 92121

JOSEPH L. BUTLER, Laboratory of Immunoregulation, National Institute of Allergy and Infectious Disease, National Institutes of Health, Bethesda, Maryland 20205. *Present address:* Division of Pediatric Rheumatology, University of Alabama in Birmingham, Birmingham, Alabama 35294

BARBARA G. CAMPLING, Department of Medicine and Radiation Oncology, Queen's University, Kingston, Ontario, Canada K7L 3N6

DENNIS A. CARSON, Scripps Clinic and Research Foundation, La Jolla, California 92037

TONY CHAN, Cetus Immune Research Laboratories, Palo Alto, California 94303

SUSAN P. C. COLE, Department of Microbiology and Immunology, Queen's University, Kingston, Ontario, Canada K7L 3N6

RICHARD J. COTE, Memorial Sloan-Kettering Cancer Center, New York, New York 10021

STEVEN COUTRE, Department of Pathology, Stanford University School of Medicine, Stanford University Medical Center, Stanford, California 94305

DOROTHY H. CRAWFORD, Department of Haematology, Faculty of Clinical Sciences, University College London, London WCIE 6HX, England

CARLO M. CROCE, The Wistar Institute of Anatomy and Biology, Philadelphia, Pennsylvania 19104

KATHLEEN A. DENIS, Departments of Microbiology and Immunology, UCLA School of Medicine, Los Angeles, California 90024

BRADLEY J. DYER, Cetus Immune Research Laboratories, Palo Alto, California 94303

AUDREY M. EATON, Cetus Immune Research Laboratories, Palo Alto, California 94303

EDGAR G. ENGLEMAN, Department of Pathology, Stanford University School of Medicine, Stanford University Medical Center, Stanford, California 94305

KARIM ESSANI, Laboratory of Oral Medicine, National Institute of Dental Research, National Institutes of Health, Bethesda, Maryland 20205

ANTHONY S. FAUCI, Laboratory of Immunoregulation, National Institute of Allergy and Infectious Disease, National Institutes of Health, Bethesda, Maryland 20205

BRIAN M. FENDLY, Cetus Immune Research Laboratories, Palo Alto, California 94303

DIANNE FISHWILD, Department of Pathology, Stanford University School of Medicine, Stanford University Medical Center, Stanford, California 94305

STEVEN K. H. FOUNG, Department of Pathology, Stanford University School of Medicine, Stanford University Medical Center, Stanford California 94305

KIRK E. FRY, Cancer Biology Research Laboratory, Department of Radiology, Stanford University School of Medicine, Stanford, California 94305

CARLO GARZELLI, Laboratory of Oral Medicine, National Institute of Dental Research, National Institutes of Health, Bethesda, Maryland 20205

MARK C GLASSY, Cancer Center, University of California, San Diego, and Veterans Administration Medical Center, San Diego, California 92103

C. GRAVEKAMP, Rotterdam Radiotherapeutic Institute, Rotterdam, The Netherlands

F. CARL GRUMET, Department of Pathology, Stanford University School of Medicine, Stanford University Medical Center, Stanford, California 94305

A. HAGEMEIJER, Department of Cell Biology and Genetics, Erasmus University, Rotterdam, The Netherlands

HAROLD H. HANDLEY, Cancer Center, University of California, San Diego, and Veterans Administration Medical Center, San Diego, California 92103

WOLF HANISCH, Cetus Corporation, Emeryville, California 94608.

SARAH M. HART, Cetus Immune Research Laboratories, Palo Alto, California 94303

JOAN M. HEBERT, Cancer Biology Research Laboratory, Department of Radiology, Stanford University School of Medicine, Stanford, California 94305

MASAHIRO HIGUCHI, Division of Chemical Toxicology and Immunochemistry, Faculty of Pharmaceutical Sciences, University of Tokyo, Tokyo 113, Japan

JOHN A. HIRST, Memorial Sloan-Kettering Cancer Center, New York, New York 10021

MICHAEL K. HOFFMANN, Memorial Sloan-Kettering Cancer Center, New York, New York 10021

ELIZABETH HORNBERGER, Centocor, Malvern, Pennsylvania 19355

ALAN N. HOUGHTON, Memorial Sloan-Kettering Cancer Center, New York, New York 10021

SYLVIA T. HSIEH-MA, Cetus Immune Research Laboratories, Palo Alto, California 94303

MARK C. JAHNSEN, Cetus Immune Research Laboratories, Palo Alto, California 94303

JEFFREY A. KASSEL, Cetus Immune Research Laboratories, Palo Alto, California 94303

YOSHIRO KOBAYASHI, Division of Chemical Toxicology and Immunochemistry, Faculty of Pharmaceutical Sciences, University of Tokyo, Tokyo 113, Japan

DANUTA KOZBOR, The Wistar Institute of Anatomy and Biology, Philadelphia, Pennsylvania 19104

PATRICK C. KUNG, Centocor, Malvern, Pennsylvania 19355. *Present address:* T cell Sciences, Inc., Lexington, MA 02173

KIT S. LAM, Cancer Biology Research Laboratory, Department of Radiology, Stanford University School of Medicine, Stanford, California 94305

JAMES W. LARRICK, Cetus Immune Research Laboratories, Palo Alto, California 94303

JUNMING LE, Department of Microbiology, New York University School of Medicine, New York, New York 10016

JULIA P. LEUNG, Hybritech, San Diego, California 92121

JEFFREY LIFSON, Department of Pathology, Stanford University School of Medicine, Stanford University Medical Center, Stanford, California 94305

DAVID LIPPMAN, Cetus Immune Research Laboratories, Palo Alto, California 94303

MARK E. LOSTROM, Genetic Systems, Seattle, Washington 98121

JOANNE MARTINIS, Hybritech, San Diego, California 92121

LLOYD MAYER, Department of Medicine, Division of Gastroenterology, Mount Sinai Medical Center, New York, New York 10029

RONALD C. McGARRY, Department of Microbiology and Immunology, Queen's University, Kingston, Ontario, Canada K7L 3N6

NAHID MOHAGHEGHPOUR, Department of Pathology, Stanford University School of Medicine, Stanford University Medical Center, Stanford, California 94305

RICHARD MOSS, Children's Hospital at Stanford, Palo Alto, California 94305

ABNER LOUIS NOTKINS, Laboratory of Oral Medicine, National Institute of Dental Research, National Institutes of Health, Bethesda, Maryland 20205

LENNART OLSSON, Cancer Biology Laboratory, State University Hospital (Rigshospitalet), DK-1200 Copenhagen, Denmark

TOSHIAKI OSAWA, Division of Chemical Toxicology and Immunochemistry, Faculty of Pharmaceutical Sciences, University of Tokyo, Tokyo 113, Japan

SUSAN PERKINS, Department of Pathology, Stanford University School of Medicine, Stanford University Medical Center, Stanford, California 94305

WOLF PRENSKY, Department of Hematology-Oncology, Hahnemann University Hospital, Philadelphia, Pennsylvania 19102

ANDREW A. RAUBITSCHEK, Cetus Immune Research Laboratories, Palo Alto, California 94303. *Present address:* Radiation Oncology Branch, National Cancer Institute, National Institutes of Health, Bethesda, Maryland 20205.

GREGORY R. REYES, Cancer Biology Research Laboratory, Department of Radiology, Stanford University School of Medicine, Stanford, California 94305

DAVID B. RING, Cetus Immune Research Laboratories, Palo Alto, California 94303

JOHN C. RODER, Department of Microbiology and Immunology, Queen's University, Kingston, Ontario, Canada K7L 3N6

IVOR ROYSTON, Cancer Center, University of California, San Diego, and Veterans Administration Medical Center, San Diego, California 92103

JO SATOH, Laboratory of Oral Medicine, National Institute of Dental Research, National Institutes of Health, Bethesda, Maryland 20205

ANDREW SAXON, Department of Medicine, UCLA School of Medicine, Los Angeles, California 90024

JIM SCHRODER, Folkhalsan Institute of Genetics, Helsinki 10, Finland

ROBERT S. SCHWARTZ, Hematology-Oncology Division, New England Medical Center, Boston, Massachusetts 02111

GEORGE SENYK, Cetus Immune Research Laboratories, Palo Alto, California 94303

JERRY W. SHAY, Department of Cell Biology, University of Texas Health Science Center at Dallas, Dallas, Texas 75235

ROSY SHENG-DONG, Cetus Immune Research Laboratories, Palo Alto, California 94303

YEHUDA SHOENFELD, Department of Medicine "D" (Research Laboratory of Autoimmune Diseases), Beilinson Medical Center, Petach Tiqva, Israel

ANTHONY W. SIADAK, Genetic Systems, Seattle, Washington 98121

FLOYD TAUB, Laboratory of Oral Medicine, National Institute of Dental Research, National Institutes of Health, Bethesda, Maryland 20205

NELSON N. H. TENG, Department of Gynecology and Obstetrics, Stanford University School of Medicine, Stanford, California 94305

FRANK TRINGALE, Cetus Immune Research Laboratories, Palo Alto, California 94303

SHU-ICHI TSUCHIYA, Division of Chemical Toxicology and Immunochemistry, Faculty of Pharmaceutical Sciences, University of Tokyo, Tokyo 113, Japan

MARY A. VALENTINE, Scripps Clinic and Research Foundation, La Jolla, California 92037

JAN VILČEK, Department of Microbiology, New York University School of Medicine, New York, New York 10016

RANDOLPH WALL, Departments of Microbiology and Immunology, UCLA School of Medicine, Los Angeles, California 90024

JANET WANG, Cetus Immune Research Laboratories, Palo Alto, California 94303

HOWARD WEINTRAUB, Cetus Immune Research Laboratories, Palo Alto, California 94303

Preface

Soon after Köhler and Milstein described the use of somatic cell hybridization for the production of murine monoclonal antibodies of desired specificity, this relatively simple technique became widely applied. Indeed, production of murine monoclonal antibodies is now considered routine by immunologists and nonimmunologists alike. However, as heterologous proteins, mouse monoclonal antibodies have one major limitation: they are immunogenic in man and, hence, their use *in vivo* is severely limited. An obvious solution to this problem is to produce human hybridomas with the same techniques used for the production of rodent hybrids. Unfortunately, the history of human hybridomas has been marked by substantive and often exasperating technical problems, and the first reports of hybrids secreting human immunoglobulin of desired specificity did not appear until 1980. These reports were met with initial enthusiasm, but it soon became apparent that while human lymphocytes might be fused, their frequency, level of Ig synthesis, and stability were such that production of human antibodies with this method was neither routine nor practical. Nonetheless, a sufficient number of investigators persevered, and during the next 5 years relatively efficient B-cell fusion partners as well as improved methods of Epstein–Barr virus transformation were developed. Generation of human T–T hybrids has also been achieved, although problems of chromosomal stability remain a substantial obstacle, more so than with B-cell lines.

In our view, sufficient progress has been made in the field to allow for the large-scale production of human hybridomas and their products, and on this basis it seemed to us an appropriate time to pool as much information as possible on the subject in the form of this monograph. Our purpose was not only to summarize the state of the art with representative examples, but, more importantly, to present sufficient methodologic detail to allow and encourage interested investigators to use these techniques. Partly because so many investigators have been frustrated in the past with attempts to produce human hybridomas, a rather detailed "how-to" appendix is included, following the pattern set in earlier monographs on mouse hybridoma technology.

We realize that some of the methods described here are likely to become obsolete, replaced by newer techniques, such as direct transformation of T cells for the generation of permanent lines and the use of recombinant DNA technology to produce human antibodies of desired specificity. In addition, as large-scale production of lymphoid products becomes a matter of routine, new challenges will emerge that relate primarily to improving product efficacy *in vivo*—for example, the need to deliver antibodies or lymphokines to particular sites or organs and the desire to combine antibodies or lymphokines with other substances (e.g., toxins, drugs, hormones) in order to increase potency or target specificity. No doubt, these topics will form the basis of an expanding research effort. More importantly, they serve to remind those of us who feel that a new era of immunodiagnosis and therapy with human lymphocyte products is close at hand that we have not quite arrived. Thus, while the contents of this book demonstrate how far we have come in learning how to produce lymphoid cell lines and their products, we do not yet know how best to use them.

Toward this end, the role of industry is large and becoming larger, as well it should be if the products are to be produced on a large scale and applied to clinical problems. This expanding industrial role is reflected by the fact that two of the four editors of this book are employed on a full-time basis at one company, and four chapters on human monoclonal antibodies were contributed by industry-based investigators. The future success of our field will depend on the continued willingness of scientists in different settings to share their findings and their know-how. So far, at least, the protection afforded by the patent process and the benefits to investigators based in either industrial or academic settings of peer recognition and participation in information exchange have been sufficient to overcome the inevitable obstacles. It is to be hoped that this trend will continue as the impact of our field increases.

Finally, we would like to acknowledge the support and patience of our respective families during the time-consuming preparation of this book. In addition, we would like to thank Kirk Jensen of Plenum Press for encouraging and facilitating this work, and we thank Dianne Jacobs and Joan Murphy for their excellent secretarial assistance.

Edgar G. Engleman
Steven K. H. Foung
James W. Larrick
Andrew A. Raubitschek

Contents

3 Production of Human Monoclonal Antibodies Using Epstein–Barr
Virus

DOROTHY H. CRAWFORD

4 The Epstein–Barr Virus-Hybridoma Technique

JOHN C. RODER, SUSAN P. C. COLE, TSEHAY ATLAW, BARBARA C.
CAMPLING, RONALD C. MCGARRY, AND DANUTA KOZBOR

5 Strategies for Stable Human Monoclonal Antibody Production:
Construction of Heteromyelomas, in Vitro Sensitization, and
Molecular Cloning of Human Immunoglobin Genes

NELSON N. H. TENG, GREGORY R. REYES, MARCIA BIEBER, KIRK
E. FRY, KIT S. LAM, AND JOAN M. HEBERT

16 Principles of *in Vitro* Immunization of Human B Lymphocytes
   MICHAEL K. HOFFMANN AND JOHN A. HIRST

E. Special Topics

17 Human–Human Hybridomas in the Study of Immunodeficiencies
   KATHLEEN A. DENIS, RANDOLPH WALL, AND ANDREW SAXON

PART II HUMAN T–T HYBRIDOMAS

18 Human T-Lymphocyte Subsets and T–T Hybridomas: An
  Overview

22 Selection of Human T-Cell Hybridomas That Produce
    Inflammatory Lymphokines by the Emetine–Actinomycin D
    Method

TOSHIAKI OSAWA, YOSHIRO KOBAYASHI, MAKOTO ASADA,
MASAHIRO HIGUCHI, AND SHU-ICHI TSUCHIYA

23 Human T–T Hybridomas Specific for Epstein-Barr Virus:
    Generation and Function

MARY A. VALENTINE AND DENNIS A. CARSON

24 Factors Generated by Human T-Cell Hybridomas Regulate B-Cell
    Activation, Polyclonal Differentiation, and Isotype Expression

1
Human Hybridomas and Monoclonal Antibodies
The Biology of Cell Fusion

Jerry W. Shay

I. Introduction

In this review I will cover, from a cell biologist's perspective, the biology of cell fusion and how the information derived from the field may be applicable to the production of human monoclonal antibodies. I will describe the development of the hybridoma technology, the advantages and disadvantages of making and using monoclonal antibodies, the methods and limitations of making human monoclonal antibodies, the freezing and thawing of hybridomas, and end with a discussion of chromosome segregation in cell hybrids.

II. Historical Development of Hybridomas

Hybridoma technology is the culmination of advances in several unrelated fields of research. The fundamental progress achieved in cell culture techniques, somatic cell genetics, and immunology provided the framework for the birth of the hybridoma field (Table I). During the 1950s cell culture techniques were becoming more routine laboratory procedures and, once in place, set the stage for the development of cell hybridization procedures. Barski and co-workers (1960) observed spontaneous fusion of mouse cells in

Jerry W. Shay • Department of Cell Biology, University of Texas Health Science Center at Dallas, Dallas, Texas 75235.

TABLE I

A. Historical development of cell culture
    1907 Harrison: First reproducible technique for growing cells *"in vitro"*
    1912 Carrel: The continuous cultivation of cells *"in vitro"*
    1943 Earle *et al.*: First continuous monolayer and suspension rodent cultures (L cells) established from single cells
    1952 Gey *et al.*: First continuous cell line derived from a human tumor (HeLa)

B. Historical development of cell fusion
    1960 Barski *et al.*: First observation of spontaneous fusion of cells in cultures
    1962 Okada and Tadokoro: First demonstration of Sendai virus-induced cell fusion
    1964 Littlefield: First description of HAT selection medium and the use of mutant cells to isolate hybrids
    1965 Harris and Watkins; Okada and Murayama; Ephrussi and Weiss: Production of hybrids by fusing cells from different species
    1967 Weiss and Green: Demonstration that both genomes are expressed in hybrids, with preferential segregation of chromosomes of one species (chromosome mapping)
    1975 Pontecorvo: Demonstration of polyethylene glycol (PEG) fusion

C. Historical development of hybridoma
    1962 Potter and Boyce: Passage of myeloma tumors in murine hosts
    1973 Cotton and Milstein: Demonstration that fusion of two antibody-producing mouse myeloma cell lines results in hybrids expressing products of both parental lines
    1973 Schwaber and Cohen: Demonstration that fusion of human lymphocytes with mouse myeloma results in hybrids that secrete myeloma- and lymphocyte-derived immunoglobulins
    1975 Köhler and Milstein: Demonstration that fusion of immunized mouse spleen cells to mouse myeloma results in hybrids that secrete antibodies determined by prior immunization (hybridoma)
    1980 Olsson and Kaplan: Fusion of human spleen cells to human myeloma to establish human–human hybridomas
    1980 Croce *et al.*: Fusion of a human lymphocyte cell line to peripheral blood cells from a patient with subacute sclerosing panencephalitis to establish human–human hybridomas

culture. Okada and Tadokoro (1962) reported that certain viruses could increase the number of fused cells from a rare, spontaneous event to a highly efficient and predictable event. Even though at this point the actual process of cell fusion was more efficient, there still was not an easy method for isolating the hybrid cells from the unfused cells. The description of the HAT selective medium and the use of mutant cell lines to isolate hybrids by Littlefield (1964) solved this problem. The principle behind HAT selection is as follows: Cells can make DNA either using a salvage pathway or by *de novo* synthesis. The drug aminopterin (the "A" in HAT) blocks *de novo* synthesis, thus requiring cells to use salvage or scavenger pathways, which depend on the presence of DNA precursors (hypoxanthine and thymidine) and the enzymes hypoxanthine-guanine phosphoribosyltransferase (HGPRT) and thymidine kinase (TK). In the presence of aminopterin and excess hypoxanthine and thymidine (HAT medium) cells will proliferate and survive as long as they have the enzymes TK and HGPRT. However, if a cell mutant is deficient in either TK or HGPRT, it will not survive in HAT medium. (See Appendix, Chapter 2 for preparation of mutant cell lines).

Littlefield took two mutant cell types, one lacking the TK enzyme but having HGPRT and the other lacking the HGPRT enzyme but having TK. These enzyme deficiencies are not detrimental to the cell under the usual culture conditions, since cells can still make DNA using folic acid via *de novo* synthesis. It is only when the *de novo* pathway is blocked with aminopterin that cells with these enzyme deficiencies cannot proliferate. Littlefield fused these enzyme-deficient cells to each other and observed that only the hybrids could grow in HAT medium. The hybrid cells survived in the selection medium because each parental cell complemented the deficiency of the other parental cell. Unfused parental cells or parental cells fused to like cells (homokaryons) did not survive, since they were still deficient in TK or HGPRT.

The method for selecting mutant cells and hybrids was adequate for cells that grew indefinitely in cell culture, but was not appropriate for normal diploid cells with a finite life in culture. The length of time required to select for cell mutants at the TK and HGPRT loci generally precludes their use in the HAT system. Davidson and Ephrussi (1965) adapted the HAT selective system to isolate hybrids by fusing a mutant cell to a normal cell containing no selectable marker. In the "half-selective" method the mutant parental cells die in the presence of HAT medium. This medium does not interfere with the growth of diploid cells, but, since they grow slowly and form a monolayer background, the hybrid cells form discrete multilayered colonies on top of the normal cells. Hybridoma technology essentially uses this same selection system (e.g., mutant myelomas fused to nonproliferating spleen cells grown in the presence of a selective agent). I will return to this selection system later in this review, when I discuss some ideas about improving hybridoma production.

While these advances in cell fusion and somatic cell genetic techniques were occurring, progress was also taking place in the field of immunology, specifically in the area of B-cell production of antibodies. Immunologists discovered that the spleen was a rich source of B cells and that some of them were producing antibodies. It was also discovered that once a particular B cell was committed to produce antibodies against a specific antigen, all descendants of that B cell produced only the one specific antibody. Thus, monoclonality of antibody production was discovered.

During this period Potter and Boyce (1962) reported the successful passaging of myeloma tumors in mice, and a few years later some of these tumors were established in cell culture. Some of these cell lines were mutagenized, resulting in enzyme-deficient cell lines. Cotton and Milstein (1973) demonstrated that fusion of two antibody-producing mouse myeloma cell lines resulted in hybrids expressing the products of both parental lines. In the same year Schwaber and Cohen (1973) demonstrated that fusion of human lymphocytes with mouse myeloma cells resulted in hybrids that secreted myeloma- and lymphocyte-derived immunoglobulins. Thus, the stage was set for the now classic observation of Köhler and Milstein (1975) in which they demonstrated that fusion of immunized spleen cells to mouse myeloma cells resulted in hybrids that secreted antibodies determined by prior immunization.

During the next few years, numerous refinements in this basic technique were reported. It was not until 1980 that Olsson and Kaplan (1980) and Croce and co-workers (1980), independently and by quite different approaches, described human–human hybridomas. Olsson and Kaplan fused human spleen cells to human myeloma cells and isolated hybrids secreting human antibodies determined by prior immunization. Croce and co-workers fused a human lymphoblastoid cell line to peripheral blood cells from a patient with subacute sclerosing panencephalitis and isolated hybrids secreting human antibodies.

Hybridoma technology has clearly had a major impact in many aspects of the basic sciences and in clinical medicine. However, along with the numerous advantages and benefits of this technology, some difficulties and technical problems remain to be resolved. Some of these areas will be discussed in this chapter.

III. Problems with Conventional Immunization

In the simplest terms, when a complex antigen, such as a protein, is introduced into an animal, it contains many antigenic determinants. The result is that many B cells will be stimulated to produce antibodies directed against the antigen. This occurs even when a highly purified antigen is used as an immunizing agent. The result is that sera obtained from immunized animals are heterogeneous. This can be reduced, but not eliminated, by appropriate absorptions. The main problems with conventional immunization are: (1) the unpredictability of the immune response (low titers, immunogenic to minor contaminants, weak or lack of antibody production of some antigens); (2) the heterogeneity of even highly specific antibodies (cross-reactivity, variations in affinity and in class and subclass); (3) the supply is often limited; (4) the identical antibody cannot be made in a new animal or from a second or third bleeding of the same animal (every bleeding is a new reagent); and (5) the procedure is relatively expensive and time-consuming.

IV. Advantages of the Monoclonal Antibody Technology

The monoclonal antibody technology provides a tool to overcome most but not all of the limitations of conventional immunization. These advantages and benefits of hybridoma technology include: (1) the monoclonal antibody is obtained from one isolated clone and is therefore homogeneous and predictable; (2) pure antibodies can be made to impure (even unknown) antigens; (3) theoretically unlimited amounts of antibody can be obtained (10–100 μg/ml from cell cultures, 1–10 mg/ml when grown in mouse ascites); (4) one can detect components in a mixture that are present in small quantities not detectable by conventional antisera; (5) the monoclonal antibody is available when needed and indefinitely; and (6) the technology is less expensive and may be less time-consuming than conventional immunization.

V. Difficulties and Technical Problems in the Production of Monoclonal Antibodies

Monoclonal antibodies are not without their problems and should not be considered better than conventional (polyclonal) antisera for all occasions. For example, some problems that were not initially appreciated include: (1) cell culture contamination [bacteria, fungi, yeast, or mycoplasma (see Appendix, Chapter 4, for mycoplasma testing and eradication procedures)]; (2) sluggish growth or even lack of growth of isolated colonies; (3) problems inherent in homogeneity (limited biological function, unusual sensitivity to inactivation by changes in pH, temperature, salt concentration, freezing, and thawing); (4) difficulty in obtaining monoclonals against weak immunogens; (5) lack of agglutinating and precipitatory properties; and (6) loss of antibody production (often occurs in 50% of the original positive clones).

Some of these problems are avoided by improved sterile techniques and by isolating enough positive colonies to allow the investigator simply to ignore colonies that do not perform as expected. However, a few aspects of this technology are potentially troublesome. For instance, a monoclonal antibody may bind to an epitope (the site on the antigen that forms the antigenic-determinant structure) shared by several antigens and thus may result in more cross-reactions than do polyclonal antibodies. For example, Lee et al. (1984) reported that in a single fusion experiment using glial filaments as an immunogen, clones were obtained producing monoclonal antibodies that recognized an epitope shared by glial and vimentin-type intermediate filaments. Another clone from this one fusion experiment produced an antibody that recognized a neurofilament protein. Thus, careful immunochemical and immunohistochemical characterizations of monoclonal antibodies are necessary if meaningful biological insights are to be gained. On a positive note, monoclonal antibodies that recognize unique and shared determinants from a variety of what initially appear to be different molecules may contribute new understandings of protein evolution and by that route increase our understanding of biological function.

To solve the problem of obtaining monoclonal antibodies against rare determinants when a multicomponent immunogen is used, Milstein and Lennox (1980) and Springer (1981) have described a cascading procedure to prepare antibodies directed against the rarer epitopes. Specifically, animals are immunized with the complex immunogen and cell fusion is obtained by standard techniques. The monoclonal antibodies produced by the various clones are mixed and used to prepare an affinity column. Once prepared, the affinity column is used to remove from the initial complex immunogen those epitopes to which antibodies have been made. The components that do not bind to the affinity column (e.g., the rarer epitopes) are now used as immunogens and reinjected into animals. A second group of monoclonal antibodies is then produced against determinants not recognized in the initial experiments. Theoretically, this procedure can be repeated several times until monoclonal antibodies are obtained against progressively rarer determinants (Payne, 1983).

Another problem that may occur from the use of monoclonal antibody technology is that the antibody may have a low and fixed affinity, which may not produce the identifying reaction pattern obtained with a polyclonal serum, and therefore make the antibody unsuitable for use in a sensitive assay system. Ehrlich *et al.* (1982, 1983) have reported that mixing of two monoclonal antibodies directed against different epitopes yielded up to tenfold enhanced affinity for antigen, so as to circumvent this problem. Even though some basic problems need further study, monoclonal antibody technology is enormously powerful and will be most effective when used in combination with, rather than in place of, the conventional production of polyclonal antibodies.

VI. Human Hybridomas and Monoclonal Antibodies

Monoclonal antibody technology has proven useful in several areas, including: (1) routine serology and tissue typing; (2) diagnosis and epidemiology of infectious agents; (3) identification of tumor antigens and tumor origins; and (4) identification of functional subpopulations of lymphoid cells. Almost all of these uses of the monoclonal antibody technology are based on mouse or rat hybrids. However, in order to use this technology to its fullest clinical potential in such areas as passive immunization or delivery of diagnostic or therapeutic agents in humans, it will be necessary to develop systems for reliability producing human monoclonal antibodies. As recently reported by Nose and Wigzell (1983) and reviewed by Larrick and Buck (1984), human monoclonal antibodies have species-specific carbohydrates, which are important in several antibody effector functions. Therefore, mouse monoclonal antibodies would appear to be of limited usefulness in treating humans. In addition, anti-mouse immunoglobulin responses in many cancer patients have limited the usefulness of mouse monoclonal antibodies (Levy and Miller, 1983; Miller *et al.*, 1983).

Thus, we come to the challenge of today, which is to make human hybridomas. As I mentioned earlier (Table I), the first reports of human monoclonals occurred in 1980. Human monoclonals have been obtained by several methods, but, unfortunately, they all have limitations that at present impede their usefulness in treating patients.

VII. Methods for Making Human Monoclonal Antibodies

There are basically two methods for producing human monoclonal antibodies: (1) cell hybridization and (2) viral transformation. Cell hybridization can be divided into two subcategories: (1) mouse–human hybrids and (2) human–human hybrids. Human–human hybrids can be produced by fusing immunized B lymphocytes to either human myeloma [Epstein–Barr virus (EBV)-negative] or human B-cell lymphoblastoid cells (EBV-positive). The second method to produce human monoclonal antibodies is *in vitro* viral transformation by SV40 or EBV of sensitized lymphocytes into permanent monoclonal antibody-producing cell lines.

VIII. Limitations in Making Human Monoclonal Antibodies

The principal problem with mouse myeloma fused to sensitized human lymphocytes is the instability of these hybrids. For years it has been known that in mouse–human hybrids, human chromosomes are preferentially segregated (eliminated), so that extensive subcloning is required to obtain stable antibody-producing hybrids. An area of basic research that has been surprisingly neglected concerns why human chromosomes are eliminated in mouse–human hybrids. I will return to a discussion of this topic later and propose experiments that may improve this method for the production of human monoclonal antibodies.

The main limitation with human myeloma fused to sensitized human lymphocytes can be summarized in one sentence: There is a severe lack of suitable human myeloma cell lines. Murine myeloma cells have been the subject of investigation for more than 20 years, whereas human myelomas have only rarely been established in culture. Considerable effort is in progress to develop human myeloma cell lines that will be suitable as the tumor fusion partner in making human hybridomas, which should greatly improve this approach in the future. In the meantime, an alternative to human myeloma cell lines is the use of B-cell lymphoblastoid cell lines (EBV$^+$) as the tumor fusion partner. Even though these cells grow well and can be fused to sensitized lymphocytes, the resulting hybridomas secrete only small amounts of immunoglobulin. This area remains promising, and a list of various human tumor cell lines currently in use as well as their source is compiled in the Appendix, Chapter 1.

Some hybridoma researchers believe that entirely too much attention has been directed to finding appropriate human tumor cell lines (Olsson et al., 1983). A different approach is to isolate donor-obtained immune lymphocytes or in vitro sensitized lymphocytes and to eternalize the antibody-producing cells by infection with EBV. (See Appendix, Chapter 11 and Crawford, this volume, Chapter 3, for a discussion of EBV transformation.) In theory this appears to be a good idea, but there are several limitations, which include: (1) the eternalized cells only produce low levels of antibody as compared with hybrids, (2) the cells often lose the ability to produce antibody; (3) the antibody is usually of the IgM class; and (4) only a small percentage of sensitized lymphocytes are eternalized by EBV transformation. This inability to obtain sufficient numbers of sensitized lymphocytes is perhaps the biggest obstacle in producing human hybridomas.

IX. Enrichment for Sensitized Lymphocytes and in Vitro Stimulation of Lymphocytes

Enrichment for appropriately sensitized B lymphocytes and/or in vitro stimulation of B lymphocytes is necessary for successful production of human monoclonal antibodies. Even though enriched lymphocytes have been obtained from lymph nodes, tonsils, and spleen, in most instances these approaches would not be appropriate in the clinical setting. Enrichment protocols for obtaining sensitized lymphocytes from peripheral blood mononuclear cells have been reported, including T-cell depletion (removal of suppressor lymphocytes) and precursor enrichment by rosetting or panning (Winger et al., 1983). Since there are relatively few circulating memory B lymphocytes in human peripheral blood, short-term expansion of B lymphocytes and/or EBV immortalization of the enriched precursors may be sufficient to increase the number of sensitized lymphocytes for cell hybridization. In vitro exposure of lymphocytes to antigen during short-term expansion followed by EBV transformation or hybridization may be the most effective approach. Various mitogens, lipopolysaccharides, and growth factors can stimulate lymphocyte growth in vitro without the use of viral agents, and basic research in this area appears promising.

line with the hypomethylating drug 5-azacytidine (J. W. Shay, unpublished observations). 5-Azacytidine induces various cell types to differentiate by an epigenetic modification of the methylation patterns of nuclear DNA. After treatment of the human cell line HT1080 with 5-azacytidine (5 μg/ml for 24 hr), we fused mouse LMTK$^-$ cells to the treated human cells and observed that the mean number of human chromosomes permanently retained in the hybrids significantly increased.

In support of this observation, Pravtcheva and Ruddle (1983) reported that the mouse X chromosome has the ability to switch the direction of chromosome segregation in mouse–Chinese hamster somatic cell hybrids and they suggested that there may be segregation reversal genes on the X chromosome. It could be proposed that in most hybridomas the loss of spleen cell chromosomes is an important cause of unstable antibody production and that, by activating certain genes via hypomethylation or by some other mechanism, one may improve the stability of the hybridomas. It has been demonstrated in hybridomas that heavy chain synthesis is lost before light chain synthesis and that these losses are correlated with the elimination of spleen cell chromosomes encoding the immunoglobulin genes. Use of HAT selection medium causes a large number of hybridomas to lose the X chromosome, which may account, in part, for the loss of the immunoglobulin gene. Thus, methods for selecting hybridomas that do not use HAT selection (Wright, 1978; Taggart and Samloff, 1983) may promote the growth of those hybridomas retaining spleen cell immunoglobulin genes.

Finally, recombinant DNA technologies may offer promise in the hybridoma field. Ochi *et al.* (1983) reported functional immunogloblin production after transfection of cloned immunoglobulin genes in lymphoid cells. If translation of immunoglobulin genes can be accomplished in bacterial host cells, then large-scale production of human monoclonal antibodies may become economically more feasible.

ACKNOWLEDGMENTS

This work was supported by grant PCM-8317788 from the NSF. I thank Dr. W. Wright for his helpful discussions.

References

Barski, G., Sorieul, S., and Cornefert, F., 1960, Production dans des cultures *in vitro* de deux souches cellulaires en association, de cellules de caractere "hybride," *C. R. Acad. Sci. Paris* **251:**1825–1827.

Brodin, T., Olsson, L., and Sjogren, H., 1983, Cloning of human hybridoma, myeloma and lymphoma cell lines using enriched human monocytes as feeder layer, *J. Immunol. Meth.* **60:**1–7.

Buttin, G., LeGuern, G., Phalente, L., Lin, E. C. C., Medrano, L., and Cazenave, P. A., 1978, Production of hybrid lines secreting monoclonal anti-idiotypic antibodies by cell fusion on membrane filters, in: *Lymphocyte Hybridoma* (I. Melchers, M. Potter, and N. L. Warner, eds.), Springer, Berlin, pp. 26–32.

Carrel, A., 1912, On the permanent life of tissues outside the organism, *J. Exp. Med.* **15**:516–528.

Clark, M. A., and Shay, J. W., 1978, Scanning electron microscopic observation on the mechanism of somatic cell fusion using polyethylene glycol, in: *Scanning Electron Microscopy/1978* (O. Johari and I. Corvin, eds.), Volume II, Chicago, Illinois, pp. 327–332.

Clark, M. A., and Shay, J. W., 1982, Long-lived cytoplasmic factors that suppress adrenal steroidogenesis, *Proc. Natl Acad. Sci. USA* **79**:1144–1148.

Clark, S. A., Stimson, W. H., Williamson, A. R., and Dick, H. M., 1981, Human hybridoma cell lines; A novel method of production, *J. Supramol. Struct. Cell Biochem. (Suppl.)* **5**:100a.

Cotton, R. G. H., and Milstein, C., 1973, Fusion of two immunoglobulin-producing myeloma cells, *Nature* **244**:42–43.

Croce, C. M., Linnenbach, A., Hall, W., Steplewski, Z., and Koprowski, H., 1980, Production of human hybridomas secreting antibodies to measles virus, *Nature* **288**:488–489.

Davidson, R. L., and Ephrussi, B., 1965, A selective system for the isolation of hybrids between L cells and normal cells, *Nature* **205**:1170–1171.

Davidson, R. L., and Gerald, P. S., 1976, Improved techniques for the induction of mammalian cell hybridization by polyethylene glycol, *Somat. Cell Genet.* **2**:165–176.

Davidson, R. L., O'Malley, K. A., and Wheeler, T. B., 1976, Polyethylene glycol-induced mammalian cell hybridization: Effect of polyethylene glycol molecular weight and concentration, *Somat. Cell Genet.* **2**:271–280.

Earle, W. R., Schilling, E. L., Stark, T. H., Straus, N. P., Brown, M. F., and Shelton, E., 1943, Production of malignancy *in vitro*. IV. The mouse fibroblast cultures and changes seen in the living cell, *J. Natl. Cancer Inst.* **4**:165–212.

Edwards, P. A. W., Smith, C. M., Neville, A. M., and O'Hare, M. J., 1982, A human/human hybridoma system based on a fast growing mutant of the ARH-77 plasma cell leukemia derived line, *Eur. J. Immunol.* **12**:641–648.

Ehrlich, P. H., Moyle, W. R., Moustafa, Z. A., and Canfield, R. E., 1982, Mixing two monoclonal antibodies yields enhanced affinity for antigen, *J. Immunol.* **128**:2709–2715.

Ehrlich, P. H., Moyle, W. R., and Moustafa, Z. A., 1983, Further characterization of cooperative interactions of monoclonal antibodies, *J. Immunol.* **131**:1906–1912.

Ephrussi, B., and Weiss, M. C., 1965, Interspecific hybridization of somatic cells, *Proc. Natl. Acad. Sci. USA* **53**:1040–1042.

Franklin, R. M., 1982, Microcomputer inventory systems for stored cell line, *J. Immunol. Meth.* **54**:141–157.

Gefter, M. C., Margulies, D. H., and Scharff, M. D., 1977, A simple method for polyethylene glycol promoted hybridization of mouse myeloma cells, *Somat. Cell Genet.* **2**:231.

Gey, G. O., Coffman, W. D., and Kubicek, M. T., 1952, Tissue culture studies of the proliferative capacity of cervical carcinoma and normal epithelium, *Cancer Res.* **12**:364–365.

Harris, H., and Watkins, J. F., 1965, Hybrid cells derived from mouse and man: Artificial heterokaryons of mammalian cells from different species, *Nature* **205**:640–646.

Harrison, R. G., 1907, Observations on the living developing nerve fiber, *Proc. Soc. Exp. Biol. Med.* **4**:140–143.

Hartwell, L. W., Bolognino, M., Bidlack, J. M., Knapp, R. J., and Lord, E. M., 1984, A freezing method for cell fusions to distribute and reduce labor and permit more thorough early evaluation of hybridomas, *J. Immunol. Meth.* **66**:59–67.

Herzenberg, L. A., Herzenberg, L. A., and Milstein, C., 1978, Cell hybrids of myelomas with antibody forming cells and T-lymphomas with T cells, in: *Handbook of Experimental Immunology*, 3rd ed. (Weir, D. M., ed.), F. A. Davis, pp. 25.1–25.7.

Jongkind, J. F., and Verkerk, A., 1982, Nonselective isolation of fibroblast heterokaryons, hybrids and cybrids by flow sorting, in: *Techniques in Somatic Cell Genetics* (J. W. Shay, ed.), Plenum Press, New York, pp. 81–100.

Jongkind, J. F., Verkerk, A., and Tanke, H., 1979, Isolation of human fibroblast heterokaryons with two-color flow sorting (FACS II), *Exp. Cell Res.* **120:**444–448.

Keeler, P. M., Person, S., and Snipes, S., 1977, A fluorescence enhancement assay of cell fusion, *J. Cell Sci.* **28:**167–177.

Köhler, G., and Milstein, C., 1975, Continuous cultures of fused cells secreting antibody of predefined specificity, *Nature* **256:**495–497.

Larrick, J. W., and Buck, D. W., 1984, Practical aspects of human monoclonal antibody production, *Bio Techniques* **1:**6–14.

Lee, V. M.-Y., Page, C. D., Wu, H.-L., and Schlaepfer, W. W., 1984, Monoclonal antibodies to gel-excised glial filament protein and their reactivities with other intermediate filament proteins, *J. Neurochem.* **42:**25–32.

Levy, R., and Miller, R. A., 1983, Tumor therapy with monoclonal antibodies, *Fed. Proc.* **42:**2650–2656.

Littlefield, J. W., 1964, Selection of hybrids from matings of fibroblasts *in vitro* and their presumed recombinants, *Science* **145:**709–710.

Mercer, W. E., and Schlegel, R. A., 1979, Phytohemagglutinin enhancement of cell fusion reduces polyethylene glycol toxicity, *Exp. Cell Res.* **120:**417–421.

Miller, R. A., Oseroff, A. R., Stratte, P. T., and Levy, R., 1983, Monoclonal antibody therapeutic trials in seven patients with T-cell lymphoma, *Blood* **62:**989–995.

Milstein, C., and Lennox, E., 1980, The use of monoclonal antibody technique in the study of developing cell surfaces, *Curr. Top. Dev. Biol.* **14:**1–32.

Norwood, T. H., Zeigler, C. J., and Martin, G. M., 1976, Dimethyl sulfoxide enhances polyethylene glycol-mediated somatic cell fusion, *Somat. Cell Genet.* **2:**263–270.

Nose, M., and Wigzeil, H., 1983, Biological significance of carbohydrate chains on monoclonal antibodies, *Proc. Natl. Acad. Sci. USA* **80:**6632–6636.

Ochi, A., Hawley, R. G., Hawley, T., Shirlman, M. J., Trauecker, A., Kohler, G., and Hozumi, N., 1983, Functional immunoglobulin M production after transfection of cloned immunoglobulin heavy and light chain genes into lymphoid cells, *Proc. Natl. Acad. Sci. USA* **80:**6351–6355.

Oi, V. T., and Herzenberg, L. A., 1980, Immunoglobulin-producing hybrid cell lines, in: *Selected Methods in Cellular Immunology* (B. B. Mishell and S. M. Shiigi, eds.), Freeman, San Francisco, pp. 351–372.

Okada, Y., and Murayama, F., 1965, Multinucleated giant cell formation by fusion between cells of two different strains, *Exp. Cell Res.* **40:**154–158.

Okada, Y., and Tadokoro, J., 1962, Analysis of giant polynuclear cell formation caused by HVJ virus from Ehrlich's tumor cells. II. Quantitative analysis of giant polynuclear cell formation, *Exp. Cell Res.* **26:**108–118.

Olsson, L., and Kaplan, H. S., 1980, Human/human hybridomas producing monoclonal antibodies of predefined antigenic specificity, *Proc. Natl Acad. Sci. USA* **77:**5429–5431.

Olsson, L., Kronstrom, H., Cambon-de Mouzon, A., Honsik, C., Brodin, T., and Jakobsen, B., 1983, Antibody producing human/human hybridomas. I. Technical aspects, *J. Immunol. Meth.* **61:**17–32.

Payne, M. R., 1983, Monoclonal antibodies to the contractile proteins, in: *Cell and Muscle Motility* (R. M. Dowben and J. W. Shay, eds.), Plenum Press, New York, pp. 137–177.

Pontecorvo, G., 1975, Production of mammalian somatic cell hybrids by means of polyethylene glycol treatment, *Somat. Cell Genet.* **1:**397–400.

Potter, M., and Boyce, C. R., 1962, Induction of plasma neoplasms in strain BALB/c mice with mineral oil and mineral oil adjuvants, *Nature* **193:**1086–1087.

Pravtcheva, D. M., and Ruddle, F. H., 1983, Normal X chromosome induced reversion in the direction of chromosome segregation in mouse–Chinese hamster somatic cell hybrids, *Exp. Cell Res.* **148:**265–272.

Schneiderman, S., Farber, J. L., and Baserga, R., 1979, A simple method for decreasing the toxicity of polyethylene glycol in mammalian cell hybridization, *Somat. Cell Genet.* **5:**263.

Schwaber, J., and Cohen, E. P., 1973, Human/mouse somatic cell hybrid clone secreting immunoglobulin of both parental types, *Nature* **244**:444–447.

Springer, T. A., 1981, Monoclonal antibody analysis of complex biological systems, *J. Biol. Chem.* **256**:3833–3839.

Taggart, R. T., and Samloff, I. M., 1983, Stable antibody-producing murine hybridomas, *Science* **219**:1228–1230.

Walker, C., and Shay, J. W., 1983, Effect of mitochondrial dosage on transfer of chloramphenicol resistance, *Somat. Cell Genet.* **9**:469–476.

Weiss, M. C., and Green, H., 1967, Human–mouse hybrid cell lines containing partial complements of human chromosomes and functional human genes, *Proc. Natl Acad. Sci. USA* **58**:1104–1111.

Winger, L., Winger, C., Shastry, P., Russell, A., and Longnecker, M., 1983, Efficient generation *in vitro*, from human peripheral blood cell, of monoclonal Epstein–Barr virus transformants producing specific antibodies to a variety of antigens without prior deliberate immunization, *Proc. Natl. Acad. Sci. USA* **80**:4484–4488.

Wright, W. E., 1978, The isolation of heterokaryons and hybrids by a selective system using irreversible biochemical inhibitors, *Exp. Cell Res.* **112**:395–407.

Zimmermann, U., and Vienken, J., 1982, Electric field-induced cell-to-cell fusion, *J. Membrane Biol.* **67**:165–182.

2

Fusion Partners for Production of Human Monoclonal Antibodies

Danuta Kozbor and Carlo M. Croce

I. Murine Plasmacytomas as Fusion Partners

The technology for production of murine monoclonal antibodies has advanced enormously since its introduction by Köhler and Milstein (1975). However, the production of human monoclonal antibodies by fusion technologies has been hampered, mainly by the current scarcity of suitable human cell lines as fusion partners. Hypoxanthine–aminopterin–thymidine (HAT)-sensitive murine plasmacytomas have been fused with human lymphocytes to yield mouse–human hybrids that secrete human antibody against the Forssman antigen (Nowinski *et al.*, 1980), keyhole limpet hemocyanin (KLH) (Lane *et al.*, 1982), tetanus toxoid (Kozbor *et al.*, 1982b; Butler *et al.*, 1983), human tumor-associated antigen (Schlom *et al.*, 1980; Sikora and Wright, 1981; Sikora and Phillips, 1981), and multiple endocrine organs (Satoh *et al.*, 1983). These interspecies hybridomas preferentially segregate human chromosomes, making it difficult to derive stable lines secreting human antibody. However, the loss of human chromosomes from mouse–human hybridomas is not random. It is known, for example, that human chromosomes 14 (heavy chain) and 22 (λ light chain) are preferentially retained, whereas chromosome 2 (κ chain) is preferentially lost (Croce *et al.*, 1979; Erikson *et al.*, 1981).

Danuta Kozbor and Carlo M. Croce • The Wistar Institute of Anatomy and Biology, Philadelphia, Pennsylvania 19104.

II. Human Plasmacytomas as Fusion Partners

Since the chromosomal constitution of intraspecific human hybrids is much more stable, human–human hybridomas are more likely to be a useful source of specific human monoclonal antibodies. However, cells of the most differentiated human lymphoid neoplasias, the plasmacytomas, seem to be among the most difficult human cells to establish in continuous culture (Kozbor and Roder, 1983). The basis for classification of these lines lies in the identity between the myeloma protein *in vivo* and the immunoglobulin synthesized *in vitro*. In addition, plasmacytoma cells have abundant rough endoplasmic reticulum (RER), few free polyribosomes, numerous mitochondria, and a well-developed Golgi apparatus. The rate of Ig secretion is high. These cells never carry Epstein–Barr virus (EBV) and are usually aneuploid (Nilsson and Pontén, 1975; Nilsson, 1978). Most of these cells have doubling times of 36–73 hr and may require a plasmacyte-stimulating factor for proliferation in tissue culture (Jobin *et al.*, 1974). Despite numerous efforts to establish long-term cultures of human plasmacytomas, to date, only a few lines fulfill the above criteria (Table I). Most myeloma, or myeloma-like, cell lines are derived from patients with very advanced disease, and are often established from

TABLE I

Characterization of Human Myeloma Cell Lines

Cell line	Tissue of origin	Karyotype	Class of Ig produced		Reference
			In vivo	*In vitro*	
RPMI-8226	Peripheral blood	Near triploid	IgG(λ)	λ	Matsuoka *et al.* (1967)
266 BL	Peripheral blood	Near diploid	IgE(λ)	IgE(λ)	Nilsson *et al.* (1970)
268 BM	Bone marrow	Near diploid	IgE(λ)	IgE(λ)	Nilsson *et al.* (1970)
LA 49	Pleural effusion	Polyploidy (23–250)	IgD(λ)	IgD(λ)	Jobin *et al.* (1974)
Oda	Subcutaneous plasmacytoma	46	IgD(λ)	IgD(λ)	Ishihara *et al.* (1977)
L363	Peripheral blood	49, X, +8M, −5, −6, +7, −8, 14q+, −22	IgG	ND[a]	Diehl *et al.* (1978)
KMM56	Pleural effusion	71 (49–144)	λ	λ	Shibuya *et al.* (1980)
Karpas 707	Peripheral blood and bone marrow	45, XY, Ph+	IgG(λ)	λ	Karpas *et al.* (1982)
KMM-1	Subcutaneous plasmacytoma	47, X, −Y 1q+, −2, +t (1:2) (cen:cen), +7, 12q+, 14q+, +mar	λ	λ	Togawa *et al.* (1982)

[a]ND, Not detected.

extramedullary sites, such as pleural effusions or subcutaneous plasmacytomas. It also appears that most of these lines are established from the more
unusual forms of myeloma, such as IgD or IgE, and it is curious that the
immunoglobulin light chain type has always been λ rather than κ.

The first reported human hybridoma produced monoclonal antibodies
against 2,4-dinitrophenyl (DNP) hapten and was obtained with the HAT-
sensitive plasma cell line U-266AR1 [later renamed SKO-007 (Olsson and
Kaplan, 1980)], derived from the IgE-producing myeloma U-266 (Table II).
The U-266AR1 cells were fused with the uninvolved splenic lymphocytes
from a Hodgkin lymphoma patient sensitized with dinitrochlorobenzene at
least 2 weeks prior to surgery. In experiments with three separate spleens,
average fusion frequencies were 37×10^{-7}. Approximately 28% of wells
containing hybrids produced IgG and 1.7% of all hybrids were specific for
DNP. Hybrids produced 3–11 µg/ml per day of monoclonal IgG, anti-DNP
antibodies. These results were not reproducible for 2 years, probably due to
mycoplasma contamination of the cells. However, on comparison of SKO-007
to another human fusion partner, a B-cell lymphoma RH-L4, the former was
found to be inferior with respect to fusion frequency (Olsson *et al.*, 1983) and
number of wells with IgG/IgM production. Abrams *et al.* (1983) derived a
second HAT-sensitive subline from the U-266 cell line and immunoglobulin-
secreting hybrids were obtained, but fusion frequencies were very low. A
third HAT-sensitive derivative of U-266, FU-266 (Teng *et al.*, 1983), has not
yet been characterized in terms of its fusion properties in human–human
hybridomas.

Another HAT-sensitive fusion partner of putative plasmacytoma origin,
8226-8AG^R (Abrams *et al.*, 1983), was derived from the RPMI-8226 line (Matsuoka *et al.*, 1967). The cells did fuse with lymphocytes from a patient with
Crohn disease, but no immunoglobulin-secreting hybrids were recovered.
Other hypoxanthine-guanine phosphoribosyltransferase (HGPRT)-deficient
cells originated from the RPMI-8226 line as potential fusion partners (Pickering and Gelder, 1982; Zeijlemaker *et al.*, 1982) have been found to be of
nonhuman origin.

III. Human Lymphoblastoid Cell Lines as Fusion Partners

The paucity of human myeloma lines prompted efforts to construct
human–human hybrids using lymphoblastoid cell lines (LCLs) as fusion partners. The LCLs established from malignant or normal hematopoietic tissue
are easily maintained in tissue culture, with population doubling times of 20–
30 hr. They show a constant association with EBV, polyclonal derivation, and
diploidy. They have numerous free polyribosomes, less well-developed RER
and Golgi apparatus, and secrete less immunoglobulin than myeloma cells.
Some of these phenotypic features are characteristic for certain stages in B-

TABLE II
Human Fusion Partners[a]

Fusion partner	Fusion partner Cell type₁[b]	Class of Ig produced	Drug resistance[c]	Source of donor lymphocytes[d]	Fusion frequency ($\times 10^{-7}$)[e]
SKO-007	Plasmacytoma	IgE(λ)	8-AG	Immune spleen (Hodgkin)	37
GM1500	LCL	IgG2(κ)	6-TG	Immune PBL (SSPE)	18
				PBL, type I diabetes	25
GM4672	LCL	IgG2(κ)	6-TG	Immune PBL, autoimmune disorders,	ND
				PBL, spleen	17
GK-5	LCL	κ	6-TG	PBL, insulin-requiring diabetes, autoimmune disorders	ND
				Myesthenia gravis	ND
LICR-LON-HMy-2	LCL	IgG1(κ)	8-AG	Normal PBL, tonsil lymph node	0.1–10
				TIL	ND
GM0467.3	LCL	IgM(λ)	8-AG	Immune tonsil (PWM)	22
H351.1	LCL	IgM(κ)	8-AG	Normal PBL, spleen (PWM)	22
LTR228	LCL	IgM(κ)	6-TG	Immune PBL, B-cell blasts	100
KR-4	LCL	IgG2(κ)	6-TG, Oua	TT–specific EBV line	112
				M. leprae–specific EBV line	36–126
				Immune PBL	
UC729-6	LCL	IgM(κ) nonsecretor	6-TG	PBL, lymphnode (cancer patients)	29
MC/CAR	LCL	IgG(κ) nonsecretor	8-AG	Immune PBL (rubella)	100
RH-L4	B-cell lymphoma	IgG(κ) nonsecretor	8-AG	PBL (PWM)	96
Heteromyelomas FU-266neo^R × X63-Ag8.653 clone D-33	Hybrid myeloma (human–mouse)	IgE(λ) nonsecretor	6-TG, Oua, G-418	Activated B cells	20–100
KR-12	Hybrid myeloma (human–human)	IgG(κ, λ)	6-TG	Immune PBL TT–specific	8
				EBV line	100

[a]ND, Not determined.
[b]LCL, Lymphoblastoid cell line.
[c]AG, azaguanine; TG, thioguanine; Oua, ouabain.
[d]PBL, peripheral blood lymphocytes; SSPE, subacute sclerosing panencephalitis; TT, tetanus toxoid; EBV, Epstein–Barr virus; TIL, tumor-infiltrating lymphocytes; PWM, pokeweed mitogen.
[e]Estimate based on assumptions made concerning the number of cells seeded per well.
[f]Cloning efficiency determined by limiting dilution.

cell differentiation and may play a crucial role in supporting the production of antibodies when fused with normal B cells.

The first LCL fusion partner was derived by Croce *et al.* (1980) from a B-cell line, GM1500, established from a patient with multiple myeloma. This line, GM1500 6TG-2, secreted IgG2(κ) and expressed the EBV-induced nuclear antigen (EBNA) (Kozbor *et al.*, 1982a). Peripheral blood mononuclear

TABLE III
Comparison of Hybridomas Constructed with Lymphoblastoid Cells
and Human Hybrid Myeloma

Cell line	Frequency of hybrid formation[a] at 10^{-6} (mean ±SEM)		Rate of Ig secretion[b] (μg/ml per 10^6 cells)	Hybridomas				
	LCL	Peripheral blood		Electron microscopy[c]	Cloning efficiency[d] (%)	Tumorigenicity[e]	Production of human Ig in ascites fluid (mg/ml)[f]	Stability (months)
KR-4	9.8 ± 2.5	0.1 ± 0.01	1–10	LCL	40–70	+	0.1–0.8	>12
KR-12	10 ± 2.2	0.8 ± 0.07	5–30	Myeloma-like	50–70	+	0.7–8.0	>10

[a]Frequency was calculated from the fraction of negative wells with the Poisson equation. Mean frequency is given for three plates. The lymphocytes and lymphoblastoid cell lines were obtained from peripheral blood of donors immunized with TT or from colorectal carcinoma patients.

[b]Secreted Ig was quantitated by a solid-phase ELISA system.

[c]In electron micrographs, well-differentiated cells with abundant RER, prominent Golgi, and condensed nuclear chromatin were considered "myelomas." Less differentiated cells with small amounts of RER, moderately developed Golgi, and extended nuclear chromatin were considered "lymphoblastoid" (LCL).

[d]Determined by limiting dilution.

[e]Human hybridomas obtained by fusion of KR-4 or KR-12 with lymphoblastoid cell line B6 were injected subcutaneously (sc) into irradiated (350 R) or unirradiated BALB/c nude mice (10^7 cells per mouse). The tumorigenic cells formed solid tumors after 2–4 weeks. The nontumorigenic variants did not form tumor even after 1–2 months from injection into irradiated animals.

[f]Tetanus-specific human hybrids, which were grown as sc tumor and then in vitro for 3–5 passages, were injected ip into irradiated or unirradiated BALB/c nude mice (10^7 cells per mouse) and ascites fluid was collected 3–6 weeks later and titered in an ELISA assay against purified human IgM and IgG standards. Ascites fluid from P3X63Ag.8 mouse myeloma was used as a negative control.

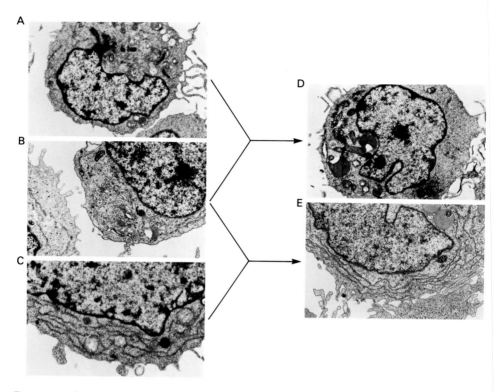

FIGURE 1. Electron micrograph of parental and hybrid cells. Cells were fixed in 3% glutaraldehyde and stained with uranyl acetate and lead citrate. Lymphoblastoid cells (A) KR-4, (B) B6, and
(D) KR-4 × B6 hybridomas show abundant polyribosomes, irregular nucleus, scant RER, prominent Golgi apparatus. Myeloma-like cells (C) KR-12 and (E) KR-12 × B6 hybrids show well-
developed RER, scattered cytoplasmic vacuoles, and mitochondria (magnification 20,000×).

hybrids (KR-12 × B6 and KR-4 × B6 cells) were grown as ascites in nude mice
after a single passage as a solid subcutaneous tumor in irradiated (350 R)
nude mice and then grown *in vitro*. Yields of human Ig in ascites fluid range
from 0.1 to 1 mg/ml for the B6 × KR-4 cell hybrids, and from 0.7 to 8 mg/ml
for hybrids constructed with the human myeloma hybrid KR-12 as a fusion
partner.

These results suggest that some characteristic(s) associated with myeloma
morphology may contribute to higher Ig production; however, the regulatory
mechanism is still unknown and, particularly with the hybrids, it can vary
from fusion to fusion. The polyploid human hybrids are not inherently unstable, but certain differentiated functions, including production of immunoglobulins, are often lost after fusion (Bengtsson *et al.*, 1975; Stanbridge *et
al.*, 1982) or can undergo more complex regulatory mechanisms (Ber *et al.*,
1978).

V. Search for Better Fusion Partners

The limitation of human hybridoma technology appears to lie in the variable and often low fusion frequency, the erratic levels of human monoclonal antibody production by these hybrids, and the presence of immunoglobulin molecules composed of heavy and/or light chains from both the myeloma (lymphoblastoid) and the B-cell parent.

In vitro stimulation of human lymphocytes by antigen prior to fusion may improve the frequency of positive hybrids: the increase in blasts after stimulation was indeed shown to be of predictive value for the successful generation of specific hybrids in the murine system (Stähli *et al.*, 1980). Various stimulators/activators, including PWM (Larrick *et al.*, 1983; Kozbor and Roder, 1984; Chiorazzi *et al.*, 1982; Shoenfeld *et al.*, 1982), antigen (Olsson and Kaplan, 1980; Chiorazzi *et al.*, 1982) and EBV (Kozbor *et al.*, 1982a; Kozbor and Roder, 1984), have been found to markedly increase fusion frequencies in a variety of human hybridoma systems. Because EBV-transformed cells can arise spontaneously from lymphocytes of patients exposed to the virus and because lymphoblastoid cell lines used as fusion partners carry the EBV genome, which may transform normal B cells, it is important to demonstrate that putative hybridomas are not just $HGPRT^+$ revertants of the fusion partner or EBV-transformed cells. This may be done by determining DNA content, karyotype, expression of HLA antigens, and class of immunoglobulin on parental and hybrids cells. Alternatively, a lymphoblastoid or myeloma cell line with a second drug marker, e.g., resistance to ouabain, may be used as a fusion partner, and the EBV-transformed or spontaneous lymphoblastoid cells can be counterselected with this drug. This greatly increases the likelihood that cells surviving the selection process are indeed hybrids.

A. Double Drug-Resistance Cell Lines

In an attempt to obtain a double drug-resistant fusion partner (KR-4), the 6-thioguanine-resistant human lymphoblastoid B-cell line GM1500 was mutagenized by low-level γ irradiation, selected for 10^{-4} M ouabain resistance, and subsequently fused with lymphocytes stimulated *in vitro* with EBV, PWM, or TT (Kozbor *et al.*, 1982a; Kozbor and Roder, 1984). Moreover, when the KR-4 cells were fused with lymphoblastoid cells, hybrids resulted that secreted antibodies against three different antigen preparations of *Mycobacterium leprae* (Atlaw *et al.*, 1984) and against colorectal carcinoma cell lines (D. Kozbor and C. M. Croce, unpublished results). The hybrids arose with a frequency of 10^{-5}, secreted 3–10 μg/ml of specific [IgM(κ)] antibodies, and were stable over a period of 12 months. Hybrid selection was done in HAT medium containing 10^{-5} M ouabain to select against the parental lines. A HAT-sensitive, ouabain-resistant fusion partner has also been derived from the LTR 288 cell line (Larrick *et al.*, 1983).

B. Non-Ig-Secreting Partners

The presence of secreted Ig molecules synthesized by the parental fusion partner dilutes the specific antibody of interest. In the murine system, this difficulty was overcome by the development of two kinds of variants: those that synthesize but do not secrete Ig (Köhler et al., 1976) and those that do not synthesize Ig (Kearney et al., 1979). Several laboratories are engaged in developing HAT-sensitive human myeloma and lymphoblastoid cells that do not secrete Ig. Glassy et al. (1983) fused the UC729-6 lymphoblastoid cell line, which does not secrete Ig but is cytoplasmic- and surface IgM(κ)-positive, with the draining lymph node cells of cancer patients. Those authors obtained two hybrids secreting 3–10 μg/ml of IgM or IgG antibody, which reacted with human tumor cell lines but not with normal cells. The UC729-6 cells were found recently to secrete low amounts of IgM [30 ng/ml per 10^6 cells (Abrams et al., 1983)].

Another LCL, MC/CAR, although reported as a nonsecretory plasmacytoid cell line, has features more characteristic of lymphoblastoid cells lines, such as expression of Epstein–Barr virus, and was found to express cytoplasmic IgG(κ) (Ritts et al., 1983). These cells were fused with mononuclear cells from a donor known to have high titers of circulating antibodies to rubella after additional in vitro stimulation with the antigen. Two out of 96 Ig-positive cultures were found to have antirubella antibody.

Larrick et al. (1983) have used the reverse-plaque technique to select for a nonproducer variant of the LTR228 lymphoblastoid cell line. Initial experiments suggest that these lines produce hybrids with an efficiency similar to that of the LTR 228 parental cells.

Most recently, Olsson et al. (1984) obtained the human–human hybrids between RH-L4 B lymphoma [IgG(κ) producer, nonsecretor] and human B lymphocytes from patients with acute myeloid leukemia (AML) to study the antigenic repertoire of the humoral immune response against the patients' own leukemia and against leukemic cells from other patients. Although Ig production (5–15 μg) was detected in more than 50% of the hybrids, only 10% of these secreted Ig specific for human leukemia cells.

C. Human Hybrid Myelomas as Fusion Partners

In another approach to obtaining a better fusion partner, Teng et al. (1983) constructed mouse–human hybrid myelomas ("heteromyelomas"), reasoning that such hybrids would retain the superior fusion characteristics of the mouse myeloma and confer greater stability to hybrids generated with them because of the presence of the human chromosomes in the heteromyeloma fusion partner. The HAT-sensitive variant of U-266 human myeloma, FU-266, was rendered resistant to the antibiotic G-418 by transfection with the recombinant plasmid vector pSV2-neo^R, and one of the resultant neo^R

clones, E-1, was subsequently fused with the non-Ig-secreting and HAT-sensitive mouse myeloma cell line X63Ag8.653 (Kearney *et al.*, 1979). Selection was done in medium containing the antibiotic G-418, to eliminate the mouse parent, and containing ouabain, to kill the human cells. Because ouabain and G-418 resistance are dominant traits, only hybrids could survive the selection. The hybrids, in addition to being ouabain- and G-418-resistant, preserved that HAT-sensitivity marker from both parents. Selected hybrid clones were then tested as fusion partners in a series of fusion with polyclonally activated human B lymphocytes, with antigen-primed human B lymphocytes, and, in some instances, after transformation of the latter with EBV. Hybrids producing $2-10$ µg/ml per 10^6 cells per day were stable for more than 6 months, and several antigen-specific monoclonal antibodies have been generated. In some instances, isolated clones have produced as much as $21-36$ µg Ig/ml per 10^6 cells per day. The frequency of hybrid formation with heteromyelomas, i.e., $6-100\%$ positive wells for hybrid outgrowth, was higher than that when human myelomas were used as fusion partners. Moreover, some of the heteromyelomas, e.g., D-33, became nonproducers after a few weeks in culture; others, e.g., D-36, ceased ε heavy chain production but retained a low level of λ light chain secretion. Although the heteromyelomas are routinely grown in the presence of G-418 to promote retention of human chromosomes with integrated bacterial genes for neomycin resistance, it is not clear how this influences the stability of new hybrids in which human chromosomes carry no drug markers and chance being segregated in the same fashion as in human–mouse hybrids. Thus, human–human hybrids are still preferable and the recently produced human hybrid myeloma KR-12 attests to the superiority of this type of hybrid.

ACKNOWLEDGMENTS

We thank Josef Weibel for preparing the electron micrographs, Marina Hoffman for editorial assistance, and Leroy Steiner for helpful discussion. This work was supported by grant CA 16685 from the National Cancer Institute to C. M. C.; D. K. is a Postdoctoral Fellow of the National Cancer Institute of Canada.

References

Abrams, P. G., Knost, J. A., Clarke, G., Wilburn, S., Oldham, R. K., and Foon, K. A., 1983, Determination of the optimal human cell lines for development of human hybridomas, *J. Immunol.* **131:**1201–1204.

Atlaw, T., Kozbor, D., and Roder, J. C., 1984, Human monoclonal antibodies against *Mycobacterium leprae, Inf. Immun.* In press.

Bengtsson, D. B., Nabholz, M., Kennett, R. H., and Bodmer, W. F., 1975, Human intraspecific somatic cell hybrids: A genetic and karyotypic analysis of crosses between lymphocytes and D98/AH-2, *Somat. Cell Genet.* **1:**41–64.

Ber, R., Klein, G., Moar, M., Povey, S., Rosén, A., Westman, A., Yefenof, E., and Zeuthen, J., 1978, Somatic cell hybrids between human lymphoma lines. IV. Establishment and characterization of a P3HR-1/Daudi hybrid, *Int. J. Cancer* **21:**707.

Butler, Y. L., Lane, H. C., and Fauci, A. S., 1983, Delineation of optimal conditions for producing mouse–human heterohybridomas from human peripheral blood B cells of immunized subjects, *J. Immunol.* **130:**165–168.

Chiorazzi, N., Wasserman, R. J., and Kunkel, H. G., 1982, Use of Epstein–Barr virus-transformed B cell lines for the generation of immunoglobulin-producing human B cell hybridomas, *J. Exp. Med.* **156:**930–935.

Croce, C. M., Shander, M., Martinis, J., Cicurel, L., D'Ancona, G. G., Dolby, T. W., and Koprowski, H., 1979, Chromosomal locations of the genes for human immunoglobulin heavy chains, *Eur. J. Immunol.* **10:**486–488.

Croce, C. M., Linnenbach, A., Hall, W., Steplewski, Z., and Koprowski, H., 1980, Production of human hybridomas secreting antibodies to measles virus, *Nature* **228:**488–489.

Diehl, V., Schaadt, M., Kirchner, H., Hellriegel, K. P., Gudat, F., Fonatsch, C., Lskewitz, E., and Guggenheim, R., 1978, Long-term cultivation of plasma cell leukemia cells and autologous lymphoblasts (LCL) *in vitro:* A comparative study, *Blut* **36:**331–338.

Dwyer, D. S., Bradley, R. J., Urguhart, C. K., and Kearney, J. F., 1983, Naturally occurring anti-idiotypic antibodies in myasthenia gravis patients, *Nature* **301:**611–614.

Edwards, P. A., Smith, C. M., Neville, A. M., and O'Hare, M. J., 1982, A human-hybridoma system based on a fast-growing mutant of the ARH-77 plasma cell leukemia-derived line, *Eur. J. Immunol.* **12:**641–648.

Eisenbarth, G. S., Linnenbach, A., Jackson, R., Scearce, R., and Croce, C. M., 1982, Human hybridomas secreting anti-islet autoantibodies, *Nature* **300:**264–267.

Erikson, J., Martinis, J., and Croce, C. M., 1981, Assignment of the genes for human λ immunoglobulin chains to chromosome 22, *Nature* **294:**173–175.

Glassy, M. C., Handley, H. H., Hagiwara, H., and Royston, I., 1983, UC 729-6, a human lymphoblastoid B-cell line useful for generating antibody-secreting human–human hybridomas, *Proc. Natl. Acad. Sci. USA* **80:**6327–6331.

Ishihara, N., Kiyofuzi, T., and Oboshi, S., 1977, Establishment and characterization of a human plasmacyte cell line derived from a patient with IgD multiple myeloma, in: *Proceedings Japanese Cancer Association, Annual Meeting,* **36:**120–126.

Jobin, M. E., Fahey, J. L., and Price, Z., 1974, Long-term establishment of a human plasmacyte cell line derived from a patient with IgD multiple myeloma. I. Requirement of a plasmacyte-stimulating factor for the proliferation of myeloma cells in tissue culture, *J. Exp. Med.* **140:**494–507.

Karpas, A., Fischer, P., and Swirsky, D., 1982, Human plasmacytoma with an unusual karyotype growing *in vitro* and producing light-chain immunoglobulin, *Lancet* **i:**931–933.

Kearney, J. F., Radbrusch, A., Liesegang, B., and Rajewski, K., 1979, A new mouse myeloma cell line that has lost immunoglobulin expression but permits the construction of antibody-secreting hybrid cell lines, *J. Immunol.* **1231:**1548–1550.

Köhler, G., and Milstein, C., 1975, Continuous cultures of fused cells secreting antibody of predefined specificity, *Nature* **256:**495–497.

Köhler, G., Howe, S. C., and Milstein, C., 1976, Fusion between immunoglobulin-secreting and non-secreting myeloma cell lines, *Eur. J. Immunol.* **6:**292–295.

Kozbor, D., and Roder, J. C., 1981, Requirements for the establishment of high-titered human monoclonal antibodies against tetanus toxoid using the Epstein–Barr virus technique, *J. Immunol.* **127:**1275–1280.

Kozbor, D., and Roder, J. C., 1983, Monoclonal antibodies produced by human lymphocytes, *Immunol. Today* **4**(3):72–79.

Kozbor, D., and Roder, J. C., 1984, *In vitro* stimulated lymphocytes as a source of human hybridomas, *Eur. J. Immunol.* **14**:23–27.

Kozbor, D., Lagarde, A. E., and Roder, J. C., 1982a, Human hybridomas constructed with antigen-specific Epstein–Barr virus-transformed cell lines, *Proc. Natl. Acad. Sci. USA* **79**:6651–6655.

Kozbor, D., Roder, J. C., Chang, T. H., Steplewski, Z., and Koprowski, H., 1982b, Human anti-tetanus toxoid monoclonal antibody secreted by EBV-transformed human B cells fused with the murine myeloma, *Hybridoma* **1**(3):323–328.

Kozbor, D., Dexter, D., and Roder, J. C., 1983, A comparative analysis of the phenotypic characteristics of available fusion partners for the construction of human hybridomas, *Hybridoma* **2**(1):7–16.

Kozbor, D., Tripputi, P., Roder, J. C., and Croce, C. M., 1984, A human hybrid myeloma for production of human monoclonal antibody, *J. Immunol.,* **133**:3001–3005.

Lane, H. C., Shelhamer, J. H., Motowski, H. S., and Fauci, A. S., 1982, Human monoclonal anti-keyhole limpet hemocyanin antibody-secreting hybridoma produced from peripheral blood B lymphocytes of a keyhole limpet hemocyanin-immune individual, *J. Exp. Med.* **155**:333–337.

Larrick, J. W., Truitt, K. E., Raubitschek, A. A., Senyk, G., and Wang, J. C. N., 1983, Characterization of human hybridomas secreting antibody to tetanus toxoid, *Proc. Natl. Acad. Sci. USA* **80**:6376–6380.

Matsuoka, Y., Moore, G. E., Yagi, Y., and Pressman, D., 1967, Production of free light chains of immunoglobulin by a hematopoietic cell line derived from a patient with multiple myeloma, *Proc. Soc. Exp. Biol.* **125**:1246–1250.

Nilsson, K., 1978, Established human lymphoid cell lines as model for B-lymphocyte differentiation, in: *Human Lymphocyte Differentiation: Its Application to Cancer* (B. Serrou and C. Rosenfeld, eds.), Elsevier/North-Holland, Amsterdam, pp. 307–317.

Nilsson, K., and Pontén, J., 1975, Classification and biological nature of established human hematopoietic cell lines, *Int. J. Cancer* **15**:321–341.

Nilsson, K., Bennich, H., Johansson, S. G. O., and Pontén, J., 1970, Established immunoglobulin producing myeloma (IgE) and lymphoblastoid (IgG) cell lines from an IgE myeloma patient, *Clin. Exp. Immunol.* **7**:477–489.

Nowinski, R., Berglund, C., Lane, Y., Lostrom, M., Bernstein, I., Young, W., Hakomori, S., Hill, L., and Cooney, M., 1980, Human monoclonal antibody against Forssman antigen, *Science* **210**:537–539.

Olsson, L., and Kaplan, H. S., 1980, Human–human hybridomas producing monoclonal antibodies of predefined antigenic specificity, *Proc. Natl. Acad. Sci. USA* **77**:5429–5431.

Olsson, L., Kronstrøm, H., Cambon-De Mouzom, A., Honsik, C., Brodin, T., and Jakobsen, B., 1983, Antibody-producing human–human hybridoma. I. Technical aspects, *J. Immunol. Meth.* **61**:17–32.

Olsson, L., Andreasen, R. B., Ost, A., Christensen, B., and Biberfeld, P., 1984, Antibody-producing human–human hybridomas. II. Derivation and characterization of an antibody specific for human leukemia cells, *J. Exp. Med.* **159**:537–550.

Osband, M., Cavagnaw, J., and Kupchick, H. Z., 1981, Biochemical analysis of specific histamine HI and H2 receptors on lymphocytes, *Blood* **60**(5, Suppl. 1):81a (abstract).

Phillips, J., Sikora, K., and Watson, J. V., 1982, Localization of glioma by human monoclonal antibody, *Lancet* **2**:1214–1215.

Pickering, J. W., and Gelder, F. B., 1982, A human myeloma cell line that does not express immunoglobulin but yields a high frequency of antibody-secreting hybridomas, *J. Immunol.* **129**:406–412.

Ritts, R. E., Jr., Ruiz-Argüelles, A., Weyl, K. G., Bradley, A. L., Weihmeir, B., Jacobsen, D. Y., and Strehlo, B. L., 1983, Establishment and characterization of a human non-secretory plasmoid cell line and its hybridization with human B cells, *Int. J. Cancer* **31**:133–141.

Satoh, J., Prabhakar, B. S., Haspel, M. V., Ginsberg-Fellner, F., and Notkins, A. L., 1983, Human monoclonal auto-antibodies that react with multiple endocrine organs, *N. Engl. J. Med.* **309:**217–220.

Schlom, T., Wunderlich, D., and Teramoto, Y. A., 1980, Generation of human monoclonal antibodies reactive with human mammary carcinoma cells, *Proc. Natl. Acad. Sci. USA* **77:**6841–6845.

Shibuya, T., Niho, Y., Yamasaki, K., Nakayama, K., Oka, Y., Arase, K., and Yanase, T., 1980, Establishment of a lambda immunoglobulin producing myeloma cell line, *Acta Haem. Jpn.* **43:**256 (In Japanese).

Shoenfeld, Y., Hsu-Lin, S. C., Gabriels, J. E., Silberstein, L, E., Furie, B. C., Furie, B., Stollar, B. D., and Schwartz, R. S., 1982, Production of auto-antibodies by human–human hybridomas, *J. Clin. Invest.* **70:**205–208.

Shoenfeld, Y., Rauch, J., Massicotte, H., Datta, S. K., Andre-Schwartz, J., Stollar, B. D., and Schwartz, R. S., 1983, Polyspecificity of monoclonal lupus auto-antibodies produced by human–human hybridomas, *N. Engl. J. Med.* **308:**414–420.

Sikora, K., and Phillips, J., 1981, Human monoclonal antibodies to glioma cells, *Br. J. Cancer* **43:**105–107.

Sikora, K., and Wright, R., 1981, Human monoclonal antibodies to lung-cancer antigens, *Br. J. Cancer* **43:**696–700.

Sikora, K., Alderson, T., Phillips, J., and Watson, J. V., 1982, Human hybridomas from malignant gliomas, *Lancet* **i:**11–14.

Stähli, Ch., Staehelin, T., Miggiano, V., Schmidt, J., and Häring, P., 1980, High frequencies of antigen-specific hybridomas: Dependence on immunization parameters and prediction by spleen cell analysis, *J. Immunol. Meth.* **32:**297–304.

Standbridge, E. J., Der, C. J., Roenson, C. J., Nishimi, R. Y., Peehl, D. M., Weissman, B. E., and Wilkinson, J. E., 1982, Human cell hybrids: Analysis of transformation and tumorigenicity, *Science* **215:**252–259.

Strike, L., Devens, B. H., and Lundak, R. L., 1982, Production of human hybridomas secreting specific immunoglobulin following *in vitro* immunization, *Immunology* **163**(2–4):272 (abstract).

Teng, N. N. H., Lam, K. S., Riera, F. C., and Kaplan, H., 1983, Construction and testing of mouse–human heteromyelomas for human monoclonal antibody production, *Proc. Natl. Acad. Sci. USA* **80:**7308–7312.

Togawa, A., Inoue, N., Miyamoto, K., Hyodo, H., and Namba, M., 1982, Establishment and characterization of a human myeloma cell line (KMM-1), *Int. J. Cancer* **29:**495–500.

Warenius, H. M., Taylor, J. W., Durack, B. E., and Cross, P. A., 1983, The production of human hybridomas from patients with malignant melanoma. The effect of pre-stimulation of lymphocytes with pokeweed mitogen, *Eur. J. Cancer Clin. Oncol.* **19:**347–355.

Zeijlemaker, W. P., Astaldi, G. C. B., Janssen, M. C., Stricker, E. A. M., and Tiebout, R. F., 1982, Production of human monoclonal antibodies, in: *Proceedings 15th International Leucocyte Culture Conference, Asilomar,* pp. 368–369.

3

Production of Human Monoclonal Antibodies Using Epstein–Barr Virus

Dorothy H. Crawford

I. Introduction

The Epstein–Barr virus (EBV) is a human lymphotrophic herpes virus that is the causative agent of infectious mononucleosis (Henle *et al.,* 1968), and is also etiologically associated with two human tumors: African Burkitt lymphoma (Epstein and Achong, 1979) and nasopharyngeal carcinoma (Epstein, 1978). When used *in vitro,* the virus infects and transforms human B lymphocytes (Pattengale *et al.,* 1973), which will thereafter grow continuously in culture as lymphoblastoid cell lines (Pope *et al.,* 1968). EBV infection also causes polyclonal activation of B lymphocytes, with the synthesis and secretion of immunoglobulin (Rosen *et al.,* 1977). The combination of these two properties of EBV makes it a useful tool for the immortalization of human antibody-secreting cells.

In this chapter I discuss the biological properties of EBV and then review its use in making stable, human monoclonal antibody-producing cell lines. The purification of antibodies produced using EBV for eventual clinical use is also discussed. Since many difficulties are encountered in the methodology currently available, I have paid particular attention to these difficulties and to suggesting methods by which they may be overcome.

DOROTHY H. CRAWFORD • Department of Haematology, Faculty of Clinical Sciences, University College London, London WC1E 6HX, England.

II. The Biological Properties of Epstein–Barr Virus

A. Transformation

The word "transformation" is used by EB virologists to mean immortalization of cells *in vitro*, rather than the transient transformation described by immunologists following mitogen stimulation of lymphocytes. It has been known for many years that all peripheral blood B lymphocytes have a receptor for EBV (Greaves *et al.*, 1975) and that when infected these cells are transformed by the virus, with the accompanying expression of the EBV nuclear antigen (EBNA) (Reedman and Klein, 1973). This antigen has become the hallmark of EBV infection. Recently, limiting dilution experiments have shown that, although all peripheral blood B cells may be infected by EBV, only a subset (around 20%) are actually immortalized *in vitro* (Henderson *et al.*, 1977; Katsuki *et al.*, 1977). Other workers, using step gradients to separate subsets of B cells, have identified the susceptible subset as the most dense (smallest) B cells, and have shown that the larger activated cells are resistant to transformation (Aman *et al.*, 1984). These data, taken in conjunction with the fact that plasma cells lack the receptor for EBV, indicate an increasing resistance of B cells to EBV transformation as they mature into plasma cells following antigen or mitogen stimulation.

1. Source of Infectious EBV

Wild-type EBV can be found in an infectious form in the saliva or throat washings of infectious mononucleosis patients (Miller *et al.*, 1973) and intermittently from the same source in normal seropositive individuals (Golden *et al.*, 1973). In most laboratories, however, the cell line B95-8 is used as a source of virus (Miller *et al.*, 1972). This is a cell line derived from cotton-topped marmoset peripheral blood mononuclear cells by *in vitro* infection with wild-type virus from an infectious mononucleosis patient. The cell line contains 10–20% of cells that are undergoing a lytic viral infection at any one time, and this percentage can be much increased (up to 80%) by treatment of the cells with various inducing agents, such as bromodeoxyuridine (Gerber, 1972), iododeoxyuridine (Fresen and Zur Hausen, 1976), phorbol esters (Zur Hausen *et al.*, 1978) and *n*-butyrate (Luka *et al.*, 1979). The virus particles are released into the culture supernatant and can be harvested by centrifuging at $400 \times g$, followed by filtering through a 0.45-μm filter, which removes cells but allows passage of the enveloped, infectious virus particles. Culture supernatant from a healthy culture of B95-8, which has grown up to a cell density of around 10^6/ml, prepared in this way should have a transforming titer of around 10^{-3} when used to infect human cord blood cells. The viral infectivity falls off when preparations are stored at temperatures above $-70°C$, but will be preserved almost indefinitely at or below this temperature. In order to increase the transforming titer, the culture supernatant can be centrifuged at 13,000 × g (17,000 rpm) for 2 hr at 4°C. The resulting pellet is resuspended in 1 ml of culture medium and stored. B95-8 cells obtained from most laboratories are contaminated with mycoplasma and thus many cell lines derived using cell-free B95-8 virus are also contaminated. Some workers have suggested that this contamination reduces the efficiency of transformation and cloning (Doyle *et al.*, 1984) and thus the likelihood of establishing antibody-producing cell lines; however, this has not been our experience.

2. EBV Infection of B Lymphocytes

In order to establish a B-cell line from peripheral blood B lymphocytes, neat, filtered culture supernatant medium from the B95-8 cell line contains sufficient infectious virus particles. However, it has been shown by analysis of virus dose–response curves that increasing the virus dose increases the number of cells infected by the virus (Zerbini and Emberg, 1983). Thus, if a high yield of infected cells is required, it is advisable to use concentrated virus preparations. Routinely, infection is carried out by resuspending pellets of up to 10^7 cells in 1 ml of B95-8 culture supernatant and incubating at 37°C for 1 hr. This time allows attachment of the virus to specific receptors on B cells and penetration into the cell. The latter is an active process requiring a temperature of 37°C. Gentle agitation of the container prevents the cells from sedimenting during the incubation. Following this, the cells are pelleted, the supernatant removed, and the cells cultured as required.

3. Cell Culture

When EBV infection of peripheral blood mononuclear cells (PBMs) is being used to obtain a long-term cell line, two points must be remembered:
1. PBMs from individuals who are seropositive for antibodies to EBV antigens (this includes 90% of the adult population worldwide) contain memory T cells that, when stimulated in culture, become specifically cytotoxic for EBV-transformed, autologous B cells (Rickinson *et al.*, 1979). Thus, in cultures seeded at high density (10^6 to $2 × 10^6$/ml) proliferating foci of B cells regularly regress after 3–4 weeks and no cell lines are obtained (Moss *et al.*, 1978). This phenomenon can be overcome in one of three ways: Cells may be seeded at low cell densities (10^5 to $5 × 10^5$/ml) (Rickinson *et al.*, 1979); T cells may be removed from the mononuclear cell pellet by density gradient separation of E-rosetted cells (Kaplan and Clark, 1974); or cyclosporin A (1 μg/ml) may be added to the culture medium for 2–3 weeks in order to inhibit T-cell activity (Crawford, 1981).
2. In order to transform and proliferate in culture, B lymphocytes require a cell feeder layer (Pope *et al.*, 1974). When PBM, or E-rosette-depleted PBMs are used, the monocytes in these preparations act efficiently to this purpose. However, if subsets of B cells are being purified prior to infection

with EBV, it is necessary to add a feeder layer to the culture in order to obtain efficient transformation. The active factors involved in this cellular interaction have not been isolated, but the phenomenon shows no genetic restriction, and many cell types have been used. These include fetal fibroblasts (Rosen *et al.*, 1983), allogeneic PBMs (Crawford *et al.*, 1983b), and cord blood PBMs (Stein and Sigal, 1983), all of which are X-irradiated prior to plating.

Cultures are incubated at 37°C in a humidified atmosphere containing 5% CO_2 in air, and should be fed weekly by replacement of half the medium without disturbing the cell layer. Cultures visualized using an inverted microscope will contain proliferating foci of transformed B cells after 1–2 weeks, which will thereafter continue to proliferate on subculturing. *In vitro* EBV-transformed cell lines show variable growth characteristics, but usually grow well at a cell density of 10^5–10^6/ml, have a doubling time of 48–72 hr (Fig. 2A), and grow in round clumps of cells, which individually show "handmirror" morphology (Nilsson and Pontén, 1975).

4. Handling of EBV in the Laboratory

Recently the more generalized use of EBV-transformed cell lines and of EBV as a tool for immortalizing cells has led to growing general concern as to the safety precautions necessary for handling this type of material. It must be remembered in this context that up to 90% of the adult population will have been infected with the virus and will carry it as a lifelong infection in lymphoid cells as well as intermittently secreting infectious virus particles into the oropharynx. Furthermore, EBV is of low infectivity and no authenticated cases of laboratory-contracted infection have been reported. It is therefore reasonable to handle EBV-transformed cell lines (most of which produce small quantities of infectious virus) according to routine microbiological laboratory practice, and to use a safety cabinet when highly concentrated virus is being handled.

B. Polyclonal Activation

On infection, EBV activates B lymphocytes to produce immunoglobulin (Ig) in a T-cell-independent manner (Rosen *et al.*, 1977). Although the actual mechanism by which EBV causes polyclonal activation is unknown, it has been shown that UV-irradiated (inactivated) virus does not cause Ig synthesis, indicating a mechanism actively associated with B-cell infection. Around 1% of infected B cells are activated to produce Ig (Henderson *et al.*, 1977; Yarchoau *et al.*, 1983). Immunoglobulin can be measured in the supernatant medium of cultures of recently infected B cells (Fig. 1A) or can be monitored as numbers of plaque-forming cells or cells showing cytoplasmic staining with anti-Ig reagents (Fig. 1B). Although all classes of Ig can be detected, IgM usually predominates. IgM, IgG, and IgA can be measured in microgram quantities in the culture supernatant for the first 4–8 weeks of the culture period.

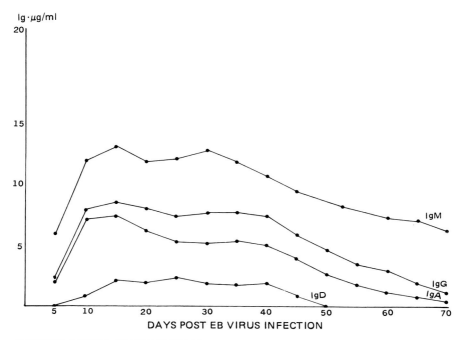

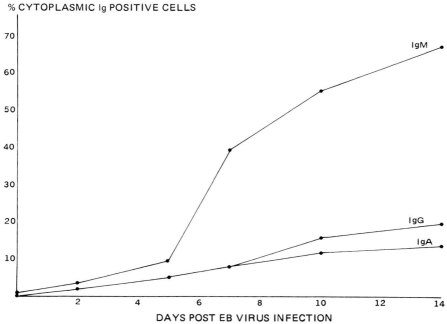

FIGURE 1. Immunoglobulin production by EBV-transformed, E-rosette-depleted PBMs. (A) IgM, IgG, and IgA levels measured in µg/ml in the culture supernatant medium over a 70-day period following EBV infection. (B) Numbers of cytoplasmic IgM-, IgG-, and IgA-containing cells in cultures over a 14-day period following EBV infection.

Following this, in uncloned cell lines, Ig levels tend to fall off and eventually reach a low steady state in which Ig of one particular class persists. These findings could be the result of one of several mechanisms:

1. The stimulation of Ig production caused by EBV transformation may be transient, and infected cells may revert to a stable state of low level production in long-term culture.
2. EBV-transformed, high-level Ig-producing cells may be intrinsically short-lived and may die out early in the culture period.
3. Ig-producing cells may have a selective disadvantage in the culture, either because they are slower growing or because they have more stringent nutrient requirements. This would lead to the eventual over-growth of nonproducer or low-level Ig-producing cells.

Of these three possibilities, the last seems to be the most likely, since cloning of cells early in the culture period allows the selection of cell lines that produce high levels of Ig in a stable manner.

III. Human Monoclonal Antibody Production

The first report of the successful immortalization of specific antibody-producing cells *in vitro* using EBV was by Steinitz *et al.* (1977). Since that time monoclonal antibodies directed against a wide variety of antigens have been produced by this method. These include antibodies to hapten molecules (Kozbor *et al.*, 1979; Steinitz *et al.*, 1979), autoantigens (Steinitz *et al.*, 1980; Kamo *et al.*, 1982), viral (Crawford *et al.*, 1983a; Seigneurin *et al.*, 1983), bacterial (Rosen *et al.*, 1983; Steinitz *et al.*, 1984; Kozbor and Roder, 1981), and protozoal (Lundgren *et al.*, 1983) antigens, blood group antigens (Craw-ford *et al.*, 1983b; Doyle *et al.*, 1984), and tumor-associated antigens (Irie *et al.*, 1982). However, the fact that only between 20 and 30 reports of EBV-trans-formed cloned cell lines that produce specific antibody have appeared in the literature since 1977 reflects the fact that certain problems encountered in the technology of producing human monoclonal antibodies by this method re-main unresolved. The main area of difficulty is that of retaining antibody production in culture for prolonged periods of time. Following EBV infection of peripheral blood B lymphocytes from an individual who has serum anti-bodies to a specific antigen, it is relatively common to be able to detect specific antibody in the supernatant medium after 2–3 weeks of culture. However, with continued growth of the culture, specific antibody levels invariably fall and become undetectable by 12–20 weeks. As discussed previously, this is probably due to the overgrowth of the culture with non-Ig-producing cells. For this reason the selection procedures for specific antibody-producing cells both prior to and following EBV transformation are essential steps in the successful production of long-term monoclonal antibody-producing cell lines.

A. Enrichment of Specific Antibody-Producing Cells

Because of the small number of specific antibody-producing cells among an unselected B-cell population, it is necessary to enrich for the desired antibody-bearing cells prior to EBV infection. This can be done first at the level of the lymphocyte donor. Since specific antibody-producing cells or memory B cells are not regularly present in the circulation even in individuals with high-titer specific serum antibody, it is preferable to use a donor who has been recently immunized to the antigen concerned. This immunization may take the form of a natural primary infection, as used by Rosen *et al.* (1983) to produce an antibody to a chlamydial antigen. Alternatively, individuals who are seropositive for an antigen may be given an antigenic boost prior to bleeding. We have used this approach successfully to produce an antibody (UCH D4) to the rhesus D blood group antigen (Crawford *et al.*, 1983b) and Kozbor and Roder (1981) also used a boosted donor to produce antibodies to tetanus toxoid. They showed that the specific Ig-producing cells are only detectable in the circulation temporarily, reaching a peak 14 days after secondary immunization.

Once the donor has been selected, it is necessary to devise a method for preselecting specific antibody-bearing B cells from PBMs. This has most often been carried out by rosetting with antigen-coated red cells (Steinitz *et al.*, 1979, 1980), which is, of course, the method of choice when cells producing antibodies to red cell antigens are being purified (Crawford *et al.*, 1983b). Papain treatment of human red cells increases the number of rosettes by removing negatively charged, surface sialic acid residues and allowing closer contact between the red cells. For other antigens chromic chloride can be used to attach other antigens to red cells prior to rosetting. Rosettes are formed by mixing equal volumes of a 4% red cell suspension, lymphocytes at 10^7/ml, and fetal calf serum, followed by centrifugation at 800 rpm for 10 min and incubation on ice for 1–2 hr. Following gentle resuspension of the cell pellet, the rosettes are separated on a Percoll gradient (Kaplan and Clark, 1974), and the contaminating red cells lysed with distilled water or ammonium chloride. Starting with E-rosette-depleted PBM populations of cells from rhesus D antigen-boosted donors, we regularly see 1–5% of cells rosetting with rhesus D-positive cells using this technique.

Another method that has been used successfully to enrich for specific antibody-producing cells in PBMs involves panning on antigen-coated plates, which Winger *et al.* (1983) used to select cells specific for sperm antigens. Kozbor and Roder (1981) used an indirect method in which PBMs were first incubated with tetanus toxoid, which bound to, and was subsequently capped from, specific antibody-bearing B cells, leaving them without surface Ig. Those cells that still expressed surface Ig after this procedure were rosetted with sheep red cells coupled to rabbit anti-human Ig, separated, and discarded, leaving the cells specific for tetanus toxoid antigens enriched.

Another approach to the selection procedure is to stimulate specific antibody-producing cells *in vitro* by culturing PBMs from a seropositive donor with antigen. This has been used successfully with influenza virus (Crawford *et al.*, 1983a), where a method for specific stimulation of memory B cells from seropositive individuals has been previously published (Callard, 1979). Time course studies using this system showed that although maximum antibody responses were obtained 6–7 days after stimulation with antigen, by this time the ability of B cells to be transformed by EBV was much reduced. This is presumably due to the previously noted (Section II.A) fact that activated B cells are resistant to EBV transformation. Thus, a 3-day incubation period with antigen prior to EBV infection was the time that led to the successful production of a monoclonal antibody. The specific antigen stimulation described by Callard (1979) is a T-cell-dependent system, and therefore T cells must be removed after the antigen incubation prior to EBV transformation in order to prevent cytotoxic T cells specific for EBV-transformed cells from arising in the culture (Moss *et al.*, 1978). Specific *in vitro* antigen stimulation of seropositive PBMs can also be achieved with other viral antigens, in particular herpes zoster virus (Souhami *et al.*, 1981); however, so far we have not succeded in establishing a stable, specific anti-herpes zoster antibody-producing cell line using this technique. Finally, Winger *et al.* (1983) have reported the successful *in vitro* stimulation of primary immune responses to a variety of antigens and the EBV transformation of these cells to give antibody-producing cell lines. If this type of procedure can be regularly achieved, it will greatly ease the problem of donor selection and immunization necessary at the present time to obtain antibody-producing cell lines.

B. Cloning Methods

In my experience it is relatively easy to get to the stage of having culture wells containing EBV-transformed B cells that produce specific antibody. The major problem is to clone these cells before antibody production is lost. Successful cloning has been carried out by limiting dilution (Crawford *et al.*, 1983b) or in agar (Steinitz *et al.*, 1977; Kozbor *et al.*, 1979). Both methods need feeder cells to support the growth of cells plated at low concentrations. A variety of feeder cells have been used, including human fetal fibroblasts (Rosen *et al.*, 1983), autologous (Winger *et al.*, 1983) or allogeneic PBMs (Crawford *et al.*, 1983b), and umbilical cord blood mononuclear cells treated with phytohemagglutinin (Stein and Sigal, 1983), all of which have to be irradiated before use to prevent their continued cell growth. We have had most success using allogeneic PBMs, and in particular those from individuals who are seronegative for antibodies to EB viral antigens (Crawford *et al.*, 1983b). Using these cells at 10^4 per well in 98-well, round-bottom microtiter plates, we regularly achieve a cloning efficiency of 1–3% at one cell per well. Cloning should be carried out as early in the culture period as possible. In practice this means screening the wells as soon as proliferating foci of cells are seen at 10–14 days, and cloning positive wells immediately. Alternatively, we (Crawford *et al.*, 1983b) and other workers (Winger *et al.*, 1983) have had success by plating cells out at limiting dilution on a feeder layer immediately after EBV infection. At this stage cells generally will not grow at concentrations less than 10^2 per well.

C. Stability of Clones

Once cell lines have been cloned twice at ten cells per well and once at one cell per well, they have remained stable in our hands and those of other workers. Our longest growing cell line has continued to grow and produce antibody in culture for 3 years (Crawford *et al.*, 1983a,b) and those of Steinitz *et al.* (1977, 1980) have remained stable for longer periods of time. On occasions, however, cloned cell lines have grown for 3–6 months in culture and then died. The reason for this cell death is not clear, but it may be that this represents a natural senescence in a particular subpopulation of B cells, and stresses once again the heterogeneity among B cells with regard to their immortalization by EBV.

D. Antibody Production by Cloned Cell Lines

The majority of antibody-producing cell lines transformed by EBV produce IgM class of antibody, although several IgG-producing lines have now been reported, and we have one that produces an IgA class of antibody (D. H. Crawford, unpublished observation). It has been suggested that the predominance of IgM-producing cells in transformed cell populations indicates a preference of the virus for infecting IgM-bearing B cells (Katsuki *et al.*, 1977). However, since no difference has been found in EBV receptor density between different B-cell subpopulations (Aman *et al.*, 1984), the finding may just reflect the proponderance of IgM-bearing cells in the PBM population.

Reported levels of antibody produced by cloned cell lines vary from low levels of 10 ng/ml (Zurawski *et al.*, 1981) to levels equivalent to the rodent hybridoma system of 10–20 μg/ml. However, figures from different laboratories are difficult to compare since there is no standardization of cell numbers or culture conditions. Our cell lines, when grown to maximum cell density [about $(1–2) \times 10^6$ cells/ml] under standard culture conditions, produce around 10–20 μg/ml of specific antibody into the culture supernatant medium (Figs. 2B and 2C). This level of antibody has been increased to 43 μg/ml by bulk culture using an air-lift system, where higher cell densities can be achieved (K. Lambert, unpublished observation). Our cell lines regularly contain 10% of cells that express cytoplasmic IgG at any one time. We have tried to increase this level of Ig-producing cells in various ways. It has been reported that antibodies to HLA DR determinants will induce Ig secretion in

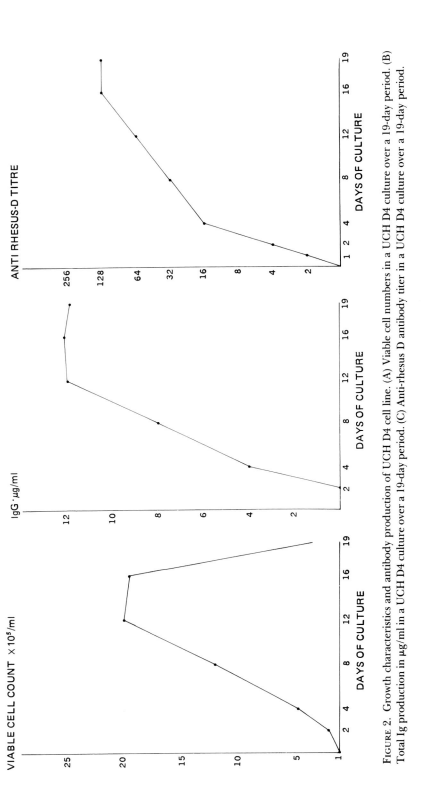

FIGURE 2. Growth characteristics and antibody production of UCH D4 cell line. (A) Viable cell numbers in a UCH D4 culture over a 19-day period. (B) Total Ig production in μg/ml in a UCH D4 culture over a 19-day period. (C) Anti-rhesus D antibody titer in a UCH D4 culture over a 19-day period.

resting B cells and B-cell lines (Palacios *et al.*, 1983), but three such antibodies had no effect on numbers of cytoplasmic Ig-containing cells or Ig production by our cell lines (I. Ando, unpublished observation). Similarly, we have attempted to influence antibody production of our anti-influenza virus nucleoprotein antibody-producing cloned cell line using HLA DR-matched, helper T-cell clones specific for the same influenza viral antigen, without success (J. Lamb unpublished observation). Other workers, however, have reported an increase in antibody production from a cell line secreting IgG specific for influenza A virus when supernatant medium from mitogen-stimulated tonsillar cells was added to the culture (M. H. Brown, unpublished observation). These, and similar results with the EBV-transformed CESS cell line (Muraguchi *et al.*, 1981), suggest that contrary to general belief, EBV-transformed cells are not "frozen" irrevocably at the stage of B-cell differentiation between an activated B cell and a plasma cell, but can be influenced by certain B-cell growth and differentiation factors.

E. Purification of Antibody for Clinical Use

Some workers have expressed doubts as to whether antibody produced by EBV genome-carrying cell lines can ever be used safely *in vivo* in humans (Netzer, 1983). This is because of the etiologic association of EBV with two geographically restricted human malignancies, African Burkitt lymphoma (Epstein and Achong, 1979) and nasopharyngeal carcinoma (Epstein, 1978), and also the ability of the virus to confer immortality on B lymphocytes *in vitro* (Pope *et al.*, 1968). It has been suggested that antibody purified from the culture supernatant medium of an EBV-transformed cell line carries an unacceptable risk of oncogenesis due to possible contamination with EBV particles or viral DNA. We have argued (Crawford *et al.*, 1983c), however, that EBV is a ubiquitous agent, which is carried as a silent infection by the vast majority of the adult population worldwide. Thus, most individuals will have had a subclinical infection during childhood. In a few cases occurring mostly during late adolescence, primary infection will have been manifest as acute infectious mononucleosis (Miller, 1975). Following primary infection, be it subclinical or not, the virus remains in the body in a latent form, carried in B lymphocytes (Nilsson *et al.*, 1971) and secreted intermittently into the saliva (Golden *et al.*, 1973). It therefore follows that EBV particles and viral DNA from cellular debris must be present in most blood donor units used for transfusion. Apart from the very rare cases of transfusion mononucleosis occurring when several units of fresh blood have been transfused into seronegative recipients (Gerber *et al.*, 1969), no ill effect attributable to EBV, and in particular no increased incidence of lymphomas, have been noted following blood transfusion. Furthermore, antibodies for injection, such as antimeasles, anti-varicella zoster, anti-hepatitis B, and anti-rhesus D, are prepared from pooled human serum by cold ethanol precipitation (Kistler and Nitschmann, 1962). These serum donors are not selected as EBV antibody-negative individuals, and yet no ill effect is noted even when these products are given to immunocompromised individuals. Thus the widespread use of blood products has proved that possible EBV-containing material administered in this way is harmless.

We have devised a scheme for the purification of UCH D4 antibody from culture supernatant medium to remove extraneous proteins, virus particles, and DNA (Crawford et al., 1983c). The protocol is shown in Table I. The culture fluid is double filtered to remove infectious EBV particles and treated with DNase (bovine pancreas DNase; Sigma Chemical Co. London) to digest DNA to less than gene-sized fragments. Following this, adherence of the IgG antibody to an anti-human IgG column allows the passage and removal of all other unwanted constituents of the culture supernatant medium. The antibody is eluted from the column with acid and dialyzed against injectable-grade isotonic saline in pyrogen-free glassware, concentrated to the desired strength, filtered to sterilize, and stored in 1-ml glass, pyrogen-free vials. A sample from each batch of purified antibody produced has been pyrogen-tested in rabbits (Safepham, Derby, England) and always found to be pyrogen-free.

In order to test the efficiency of this purification schedule for removing infectious EBV particles and DNA from the culture supernatant medium, we have carried out spiking experiments in which known amounts of EBV or DNA were added to UCH D4 culture supernatant prior to purification and their presence sought in the final concentrated product (Crawford et al., 1984). When 10^{-3} g/ml of DNA was used this was reduced to less than 10^{-8} g/ml in the purified product. Since UCH D4 supernatant medium actually contains around 10^{-6} g/ml of DNA, this would be purified by the same procedure to 10^{-11} g/ml DNA. Knowing that UCH D4 cell line contains approximately 20 EBV genomes/cell, we can determine that a 1-ml dose (100 μg) of the final purified product would contain less than one EBV genome worth of DNA.

TABLE I

Purification Scheme for Human
Monoclonal Antibody from Culture
Supernatant Medium

1. Pass through 0.22-μm filter
2. Pass through 0.1-μm filter
3. Treat with DNase 1 hr, 37°C
4. Pass down anti-human IgG column
5. Elute with 0.5% acetic acid
6. Dialyze against isotonic saline
7. Concentrate using Amicon filter
8. Pass through 0.22-μm filter
9. Pyrogen test in rabbits

When 5 ml of concentrated EBV prepared from culture supernatant medium of the B95-8 cell line with a transforming titer of over 10^{-3} was added to 100 ml of UCH D4 culture supernatant medium, transforming EBV was easily detectable. No transforming virus was detectable in the final purified product of UCH D4 antibody. These results encouraged us to use our purified UCH D4 antibody in *in vivo* trials in human adult volunteers.

F. Clinical Testing of Antibodies

Human antibodies prepared from immune serum are used clinically for the prevention of many diseases, particularly infectious diseases in immunosuppressed individuals, and in the prevention of rhesus disease of the newborn. In most cases antibodies are in short supply and the unlimited supply of a standardized, safe, monoclonal reagent would be an obvious advantage. In the case of anti-rhesus D antibody at the present time male rhesus-negative volunteers are immunized with rhesus D-positive cells in order to supply the demand. IgG antibody purified from this hyperimmune serum is given to rhesus-negative mothers at the time of birth of a rhesus-positive baby, when rhesus-positive red cells may enter the circulation and cause the production of an anti-rhesus D antibody (Clarke *et al.*, 1963). This antibody is usually of the IgG class, which can cross the placenta and cause destruction of the red cells of a subsequent rhesus-positive fetus. It is not known exactly how the passive administration of anti-D antibody works to prevent this immune response, but it is suggested that coating of the antigenic sites on the positive red cells followed by their rapid removal from the circulation to the spleen may prevent their recognition by the immune system. We are at present testing UCH D4 for its ability to prevent an immune response when given to rhesus-negative volunteers subsequently challenged with rhesus-positive red cells.

IV. Future Perspectives

At the present time there is no method for making human monoclonal antibodies *in vitro* that compares in efficiency with the mouse or rat hybridoma technique (Köhler and Milstein, 1975). It is clear that both the use of EBV transformation of B cells and the application of the hybridoma technology to make cell lines producing human monoclonal antibodies must be much improved before they can be recommended for routine use. One of the main problems common to both these systems is that of donor selection, since humans, unlike rodents, cannot be hyperimmunized, and spleen tissue, where most antibody-producing cells probably reside, is not usually available. The further study of *in vitro* stimulation of B cells with specific antigen may at least partly overcome this problem.

It is still unclear which subset of human B lymphocytes is infected, immortalized, and activated to produce Ig by EBV; the isolation of such a subset would greatly ease the initial stages in the preparation of monoclonal antibody-producing cell lines, when overgrowth by unwanted cells is a constant problem. It may be that such cells exist in higher concentrations in human lymphoid tissue, and a thorough study of the susceptibility to EBV transformation of B-cell populations in human tonsil, spleen, and lymph node material may yield profitable results.

Another method for increasing the yield of monoclonal antibody-producing clones is to use EBV initially to amplify the few specific antibody-producing cells in PBMs, and then fuse these cells to immortalized cell lines bearing two selectable features (J. C. Roder, *et al.,* this volume, Chapter 4). In this way the stability of the clone may be improved, and it is also stated that Ig production can be increased (Kozbor *et al.,* 1982). Thus, much investigation is necessary in order to define the best system for the use of EBV as a tool to make human monoclonal antibody-producing cell lines, but the fact that so many stable lines have already been produced encourages us to continue in the search for the ideal system.

ACKNOWLEDGMENTS

I thank N. Mulholland for technical help, Dr. S. Pereira for measurements of Ig levels (Fig. 1), and K. Brickenden for clerical assistance.

References

Aman, P., Ehlin-Henriksson, B., and Klein, G., 1984, Epstein–Barr virus susceptibility of normal human B lymphocyte populations, *J. Exp. Med.* **159**:208–220.

Callard, R. E., 1979, Specific *in vitro* antibody response to influenza virus by human blood lymphocytes, *Nature* **282**:734–736.

Clarke, C. A., Donohue, W. T. A., McConnell, R. B., Woodrow, J. C., Finn, R., Krevans, J. R., Kulke, W., Lehare, D., and Sheppard, P. M., 1963, Further experimental studies on the prevention of Rh haemolytic disease, *Br. Med. J.* **i**:979.

Crawford, D. H., 1981, Lymphomas after cyclosporin A treatment, in: *Transplantation and Clinical Immunology XIII* (J. T. Touraine, J. Traeger, H. Betuel, J. Brochier, J. M. Dubernard, J. P. Revillard, and R. Triau, eds.), Excerpta Medica, Amsterdam pp. 48–52.

Crawford, D. H., Callard, R. E., Muggeridge, M. I., Mitchell, D. M., Zanders, E. D., and Beverley, P. C. L., 1983a, Production of human monoclonal antibody to X31 influenza virus nucleoprotein, *J. Gen Virol.* **64**:697–700.

Crawford, D. H., Barlow, M. J., Harrison, J. F., Winger, L., Huehns, E. R., 1983b, Production of human monoclonal antibody to rhesus D antigen, *Lancet* **i**:386–388.

Crawford, D. H., Huehns, E. R., and Epstein, M. A., 1983c, Therapeutic use of human monoclonal antibodies, *Lancet* **i**:1040.

Crawford, D. H., Barlow, M. J., Mulholland, N., McDougall, D. C. J., Zanders, E. D., Tippett, P., and Huehns, E. R., 1984, The production and characterisation of a human monoclonal antibody to the rhesus D antigen, *Proc. Br. Blood Transfusion Soc.* **1**:113–121.

Doyle, A., Jones, T., Bidwell, J., and Bradley, B., *In vitro* production of human monoclonal antibody producing plasmacytoma, *Hum. Immunol.* In press.

Epstein, M. A., 1978, Epstein–Barr virus—Discovery, properties and relationship to nasopharyngeal carcinoma, in: *NasoPharyngeal Carcinoma; Aetiology and Control* (G. de-The, Y. Ho, and W. Davis, eds.), IARC, Lyon, pp. 333–345.

Epstein, M. A., and Achong, B. G., 1979, The relationship of the virus to Burkitt's lymphoma, in: *The Epstein–Barr Virus* (M. A. Epstein and B. G. Achong, eds.), Springer, Berlin, pp. 321–337.

Fresen, U., and Zur Hausen, H., 1976, Establishment of EBNA-expressing cell lines by infection of Epstein–Barr virus (EBV)-genome-negative human lymphoma cells with different EBV strains, *Int. J. Cancer* **17**:161–166.

Gerber, P., 1972, Activation of Epstein–Barr virus by 5-bromodeoxyuridine in virus-free human cells, *Proc. Natl. Acad. Sci. USA* **69**:83–85.

Gerber, P., Walsh, J. H., Rosenblum, E. N., and Purcell, R. H., 1969, Association of EB-virus infection with the post-perfusion syndrome, *Lancet* **i**:593–596.

Golden, H. D., Chang, R. S., Prescott, W., Simpson, E., and Cooper, T.Y., 1973, Leukocyte-transforming agent: Prolonged excretion by patients with mononucleosis and excretion by normal individuals, *J. Infect. Dis.* **127**:471–473.

Greaves, F. M., Brown, G., and Rickinson, A. B., 1975, Epstein–Barr virus binding sites on lymphocyte subpopulations and the origin of lymphoblasts in cultured lymphoid cell lines and in the blood of patients with infectious mononucleosis, *Clin. Immunol. Immunopathol.* **3**:514.

Henderson, E., Miller, G., Robinson, J., and Heston, L., 1977, Efficiency of transformation of lymphocytes by Epstein–Barr virus, *Virology* **76**:152–163.

Henle, G., Henle, W., and Diehl, V., 1968, Relation of Burkitt's tumour-associated herpes-type virus to infectious mononucleosis, *Proc. Natl. Acad. Sci. USA* **59**:94–101.

Irie, R. F., Sze, L. L., and Saxton, R. E., 1982, Human antibody to OFA-1, a tumour antigen, produced *in vitro* by Epstein–Barr virus-transformed human B-lymphoid cell lines, *Proc. Natl. Acad. Sci. USA* **79**:5666–5670.

Kamo, I., Furukawa, S., Tada, A., Mano, Y., Iwasaki, Y., and Furuse, T., 1982, Monoclonal antobody to acetylcholine receptor: Cell line established from thymus of patient with myasthenia gravis, *Science* **215**:995–997.

Kaplan, M. E., and Clark, C., 1974, An improved rosetting assay for detection of human T lymphocytes, *J. Immunol. Meth.* **5**:131–135.

Katsuki, T., Hiruma, Y., Yamamoto, N., Abo, T., and Kumagai, K., 1977, Identification of the target cells in human B lymphocytes for transformation by Epstein–Barr virus, *Virology* **83**:287–294.

Kistler, P., and Nitschmann, H., 1962, Large scale production of human plasma fractions, *Vox Sang.* **7**:414–424.

Köhler, G., and Milstein, C., 1975, Continuous cultures of fused cells secreting antibody of predefined specificity, *Nature* **256**:496.

Kozbor, D., and Roder, J. C., 1981, Requirements for the establishment of high-titred human monoclonal antibodies against tetanus toxoid using the Epstein–Barr virus technique, *J. Immunol.* **127**:1275–1280.

Kozbor, D., Steinitz, M., Klein, G., Koskimies, S., and Makela, O., 1979, Establishment of anti-TNP antibody producing human lymphoid lines by preselection for hapten binding followed by EBV transformation, *Scand. J. Immunol.* **10**:187–194.

Kozbor, D., Lagarde, A. E., and Roder, J. C., 1982, Human hybridomas constructed with antigen-specific Epstein–Barr virus-transformed cell lines, *Proc. Natl. Acad. Sci. USA* **79**:6651–6655.

Luka, J., Kallin, B., and Klein, G., 1979, Induction of the Epstein–Barr virus (EBV) cycle in latently infected cells by *n*-butyrate, *Virology* **94**:228–231.

Lundgren, K., Wahlgren, M., Troye-blomberg, M., Berzins, I. C., Perlmann, H., and Perlmann, P., 1983, Monoclonal anti-parasite and anti-RBC antibodies produced by stable EBV-transformed B cell lines from malaria patients, *J. Immunol.* **131:**2000–2003.

Miller, G., 1975, Epstein–Barr herpes virus and infectious mononucleosis, *Progr. Med. Virol.* **20:**84–112.

Miller, G., Shope, T., Lisco, H., Stitt, D., and Lipman, M., 1972, Epstein–Barr virus: Transformation cytopathic changes and viral antigens in squirrel monkey and marmoset leucocytes, *Proc. Natl. Acad. Sci. USA* **69:**383–387.

Miller, G., Niederman, J. C., and Andrews, L. L., 1973, Prolonged oropharyngeal excretion of Epstein–Barr virus after infectious mononucleosis, *N. Eng. J. Med.* **288:**229–232.

Moss, D. J., Rickinson, A. B., and Pope, J. H., 1978, Long-term T-cell-mediated immunity to Epstein–Barr virus in man. I. Complete regression of virus-induced transformation in cultures of seropositive donor leucocytes, *Int. J. Cancer* **22:**662–668.

Muraguchi, A., Kishimoto, T., Miki, Y., Kuritoni, T., Kaieda, T., Yoskizaki, K., and Yamamura, Y., 1981, T Cell-replacing factor (TRF) induced IgG secretion in a human B blastoid cell line and demonstrations of acceptors for TRF, *J. Immunol.* **127:**412–416.

Netzer, W., 1983, Monotech patents method for human–human hybridomas, *Gene. Eng. News* **1983**(January/February):1.

Nilsson, K., and Pontén, J., 1975, Classification and virological nature of established human haemopoetic cell lines, *Int. J. Cancer* **15:**321–341.

Nilsson, K., Klein, G., Henle, W., and Henle, G., 1971, The establishment of lymphoblastoid lines from adult and foetal human lymphoid cells and its dependence on EBV, *Int. J. Cancer* **8:**443–450.

Palacios, R., Martinez-Maza, O., and Guy, K., 1983, Monoclonal antibodies against HLA DR antigens replace T helper cells in activation of B lymphocytes, *Proc. Natl. Acad. Sci. USA* **80:**3456–3460.

Pattengale, P. K., Smith, R. W., and Gerber, P., 1973, Selective transformation of B lymphocytes by EB virus, *Lancet* **ii:**93–94.

Pope, J. H., Horne, M. K., and Scott, W., 1968, Transformation of foetal human leucocytes *in vitro* by filtrates of a human leukaemia cell line containing herpes-like virus, *Int. J. Cancer* **3:**857–866.

Pope, J. H., Scott, W., and Moss, D. J., 1974, Cell relationships in transformation of human leucocytes by Epstein–Barr virus, *Int. J. Cancer* **14:**122–129.

Reedman, B. M., and Klein, G., 1973, Cellular localisation of an Epstein–Barr virus (EBV)-associated complement-fixing antigen in producer and non-producer lymphoblastoid cell lines, *Int. J. Cancer* **2:**499–520.

Rickinson, A. B., Moss, D. J., and Pope, J. H., 1979, Long-term T-cell mediated immunity to Epstein–Barr virus in man. II Components necessary for regression in virus infected leucocyte culture, *Int. J. Cancer* **23:**610–617.

Rosen, A., Gergely, P., Jondal, M., Klein, G., and Britton, S., 1977, Polyclonal Ig production after Epstein–Barr virus infection of human lymphocytes *in vitro*, *Nature* **267:**52–54.

Rosen, A., Persson, K., and Klein, G., 1983, Human monoclonal antibodies to a genus-specific chlamydial antigen, produced by EBV-transformed B cells, *J. Immunol.* **130:**2899–2902.

Seigneurin, J. M., Desgranges, C., Seigneurin, D., Paine, J., Renversez, J. C., Jacquemond, B., and Micouin, C., 1983, Herpes simplex virus glycoprotein D: Human monoclonal antibody produced by bone marrow cell line, *Science* **221:**173–175.

Souhami, R. L., Babbage, J., and Callard, R. E., 1981, Specific *in vitro* antibody response to varicella zoster, *Clin. Exp. Immunol.* **46:**98–105.

Stein, L. D., and Sigal, N. H., 1983, Limiting dilution analysis of Epstein–Barr virus-induced immunoglobulin production, *Cell. Immunol.* **79:**309–319.

Steinitz, M., Klein, G., Koskimies, S., and Makela, O., 1977, EB virus induced B lymphocyte cell lines producing specific antibody, *Nature* **269:**420–422.

Steinitz, M., Koskimies, S., Klein, G., and Makela, O., 1979, Establishment of specific antibody producing human lines by antigen preselection and Epstein–Barr (EBV) transformation, *Clin. Lab. Immunol.* **2:**1–7.

Steinitz, M., Izak, G., Cohen, S., Ehrenfeld, M., and Flechner, I., 1980, Continuous production of monoclonal rheumatoid factor by EBV-transformed lymphocytes, *Nature* **287:**443–445.

Steinitz, M., Tauier, S., and Goldfarb, A., 1984, Human anti-pneumococci antibody produced by an Epstein–Barr virus (EBV)-immortalised cell lines, *J. Immunol.* **132:**877–882.

Winger, L., Winger, C., Shastry, P., Russell, A., and Longenecker, M., 1983, Efficient generation *in vitro* of monoclonal Epstein–Barr virus-transformants producing specific antibody to a variety of antigens, without prior deliberate immunisation, *Proc. Natl. Acad. Sci. USA* **80:**4484–4488.

Yarchoau, R., Tosato, G., Blaese, R. A., Simon, R. M., and Nelson, D. L., 1983, Limiting dilution analysis of Epstein–Barr virus-induced immunoglobulin production by human B cells, *J. Exp. Med.* **157:**1–14.

Zerbini, M., and Emberg, I., 1983, Can Epstein–Barr virus infect and transform all the B-lymphocytes of human cord blood?, *J. Gen. Virol.* **64:**539–547.

Zurawski, V. R., Spedden, S. E., Black, P. H., and Haber, E., 1978, Clones of human lymphoblastoid cell lines producing antibody to tenanus toxoid, in: *Lymphocyte Hybridomas, Volume 81* (F. Melchers, M. Potter, N. Warner, eds.), Springer, Berlin, pp. 152–155.

Zur Hausen, H., O'Neill, F. J., Freese, U. K., and Hecker, E., 1978, Persisting oncogenic herpes virus induced by the tumor promoter TPA, *Nature* **272:**373–375.

4

The Epstein–Barr Virus-Hybridoma Technique

JOHN C. RODER, SUSAN P. C. COLE,
TSEHAY ATLAW, BARBARA G. CAMPLING,
RONALD C. MCGARRY, AND DANUTA KOZBOR

I. Epstein–Barr Virus Technology

A. Immortalization

Several years before the application of Köhler and Milstein's (1975) hybridoma technology to the production of human monoclonal antibodies, human lymphoid lines producing antibody with defined antigenic specificity were established by Epstein–Barr virus (EBV) "immortalization" (Steinitz *et al.*, 1977). EBV is a lymphotropic herpes virus, which transforms normal B lymphocytes and makes it possible to culture these cells as permanent lines. Rosen *et al.* (1977) demonstrated that direct infection of purified human blood lymphocytes with EBV *in vitro* induced polyclonal secretion of immunoglobulins. Culture supernatants assayed by immunoassay contained a heterogeneous assortment of immunoglobulin isotypes and antibodies specific for various randomly selected antigens. It became obvious, then, that if monospecific B cells could be transformed *in vitro* into continuous cell lines by EBV and if

JOHN C. RODER, SUSAN P. C. COLE, TSEHAY ATLAW AND RONALD C. MCGARRY • Department of Microbiology and Immunology, Queen's University, Kingston, Ontario, Canada K7L 3N6. BARBARA G. CAMPLING • Department of Medicine and Radiation Oncology, Queen's University, Kingston, Ontario, Canada K7L 3N6. DANUTA KOZBOR • The Wistar Institute of Anatomy and Biology, Philadelphia, Pennsylvania 19104.

these "immortalized" cells could be triggered to produce antibodies, permanent lines of B lymphocytes might be established that were capable of producing specific monoclonal antibodies against any appropriate antigen.

B. Selection of Antigen-Specific Cells

In the EBV technique, as in the hybridoma procedure, it is important to use lymphocytes of individuals who have previously been immunized with the antigens and have increased numbers of specific antibody-producing cells. The procedure involves two steps: (1) the enrichment of cells with receptors for the given antigen; and (2) "immortalization" of these cells by EBV infection. Preselection of antigen-specific cells may facilitate the establishment of specific cell lines, since even after immunization in vivo, only a small fraction of the B lymphocytes produce the desired antibody. Several methods of preselection have been tried: (1) antigen-specific lymphocytes were enriched by rosetting with antigen-coupled erythrocytes (Steinitz et al., 1977, 1979, 1980; Steinitz and Tamir, 1982; Kozbor et al., 1979; Koskimies, 1979; Boylston et al., 1980), (2) fluorescence-labeled antigen was bound to the surface of the antigen-specific cells, which were subsequently separated on the fluorescence-activated cell sorter (FACS) (Kozbor and Roder, 1981), (3) antigen was bound to solid surfaces in a panning technique (Winger et al., 1983), and (4) cells that did not bind antigen were removed (Kozbor and Roder, 1981). This negative preselection technique was first performed in the mouse by Walker et al. (1977) and is based on the observation that B cells, upon binding to antigen, usually shed their surface Ig receptors and become nude (stripped) (Kozbor and Roder, 1981). In the human, the B-cell-enriched fractions were obtained by the removal of monocytes and cells rosetting with sheep red blood cells (SRBC). Those B cells not binding antigen, and therefore maintaining their surface Ig, are removed by rosetting with $F(ab')_2$ anti-human Ig-coated SRBC. The remaining nonrosetting B cells are then EBV-infected and the resulting antigen-specific cell line is cloned by limiting dilution on a feeder layer.

However, despite the occasional success of these techniques, it is not yet clear which type of B cell can be infected and triggered by EBV to secrete immunoglobulin, and therefore some methods of enrichment for antigen-binding cells may lead to the selection of cells that are at an inappropriate stage of maturation for Ig secretion after EBV transformation under the conditions employed. An alternative strategy involves the transformation of the total B-cell population with subsequent cloning and testing for antibody-producing cultures (Zurawski et al., 1978a,b; Yoshie and Ono, 1980; Tsuchiya et al., 1980; Kamo et al., 1982; Irie et al., 1982; D. B. Watson et al., 1983; Rosen et al., 1983; Crawford et al., 1983b; Seigneurin et al., 1983).

C. Limitations of the System

Using the EBV technique, several cell lines have been established and a variety of antibodies obtained: IgM anti-NNP (4-hydroxyl-3,5-dinitrophenacetic acid) (Steinitz et al., 1977); IgM anti-DNP (trinitrophenyl hapten) (Kozbor et al., 1979); IgM anti-streptococcal carbohydrate (Steinitz et al., 1979); IgG anti-tetanus toxoid (Zurawski et al., 1978a,b), IgG and IgM anti-rhesus antigen D (Koskimies, 1979; Boylston et al., 1980; Crawford et al., 1983a); IgM phosphorylcholine (Yoshie and Ono, 1980); IgM anti-IgG complexed with antigens [e.g., rheumatoid factor (Steinitz et al., 1980)]; IgM anti-tetanus toxoid (Kozbor and Roder, 1981), and antibodies against diptheria toxoid (Tsuchia et al., 1980), acetylcholine receptor (Kamo et al., 1982), melanoma antigens (Irie et al., 1982; D. B. Watson et al., 1983), bacterial antigens (Rosen et al., 1983), viral antigens (Crawford et al., 1983b; Seigneurin et al., 1983), and DNA (Winger et al., 1983). The main limitations of the EBV technique, in general, are the low quantities of antibody produced (<1 μg/ml) and the relative instability (<8 months) of these lines. The reason for the instability of some of these lines is still unclear. In the cell lines that secrete anti-tetanus toxoid (TT), declining anti-TT antibody production was observed in uncloned bulk cultures (Kozbor and Roder, 1981). The reason for the gradual loss of antibody secretion did not reside solely in differential growth rates of producer and nonproducer cells. It is likely that more complex, intracellular changes are involved, such as the selective loss of light-chain expression that we observed in one TT-specific, cloned cell line after 8 months of continuous culture (Kozbor et al., 1982b). However, it is possible to rescue high amounts of antibody production in these declining EBV lines by somatic cell hybridization, as outlined below.

II. The Epstein–Barr Virus-Hybridoma Technique

Antibody secretion can be "rescued" in B cells at various stages of maturation. Laskov et al. (1979) reported the induction of IgM secretion in a murine B lymphoma, which expressed only surface IgM, by fusion with IgG-secreting plasmacytoma cells. Levy and Dilley (1978) have demonstrated that human neoplastic B cells that do not normally secrete Ig can be induced to secrete large amounts of Ig when hybridized to mouse plasmacytoma cells.

A. Interspecies Hybrids

These results suggested that a general approach to the establishment of human antibody-secreting lines might consist in somatic cell fusion of EBV-transformed cells with a murine plasmacytoma cell line. First, an EBV-transformed clone (B6) producing anti-tetanus toxoid antibody and obtained from blood lymphocytes of a healthy TT-immunized donor was fused with a non-Ig-producing murine plasmacytoma P3X63Ag.8 v.653 and selected in HAT medium containing 10^{-5} M ouabain (Oua), since the EBV-infected lymphocytes used for fusion were immortalized and could not be counterselected otherwise (Kozbor et al., 1982a). Hybrid clones were stable for 6 months of culture and produced up to 1.8 μg/ml of specific antibody on days 9 and 10 after seeding, whereas the human EBV parent produced only 0.7 μg/ml (Table I). Clones eventually lost antibody production after 6 months of continuous culture, possibly due to inherent chromosomal instability of interspecies hybrids.

B. Intraspecies Hybrids: Development of a Fusion Partner

In order to avoid this instability, the EBV-transformed, anti-TT-antibody-producing clone B6 was fused with a human partner. Because ouabain resistance is a dominant trait and mouse cells have a naturally 10,000-fold greater resistance to it than human cells, ouabain became very useful for selecting mouse–human hybrids. However, this species difference in ouabain sensitivity is of no advantage when both fusion partners are of human origin. Therefore, in order to obtain the human–human hybrids, especially since both parental cells showed indefinite outgrowth in vitro, it was necessary to select an ouabain-resistant fusion partner. A 6-thioguanine-resistant GM1500 human lymphoblastoid cell line (LCL) was mutagenized by low-level γ irradiation, selected for ouabain resistance, and fused with an EBV-transformed cell line producing anti-TT antibody (Kozbor et al., 1982b). Due to the dominance of ouabain resistance and the recessiveness of thioguanine resistance in the parental LCL, now designated KR-4, only hybrid cells derived from the fusion of KR-4 and the EBV clone could survive selection in HAT medium containing ouabain. The hybridomas produced four- to eightfold more anti-TT antibody per 10^6 cells than did the EBV parent (Table I). Biosynthetic labeling of proteins followed by SDS–PAGE of immunoprecipitates revealed that hybrids synthesized both μ and λ chains from the parental lines as well as κ light chains. The EBV-transformed parental line synthesized very little light chain in comparison to μ chain, a finding that may explain the declining anti-TT titer observed during prolonged proliferation. It is noteworthy that anti-TT production in hybridomas has remained stable throughout 24 months of continuous culture to the present time. Indeed, the karyotype analysis of human–human hybrids indicated that chromosome segregation was very limited, and in several instances a chromosome modal number close to tetraploid was found.

TABLE I

A Comparison of the EBV and EBV-Hybridoma Systems for Producing Human Monoclonal Antibodies

Lymphocyte source[a]	Selection[b]	Donor[c]	EBV-transformed[d]	Fusion partner[e]	Number of hybrids or clones screened[f]	Antigen[g]	Fusion frequency[h] (× 10^{-7})	Percent antigen-specific hybrids or clones[i]	Specific Ig-secretion[j] (μg/ml)	Ig class[k]	Cloning efficiency[l] (%)	Stability[m] (months)	Reference
PBL	+	V	+	None	96	TT	NA	3.1	0.7	IgM	30	6	Kozbor and Roder (1981)
PBL	+	V	+	P3X63Ag.8	200	TT	100	70.0[n]	1.8	IgM	ND	6	Kozbor et al. (1982a)
PBL	+	V	+	KR-4	395	TT	112	94.0	4.2	IgM	64	>24	Kozbor et al. (1982b)
PBL	−	V	+	KR-4	936	TT	36	0.7	2.6	IgM/IgG	ND	>6	Kozbor and Roder (1984)
PBL	−	V	−	KR-4	20	TT	2	0.0	0.0	—	ND	ND	Kozbor et al. (1982b), Kozbor and Roder (1984)
Tonsil	−	V	−	KR-4	32	TT	8	0.0	0.0	—	ND	ND	Kozbor and Roder (1984)
PBL	−	L	+	KR-4	4,400	Lep	126	8.2	10.0	IgM	90	>6	Atlaw et al. (1985)
PBL	−	L	−	KR-4	5	Lep	2	0.0	0.0	—	ND	ND	Atlaw et al. (1985)
PBL	−	L	+	None	10,000	Lep	NA	0.42	ND	ND	ND	2	Atlaw et al. (1985)
PBL, LN, BM, TIL, PE	−	C	+	KR-4	4,500	Tum	166	8.0	44	IgM	20	>11	Cole et al. (1984a)
PBL, LN, BM, TIL, PE	−	C	+	None	140	Tum	NA	0.7	ND	ND	1	ND	Cole et al. (1984a)
PBL	−	N	+	None	300	MAG	NA	0.6	ND	ND	ND	ND	McGarry et al. (1985)

[a] Source of lymphocytes: PBL, fresh peripheral blood lymphocytes; tonsil, pokeweed mitogen-stimulated tonsilar lymphocytes; LN, draining lymph node cells; BM, bone marrow cells; TIL, tumor-infiltrating lymphocytes; PE, pericardial effusion cells.

[b] EBV lines were selected for anti-tetanus toxoid reactivity and one clone, B6, from such a line was used on the donor cell in hybridization experiments.

[c] V, normal donors vaccinated with tetanus toxoid 2–3 weeks prior to fusions; L, lepromatous leprosy patients selected with high levels of circulating antibody against $M.$ $leprae$; C, lung cancer patients with small-cell, large-cell, adeno, squamous, and bronchoalveolar carcinoma used as lymphocyte donors; N, peripheral neuropathy patients with IgM paraproteinemia and high titers of anti-myelin-associated glycoprotein antibody used as PBL donors.

[d] Lymphocytes were transformed with Epstein–Barr virus (B95-8).

[e] Donor lymphocytes were fused with a TG^R murine plasmacytoma P3X63Ag8.653 or a TG^R, Oua^R human lymphoblastoid cell line, KR-4, for hybridoma studies or were not fused for studies of EBV clones.

[f] Number of hybrids or clones screened for reactivity with an enzyme-linked immunosorbent assay (ELISA). Hybridization was confirmed by analysis of chromosomes and codominant expression of phenotypic markers in selected hybridomas. Clonality was confirmed by isoelectric focusing of secreted immunoglobulins in selected cases.

[g] TT, Purified tetanus toxoid; Lep, glycolipid or protein extracts from $Mycobacterium$ $leprae$; Tum glutaraldehyde-fixed human lung tumor cells; MAG, purified human myelin-associated glycoprotein (molecular weight 110,000).

[h] Fusion frequency (ff) was calculated from the following formula using 96-well plates with less than the Poisson number (66% of wells positive for growth: ff = $[\ln(\Delta/96)]/\chi$, where Δ is the number of wells negative for growth and χ is one-half the number of cells plated per well, since equal numbers of lymphocytes and fusion partner cells were hybridized. NA, Not applicable.

[i] The proportion of all wells positive for growth that secreted antibody reacting with the antigen in question.

[j] The quantity of antigen-reactive antibody secreted from 10^5 hybridoma cells grown in a logarithmic fashion over a 7-day growth period. Values are means from several high-producing hybridomas selected for further study. ND, Not determined.

[k] Most hybridomas secreted antigen specific antibody of the IgM class, although occasionally (1/20) IgG hybridomas were also found. ND, Not determined.

[l] Cloning was performed by limiting dilution on feeder layers and cloning efficiency was calculated using the formula in footnote h. ND, Not determined.

[m] The length of time in continuous culture that hybridomas or EBV clones continued to produce specific antibody before becoming unstable and ceasing specific Ig secretion. "Greater than" signifies that an endpoint was not reached and cultures secreted antibody beyond the time indicated. ND, Not determined.

[n] Only 1/5 of these were stable for the 6-month period of study.

III. Anti-Tetanus Monoclonals from in Vitro Immunized Cultures

One limitation of human hybridoma technology is the requirement thus far to use lymphocytes from hyperimmunized donors. Sources of parental cells have included peripheral blood lymphocytes (PBLs) from measles virus-infected, subacute sclerotizing panencephalitis patients (Croce *et al.*, 1980), spleen cells from dinitrochlorobenzene-sensitized Hodgkin patients (Olsson and Kaplan, 1980), tumor-infiltrating lymphocytes (Sikora *et al,,* 1982, 1983), and tonsils from tetanus-vaccinated donors (Chiorazzi *et al.*, 1982). It is apparent that PBLs from humans offer the only readily available source of normal lymphocytes for fusion. However, the fact that only one in ten PBLs is a B cell is no small barrier to the hybridoma field. As reported by Stevens *et al.* (1979), the frequency of B cells in the circulation capable of responding to pokeweed mitogen (PWM) by producing anti-tetanus toxoid (TT) antibody of the IgG class was only 1×10^{-4} 2–4 weeks after booster injection. This low number, together with a fusion frequency of 10^{-6} and a B-cell frequency of 10^{-1}, makes the chance of obtaining a specific hybridoma on the order of 10^{-11}, or 10^{-9} if we allow for a 100-fold greater fusion frequency with antigen-stimulated B cells.

We have compared the usefulness of specific antigens (TT) and two polyclonal mitogens (PWM, EBV) in stimulating cultures of PBLs prior to fusion (Fig. 1). Stimulation with EBV yielded cells with much higher frequencies of hybrid formation (36×10^{-7}) compared to unstimulated PBL or cells cultured with PWM or TT antigen. The proportion of hybridomas (approximately 1%) producing anti-TT antibody was similar in EBV- and TT-stimu-

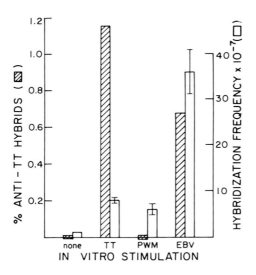

FIGURE 1. The effect of *in vitro* stimulation on hybridoma formation. PBLs of five TT-immunized donors were cultured for 5 days with tetanus toxoid (TT) (0.5 μg/ml) or PWM (1/100) or for 14 days with EBV. Cells were harvested, fused with KR-4, and seeded at 2×10^5 cells/well on feeder layers. Hybrids were selected in HAT medium containing ouabain and wells were scored for cell growth 3–4 weeks after fusion. Culture supernatants were assayed at half confluence for anti-TT production using an ELISA technique. Fusion frequency was calculated from the mean fraction of negative wells/plate using the Poisson equation. Positive hybrids all produced >100 ng/ml anti-TT antibody at a level of detection of 1 ng/ml.

lated cultures. Preselection of EBV subcultures for high anti-TT production prior to fusion resulted in a fivefold increase in TT-specific hybridomas (p <0.001). Most (20/21) specific hybrids produced IgM anti-TT, whereas only one (1/21) produced IgG anti-TT, possibly due to the immature stage of differentiation in EBV-stimulated parental cells. The ability to choose an antigen, immunize, and expand the rare antigen-specific B cells from PBL *in vitro* with EBV or antigen prior to fusion should yield an increasing spectrum of human monoclonal antibodies for diagnostic, therapeutic, or basic studies.

IV. Anti-Mycobacterium leprae Monoclonals

Human hybridomas were constructed that produce antibodies against three different antigen preparations of *Mycobacterium leprae* (Table I). EBV-transformed cell lines from lepromatous leprosy (LL) patients fused with KR-4 at frequencies of 1.26×10^{-5}. Non-EBV-transformed donor cells fused at much lower rates (2×10^{-7}). An enzyme-linked immunosorbent assay (ELISA) was used to screen for antibodies against three antigen preparations of armadillo-derived *M. leprae*, including (1) a soluble sonicate antigen, (2) an SDS extract of insoluble sonicated *M. leprae,* and (3) a phenolic glycolipid antigen. Out of a total of 4400 clones screened, 359 (8.15%) were found to secrete antibody that bound to soluble sonicate antigen and SDS extract. In another series of 168 clones, 21 (12.5%) showed positivity to the glycolipid antigen. The specificity of these monoclonal antibodies was partially determined by screening on a panel of antigens from four other mycobacteria. Nine clones out of 122 showed specificity for *M. leprae*. The predominant immunoglobulin was IgM and quantities of up to 10 µg/ml were produced. Antibody production by hybrid clones was stable in more than 75% of the clones grown in continuous culture. In comparison, 10,000 EBV-transformed lymphocyte clones from lepromatous leprosy patients were screened for anti-*M. leprae* antibody production and all the 42 clones that were initially positive in the ELISA lost their antibody-producing capabilities within 6 weeks in culture. These results suggest that a combination of EBV transformation and hybridization may be an optimal method in producing human monoclonal antibodies from leprosy patients (Atlaw *et al.*, 1984).

V. Human Monoclonal Antibodies against Lung Carcinoma Cell Lines

EBV-immortalized cell lines were established from lymphocytes derived from peripheral blood, draining lymph nodes, bone marrow aspirates, tumors, and pericardial effusions from lung cancer patients (Table I). Ten of these lines were cloned and screened against glutaraldehyde-fixed lung t.

mor cells for tumor-specific antibody production using ELISA. Only one of the 140 clones tested secreted antibody binding to tumor cells. This reaction was not tumor-specific, however, suggesting that B lymphocytes specific for tumor antigens are rare in lung cancer patients. The EBV lines from the lung cancer patients were then hybridized with KR-4 in an attempt to rescue low-frequency B-cell precursors. Supernatants from more than 4500 hybridomas surviving HAT/ouabain selection were screened against human lung tumor cells in ELISA. Over 360 hybrids showed significant levels of activity, although most were not tumor-cell-specific, since they also reacted with EBV-infected cells from the lymphocyte donor. Two hybridomas showed apparent specific binding early after fusion, but this activity was lost upon continued growth, although, in general, hybrids continued to secrete high levels (up to 50 μg/ml) of IgM, in some cases beyond 11 months in culture. The human EBV-hybridoma system described here may be useful for rescuing low-frequency tumor-reactive B-cell precursors in lung cancer patients (Cole *et al.*, 1984b).

VI. Human Monoclonal Antibodies against Myelin-Associated Glycoprotein

Myelin-associated glycoprotein (MAG) is a minor glycoprotein component of the myelin sheath, comprising less than 1% of the total protein present. It has a molecular weight of approximately 110,000 and is comprised of 30% carbohydrate. The IgM gammopathy detected in some peripheral neuropathy patients has been found to recognize an epitope on MAG, which is, in part, formed by the carbohydrate residues (P. Braun, personal communication). Peripheral blood from a well-characterized neuropathy patient (ARM; blood courtesy of Dr. P. Braun) was separated on Ficoll–Hypaque and transformed with EBV. This EBV line was cloned at ten cells/well in 96-well plates on irradiated mouse spleen cells as a feeder layer. Screening of the clones was begun at 3 weeks using an ELISA system with MAG in the solid phase as the antigen (2 μg/ml). Dilutions of ARM serum and normal serum served as controls. Positive wells were detected at 5 weeks in two out of 400 wells tested. The strongest MAG-reactive well (clone 1) was grown up and fused with KR-4. Hybrids are currently being screened (McGarry *et al.*, 1985).

VII. New Fusion Partners

Plasmacytomas represent end cells in the B-cell lineage and up to 40% of their protein synthesis is directed to an immunoglobulin product. These cells have abundant rough endoplasmic reticulum, numerous mitochondria, and a well-developed Golgi apparatus. However, human plasmacytomas are difficult to establish as cell lines, unlike the situation in mice, and only a few are available (Kozbor, Dexter, and Roder, 1983; Cole *et al.*, 1984a). These generally fuse poorly and grow at a slow rate. On the other hand, lymphoblastoid cell lines have high fusion frequencies, grow at a fast rate, and are easily established in tissue culture. We have therefore fused our lymphoblastoid cell line KR-4 with a plasmacytoma RPMI-8226 to obtain a hybrid with the combined advantages of each cell type (Kozbor *et al.*, 1984). Hybrids were back-selected for resistance to thioguanine and ouabain. Two fusion partners were obtained, KR-12 and KR-22, which produced high amounts of immunoglobulin (5–30 µg/ml) when fused with EBV-transformed donor lymphocytes. Fusion rates were high (10^{-5}) and hybrids exhibited between 100 and 140 chromosomes. The extra chromosome load in these lines may not be an impediment to stable monoclonal antibody production, since some of the most widely used mouse fusion partners were hybrids (Schulman *et al.*, 1978). Indeed, Milstein and Cuello (1983) have recently described the use of triple hybrids. In our studies, several stable (>8 months) hybridomas specific for tetanus toxoid were obtained. The parental fusion partner (KR-12) secreted γ heavy chains and both κ and λ light chains. Current efforts are directed at developing nonsecreting variants of these hybrid myeloma fusion partners.

VIII. Ascites Growth of Human Hybridomas

We have found that human hybridomas can be adapted for ascites growth in nude mice by a single prior passage as a solid subcutaneous tumor in 250-R irradiated nude mice followed by *in vitro* growth. As shown in Table II, hybrids have been found to secrete on average approximately 0.3 mg/ml ascites fluid of human immunoglobulin (mice 1–7). Repassage of ascites-recovered XY134 cells in BALB/c nude mice gave yields of human IgM in the range of 2–7 mg/ml (mice 8–11). In our studies, we have found that the appearance of subcutaneous tumors and ascites was not significantly affected by pretreatment of mice with pristane or by depletion of natural killer cells with anti-asialo GM_1. On the other hand, irradiation of the mice improved results with first passage ascites hybrids, as did the use of implanted B-estradiol pellets, in which case yields of human immunoglobulin of over 1.0 mg/ml were obtained in ascites fluid. It should be noted that rather small quantities of ascites (~1.0 ml) are obtained per mouse and often the tumor appears to grow as a solid mass within the peritoneal cavity, together with large deposits of necrotic fat.

IX. Epstein–Barr Virus-Hybridoma Protocol

A. EBV Transformation of Lymphocytes

1. Isolate lymphocytes by centrifugation on Ficoll–Hypaque (Pharmacia; density 1.077 g/ml).

TABLE II

Levels of Human Immunoglobulin in the Ascites Fluid of Nude Mice Challenged with a Human Hybridoma

Mouse no.	Nude mouse strain	Irradiation (250 R)	Concentration of human IgM (μg/ml)
1	NIH-II	+	686
2	NIH-II	+	160
3	BALB/c	+	106
4	BALB/c	+	55
5	NIH-II	−	180
6	NIH-II	−	860
7	NIH-II	−	110
8	BALB/c	−	2810
9	BALB/c	−	7420
10	BALB/c	−	6580
11	BALB/c	−	7750

[a]A tetanus toxoid-specific human hybridoma (XY134) which had previously been passed as a subcutaneous tumor and then grown *in vitro* several passages was injected ip at 2×10^7 cells per mouse into irradiated (250 R) or unirradiated nu/nu mice and ascites fluid was collected 4–8 weeks later and titered in ELISA against a purified human IgM standard ($y = 0.536X + 0.640$; $r = 0.99$). Normal mouse serum was used as a negative control and gave values of 0 μg/ml human IgM. Mice 5–11 represent a second ascites passage of XY134 hybridoma cells. Approximately one-third of the mice injected did not develop any ascites fluid for analysis.

2. Add EBV (B95-8; Showa Research Institute, Clearwater, Florida) at approximately 10^7 transforming units/10^6 cells in tissue culture medium (RPMI 1640–10% FBS).
3. Allow to grow to sufficient numbers for freezing stocks and fusion; viability should be >90% prior to fusion.

B. Cell Fusion

1. Remove drugs (ouabain, 5×10^{-4} M; 6-thioguanine 30 μg/ml) from culture medium of KR-4 (fusion partner) 24–48 hr before fusion.
2. Autoclave polyethylene glycol (PEG) 4000 (Sigma) (2 g) for 15 min and maintain at 60°C for immediate use or allow to solidify for future use (remelt at 60°C).
3. Mix 10^7 KR-4 cells and 10^7 EBV-transformed lymphocytes in a 50-ml conical centrifuge tube, centrifuge, and wash the cell pellet three times with serum-free RPMI 1640 medium; after final wash, remove medium completely.
4. Add warm (37°C) serum-free RPMI 1640 medium (2.4 ml) to the liquid PEG and mix well (45% PEG w/v); adjust pH to neutrality, if required, with sterile 0.1 M NaOH.

5. Add PEG solution (0.5 ml) over a 1-min period to the cell pellet, stirring *gently* with the pipette tip.
6. After allowing tube to sit at room temperature for an additional 90 sec with occasional gentle mixing, add pre-warmed (37°C) RPMI 1640 medium (10 ml) very slowly with gentle mixing over 6–10 min.
7. Cap the tube and incubate at 37°C for 20 min to 1 hr. (Note: additional fusions may be done at this time if desired).
8. Centrifuge the cells and wash once with RPMI 1640 medium and resuspend in RPMI 1640–20% FBS with 20 mM L-glutamine and 5 × 10⁻⁵ M 2-mercaptoethanol.
9. Plate cells into 96-well plates (Linbro 76-032-05) in a total volume of 0.1 ml per well with 3000-R-irradiated mouse spleen cells [(2–5) × 10^5/well] and mouse peritoneal exudate cells ($\leq 5 \times 10^3$/well). Plate control wells (parental cells).
10. Twenty-four hours after fusion, add 0.1 ml of 2× HAT–1× ouabain medium [4 ml 50× HAT (Flow Laboratories) and 100 μl 10 mM ouabain per 100 ml medium] to each well.
11. Three days after fusion, remove half the medium and replace with 0.1 ml 1× HAT–1× ouabain medium per well. Thereafter, feed hybrids every 4–6 days with HAT–ouabain medium; first putative hybrids may be detected microscopically 7–12 days after fusion and screened 18–30 days after fusion.

X. *The Advantages of Human Monoclonal Antibodies*

Human monoclonal antibodies are desirable and have advantages over conventional murine fusion products for several reasons.

1. Human monoclonal antibodies are preferable for γ-globulin therapy because of the risk of sensitization with xenoantisera. Almost half of the 20 patients treated to date in various centers with murine monoclonal antibodies have developed an antibody response to the mouse Ig, which prevented effective treatment (R. A. Miller and Levy, 1981; R. A. Miller *et al.*, 1981, 1982; Ritz *et al.*, 1981; Sears *et al.*, 1982; Nadler *et al.*, 1980; Dillman *et al.*, 1982). Human Ig would be far less immunogenic in humans than xenogeneic mouse Ig. In the past γ-globulin prophylaxis for infections (tetanus, rabies) was switched from horse antiserum to human antiserum, which elicits far fewer adverse reactions. Even human Ig, however, may be expected in some cases to stimulate a response to allotypic or idiotypic sites.
2. Autoantibodies or naturally occurring human antibodies could be used as antigens to select and develop human monoclonal anti-idiotypic antibodies, which would potentially be useful for suppressing the response to autoantigens or transplant antigens.

3. The human immune response would generate a wider range of antibodies against HLA and other polymorphic surface determinants than immunization across species barriers.
4. From the biological standpoint, human monoclonal antibodies would tell us more than murine monoclonal antibodies about the spectrum of the human B-cell specificity repertoire. However, the difficulties encountered in the murine hybridoma field are relevant to the human system as well.

XI. Possible Limitations

One potential limitation relates to the presence of either EBV or retroviruses in monoclonal antibody preparations intended for human use. Xenotropic retroviruses are released from many murine hybridomas or fusion partners and are known to be infectious for human cells (Weiss, 1982). This knowledge, however, has not prevented the experimental use of murine monoclonal antibodies in man (see above). Similar C-type and A-type virus particles have not yet been observed in human fusion partners or hybridomas, but the recent discovery of a human C-type virus, HTLV, in certain T-cell lymphomas (Poiesz *et al.*, 1980; Miyoshi *et al.*, 1981) warrants a closer look at human fusion partners of the B-cell lineage. The EBV used for human hybridoma work is derived from the B95-8 marmoset cell line (G. Miller and M. Lipman, 1973). This virus transforms human B lymphocytes *in vitro* and the EBV nuclear antigen (EBNA) is expressed, but the viral cycle is not completed. Consequently, infectious virus is not released, although the possibility of contaminating hybridoma supernatants with transforming viral DNA does exist at least in theory. However, virus and viral DNA can easily be inactivated or removed from antibody preparations (Crawford *et al.*, 1983c), which can be monitored by sensitive B-cell transformation tests and possibly by injection into marmosets, a species in which EBV is rapidly fatal. By analogy, hyperimmune serum from hepatitis patients is currently used for γ-globulin prophylaxis after removal of contaminating virus. As an additional safeguard, potential recipients of human monoclonal antibodies could be screened for serum antibodies to EBV. Most adults in Western countries are positive, having been exposed to infectious mononucleosis. Only in the very rare X-linked lymphoproliferative syndrome (Sullivan *et al.*, 1980) would EBV infection be life-threatening. A patient has already been exposed to EBV-carrying human hybridomas growing within implanted, cell-impermeable chambers (J. V. Watson *et al.*, 1983). As in all novel therapies, the potential benefits to the patient will have to be weighed against any potential risks. If certain monoclonal antibodies should prove efficacious in life-threatening human diseases, then a decision not to adopt them for widespread use because of unproven risks becomes ethically indefensible.

XII. Conclusions

A number of human fusion partners have been described for the production of human hybridomas, but the majority are lymphoblastoid cell lines and only two are definite plasmacytomas. A detailed comparison of hybridization frequencies, yield of antigen-specific hybridomas, immunoglobulin secretion levels, cloning efficiencies, division times, and stability (Kozbor and Roder, 1983; Cole *et al.*, 1984a) leads to the conclusion that the EBV-hybridoma system described here is near optimal and approaches the murine system in efficiency, with mean fusion frequencies of 1.54×10^{-5} in four independent studies and *in vitro* secretion levels of >5 μg/ml specific antibody (Table I). Lymphocytes from lymph nodes, tonsils, bone marrow, and peripheral blood of hyperimmune patients or *in vitro* immunized cultures (Fig. 1) have been fused effectively and human monoclonal antibodies against *M. leprae*, tetanus toxoid, lung tumor cells, and myelin-associated glycoprotein have been generated in our laboratory. A myeloma-like fusion partner has been constructed and we have successfully established our human hybridomas as ascites tumors in nude mice. We are currently developing a non-Ig-secreting fusion partner.

The EBV-hybridoma technique offers a high degree of flexibility, since the use of EBV (1) immortalizes the donor B cells for future use and repeated fusions, (2) aids the expansion of rare antigen-specific B cells in the peripheral blood prior to fusion, and (3) increases hybridization frequencies over tenfold. One limitation of the system is that only one of 21 hybridomas obtained in this way has secreted antigen-specific IgG; most (20/21) produce IgM. Recent developments may allow induction of an IgM to IgG switch in these hybrids with UV light (Rosen and Klein, 1983). We hope that human monoclonal antibodies produced by the EBV-hybridoma technique will become useful tools for the diagnosis and treatment of human disease.

References

Atlaw, T., Kozbor, D., and Roder, J. C., 1985, Human monoclonal antibodies against *Mycobacterium Leprae*, *Infect. Immun.*, in press.

Boylston, A. W., Gardner, B., Anderson, R. L., and Hughes-Jones, N. C., 1980, Production of human IgM anti-D in tissue culture by EB-virus transformed lymphocytes, *Scand. J. Immunol.* **12:**355–358.

Chiorazzi, N., Wasserman, R. L., and Kunkel, H. G., 1982, Use of Epstein–Barr virus-transformed B cell lines for the generation of immunoglobulin-producing human B cell hybridomas, *J. Exp. Med.* **156:**930–935.

Cole, S. P. C., Campling, B. G., Atlaw, T., Kozbor, D., and Roder, J. C., 1984a, Human monoclonal antibodies, *Mol. Cell. Biol.*, **62:**109–120.

Cole, S. P. C., Campling, B. G., Louwman, I. H., Kozbor, D., and Roder, J. C., 1984b, A strategy for the production of human monoclonal antibodies reactive with lung tumour cell lines, *Cancer Res.*, **44:**2750–2753.

Crawford, D. H., Barlow, M. J., Harrison, J. F., Winger, L., and Huehns, E. R., 1983a, Production of human monoclonal antibody to rhesus D antigen, *Lancet* **i:**386–388.

Crawford, D. H., Callard, R. E., Muggeridge, M. I., Mitchell, D. M., Zanders, E. D., and Beverley, P. C. L., 1983b, Production of human monoclonal antibody to X31 influenza virus nucleoprotein, J. Gen. Virol. **64**:697–700.

Crawford, D. H., Heuhns, E. R., and Epstein, M. A., 1983c, Therapeutic use of human monoclonal antibodies, Lancet **i**:1040 (letter).

Croce, C. M., Linnenbach, A., Hall, W., Steplewski, Z., and Koprowski, H., 1980, Production of human hybridomas secreting antibodies to measles virus, Nature **288**:488.

Dillman, R. O., Shawler, D. L., Sobol, R. E., Collins, H. A., Beauregard, J. C., Wormsley, S. B., and Royston, I., 1982, Murine monoclonal antibody therapy in two patients with chronic lymphocytic leukemia, Blood **59**:1036–1045.

Irie, R. F., Sze, L. L., and Saxton, R. E., 1982, Human antibody to OFA-1, a tumor antigen produced in vitro by Epstein–Barr virus-transformed human B-lymphoid cell lines, Proc. Natl. Acad. Sci. USA **79**:5666–5670.

Kamo, I., Furukawa, S., Tada, A., Mano, Y., Iwasaki, Y., and Furuse, T., 1982, Monoclonal antibody to acetylcholine receptor: Cell line established from thymus of patient with myasthenia gravis, Science **215**:995–997.

Köhler, G., and Milstein, C., 1975, Continuous cultures of fused cells secreting antibody of predefined specificity, Nature **256**:495–497.

Koskimies, S., 1979, A human lymphoblastoid cell line producing specific antibody against Rh-antigen D, Scand. J. Immunol. **10**:371 (abstract).

Kozbor, D., and Roder, J. C., 1981, Requirements for the establishment of high titered human monoclonal antibodies against tetanus toxoid using the Epstein–Barr virus technique, J. Immunol. **127**:1275–1280.

Kozbor, D., and Roder, J. C., 1983, Monoclonal antibodies produced by human lymphocytes, Immunol. Today **4**:72–79.

Kozbor, D., and Roder, J., 1984, In vitro stimulated lymphocytes as a source of human hybridomas, Eur. J. Immunol., **14**:23–27.

Kozbor, D., Steinitz, M., Klein, G., Koskimies, S., and Makela, O., 1979, Establishment of anti-TNP antibody-producing human lymphoid lines by preselection for hapten binding followed by EBV transformation, Scand. J. Immunol. **10**:187–194.

Kozbor, D., Roder, J. C., Chang, T. H., Steplewski, Z., and Koprowski, H., 1982a, Human anti-tetanus toxoid monoclonal antibody secreted by EBV-transformed human B cells fused with a murine myeloma, Hybridoma **1**:323–328.

Kozbor, D., Lagarde, A., and Roder, J. C., 1982b, Human hybridomas constructed with antigen-specific, EBV-transformed cell lines, Proc. Natl. Acad. Sci. USA **79**:6651–6655.

Kozbor, D., Dexter, D., and Roder, J. C., 1983, A comparative analysis of the phenotypic characteristics of available fusion partners for the construction of human hybridomas, Hybridoma **2**:7–16.

Kozbor, D., Tripputi, P., Roder, J. C., and Croce, C. M., 1984, A human hybrid myeloma is an efficient fusion partner that enhances monoclonal antibody production, J. Immunol. **133**:3001–3005.

Laskov, R., Kim, J. K., and Asofsky, R., 1979, Induction of amplified synthesis and secretion of IgM by fusion of murine B lymphoma with myeloma cells, Proc. Natl. Acad. Sci. USA **76**:915–919.

Levy, R., and Dilley, J., 1978, Rescue of immunoglobulin secretion from human neoplastic lymphoid cells by somatic cell hybridization, Proc. Natl. Acad. Sci. USA **75**:2411–2415.

McGarry, R., Cole, S. P. C., and Roder, J., 1985, Human hybridomas from patients with peripheral demyelination react with myelin-associated glycoprotein, manuscript in preparation.

Miller, G., and Lipman, M., 1973, Release of infectious Epstein–Barr virus by transformed marmoset leukocytes, Proc. Natl. Acad. Sci. USA **70**:190–194.

Miller, R. A., and Levy, R., 1981, Response of cutaneous T-cell lymphoma to therapy with hybridoma monoclonal antibody, Lancet **2**:226–230.

Miller, R. A., Maloney, D. G., McKillop, J., and Levy, R., 1981, In vivo effects of murine hybridoma monoclonal antibody in a patient with T-cell leukemia, Blood **58**:78–86.

Miller, R. A., Maloney, D. G., Warnke, R., and Levy, R., 1982, Treatment of B-cell lymphoma with monoclonal anti-idiotype antibody, *N. Engl. J. Med.* **306:**517–522.

Milstein, C., and Cuello, A. C., 1983, Hybrid hybridomas and their use in immunohistochemistry, *Nature* **305:**537–540.

Miyoshi, I., Kubonishi, E., Yoshimoto, S., Akagi, T., Ohtsuki, Y., Shiraishr, Y., Nagata, K., and Hinuma, Y., 1981, Type C virus particles in a cord T-cell line derived by co-cultivating normal human cord leukocytes and leukemia T cells, *Nature* **294:**770–771.

Nadler, L. M., Stashenko, P., Hardy, R., Kaplan, W. D., Button, L. N., Kufe, D. W., Atman, K. H., and Schlossman, S. F., 1980, Serotherapy of a patient with a monoclonal antibody directed against a human lymphoma-associated antigen, *Cancer Res.* **40:**3147–3154.

Olsson, L., and Kaplan, H. S., 1980, Human–human hybridomas producing monoclonal antibodies of predefined antigenic specificity, *Proc. Natl. Acad. Sci. USA* **77:**5429–5431.

Poiesz, B. J., Ruscetti, F. W., Gazdar, A. F., Bunn, P. A., Minna, J. D., and Gallo, R. C., 1980, Detection and isolation of type C retrovirus particles from fresh and cultured lymphocytes of a patient with cutaneous T-cell lymphoma, *Proc. Natl. Acad. Sci. USA* **77:**7415–7419.

Ritz, J., Pesando, J. M., Sallan, S. E., Clavell, L. A., Notis-McConarty, J., Rosenthal, P., and Schlossman, S. F., 1981, Serotherapy of acute lymphoblastic leukemia with monoclonal antibody, *Blood* **58:**141–151.

Rosen, A., and Klein, G., 1983, UV light-induced immunoglobulin heavy-chain class switch in a human lymphoblastoid cell line, *Nature* **306:**189–190.

Rosen, A., Britton, S., Gergely, P., Jondal, M., and Klein, G., 1977, Polyclonal Ig production after Epstein–Barr virus infection of human lymphocytes, *Nature* **267:**52–54.

Rosen, A., Persson, K., and Klein, G., 1983, Human monoclonal antibodies to a genus-specific chlamydial antigen, produced by EBV-transformed B cells, *J. Immunol.* **130:**2899–2902.

Schulman, M., Wilde, C. D., and Kohler, G., 1978, A better cell line for making hybridomas secreting specific antibodies, *Nature* **276:**269–270.

Sears, H. F., Atkinson, B., Herlyn, D., Ernst, C., Matteis, J., Steplewski, Z., and Koprowski, H., 1982, Phase I clinical trial of monoclonal antibody in treatment of gastrointestinal tumours, *Lancet* **i:**762–765.

Seigneurin, J. M., Desgranges, C., Seigneurin, D., Paire, J., Renversez, J. C., Jacquemont, B., and Micouin, C., 1983, Herpes simplex virus glycoprotein D: Human monoclonal antibody produced by bone marrow cell line, *Science* **221:**173–175.

Sikora, K., Alderson, T., Phillips, J., and Watson, J. V., 1982, Human hybridomas from malignant gliomas, *Lancet* **i:**11–14.

Sikora, K., Alderson, T., Ellis, J., Phillips, J., and Watson, J., 1983, Human hybridomas from patients with malignant disease, *Br. J. Cancer* **47:**135–145.

Steinitz, M., and Tamir, S., 1982, Human monoclonal autoimmune antibody produced *in vitro*: Rheumatoid factor generated by Epstein–Barr virus-transformed cell line, *Eur. J. Immunol.* **12:**126–133.

Steinitz, M., Klein, G., Koskimies, S., and Makela, O., 1977, EB virus-induced B lymphocyte cell lines producing specific antibody, *Nature* **269:**420–422.

Steinitz, M., Seppala, F., Eichman, K., and Klein, G., 1979, Establishment of a human lymphoblastoid cell line with the specific antibody production against group A streptococcal carbohydrate, *Immunobiology* **156:**41–47.

Steinitz, M., Izak, G., Cohen, S., Ehrenfeld, M., and Flechner, I., 1980, Continuous production of monoclonal rheumatoid factor by EBV-transformed lymphocytes, *Nature* **287:**443–445.

Stevens, R. H., Macy, E., Morrow, C., and Saxon, A., 1979, Characterization of a circulating subpopulation of spontaneous anti-tetanus toxoid antibody producing B cells following *in vivo* booster immunization, *J. Immunol.* **122:**2498–2504.

Sullivan, J. L., Byron, K. S., Brewster, F. F., and Purtilo, D., 1980, Deficient natural killer cell activity in X-linked lymphoproliferative syndrome, *Science* **210:**543–545.

Tsuchiya, S., Yokoyama, S., Yoshie, O., and Ono, Y., 1980, Production of diptheria antitoxin antibody in Epstein–Barr virus-induced lymphoblastoid cell lines, *J. Immunol.* **124:**1970–1976.

Walker, S. M., Meinke, G. C., and Weigle, W. O., 1977, Cell separation on antigen-coated columns. Elimination of high rate antibody-forming cells and immunological memory cells, *J. Exp. Med.* **146**:445–446.

Watson, D. B., Burns, G. F., and MacKay, I. R., 1983, *In vitro* growth of B lymphocytes infiltrating human melanoma tissue by transformation with EBV: Evidence for secretion of anti-melanoma antibodies by some transformed cells, *J. Immunol.* **130**:2442–2447.

Watson, J. V., Alderson, T., Sikora, K., and Phillips, J., 1983, Subcutaneous culture chamber for continuous infusion of monoclonal antibodies, *Lancet* **i**:99–100.

Weiss, R. A., 1982, Hybridomas produce viruses as well as antibodies, *Immunol. Today* **3**:292–294.

Winger, L., Winger, C., Shastry, P., Russell, A., and Longenecker, M., 1983, Efficient generation *in vitro*, from human peripheral blood cells, of monoclonal Epstein–Barr virus transformants producing specific antibody to a variety of antigens without prior deliberate immunization, *Proc. Natl. Acad. Sci. USA* **80**:4484–4488.

Yoshie, O., and Ono, Y., 1980, Anti-phosphorylcholine antibody producing cells in human lymphoblastoid cell lines established by transformation with Epstein–Barr virus, *Cell. Immunol.* **56**:305–315.

Zurawski, V. R., Jr., Haber, E., and Black, P. M., 1978a, Production of antibody to tetanus toxoid by continuous human lymphoblastoid cell lines, *Science* **199**:1439–1441.

Zurawski, V. R., Jr., Spedden, S. E., Black, P., and Haber, E., 1978b, Clones of human lymphoblastoid cell lines producing antibody to tetanus toxoid, *Curr. Top. Microbiol. Immunol.* **81**:152–155.

5

Strategies for Stable Human Monoclonal Antibody Production

Construction of Heteromyelomas, *in Vitro* Sensitization, and Molecular Cloning of Human Immunoglobulin Genes

NELSON N. H. TENG, GREGORY R. REYES, MARCIA BIEBER, KIRK E. FRY, KIT S. LAM, AND JOAN M. HEBERT

I. Introduction

The development of hybridoma technology by Köhler and Milstein (1975) opened a new era not only in immunology, but in all fields of biological science. Hybridoma cell lines formed by the fusion of mutant mouse myeloma cells with spleen cells from an immunized mouse assure the permanent availability of monoclonal antibody of defined specificity. The clinical use of these

---

GREGORY R. REYES, MARCIA BIEBER, KIRK E. FRY, KIT S. LAM, AND JOAN M. HEBERT • Cancer Biology Research Laboratory, Department of Radiology, Stanford University School of Medicine, Stanford, California 94305. NELSON N. H. TENG • Department of Gynecology and Obstetrics, Stanford University School of Medicine, Stanford, California 94305.
This paper is dedicated to the memory of Henry Seymour Kaplan (1918–1984), who founded this work. His passing leaves a chasm that cannot be filled. A gifted, singular intellectual giant, he represented one of the last academic aristocrats in medicine. He approached research and clinical problems with tenacious perseverance and unbridled enthusiasm. It was he who made this work possible.

xenoantibodies in human patients, however, will be limited by the fact that they themselves will be immunogenic upon repeated administration. Accordingly, for therapeutic applications in man, the availability of human monoclonal antibodies would be advantageous. The advance of human hybridoma technology has, however, been slowed by the unavailability of suitable fusion partners. Early attempts to generate immortalized human immunoglobulin-producing cells involved the fusion of human lymphoid cells with mouse myeloma cells to create chimeric hybridomas (Levy and Dilley, 1978; Schwaber, 1975; Schwaber and Cohen, 1973). Although exceptions have been reported (Schlom *et al.*, 1980; Lane *et al.*, 1982), such mouse–human hybridomas have tended to be unstable and cease immunoglobulin production due to the selective loss of human chromosomes (Weiss and Green, 1967; Nabholz *et al.*, 1969), or to disturbances of gene expression (Raison *et al.*, 1982). A second approach has involved the transformation of antigen-primed human B lymphocytes with Epstein–Barr virus (EBV) (Zurawski *et al.*, 1978; Steinitz *et al.*, 1979; Kozbor *et al.*, 1979; Hirano *et al.*, 1980; Tsuchiya *et al.*, 1980; Yoshie and Ono, 1980). This method has also had some success, but in most instances, such cultures have tended to be unstable and produce low yields of antibody (Zurawski *et al.*, 1978; Tsuchiya *et al.*, 1980).

More recently, several groups, including our own, have succeeded in fusing drug-selectable human myeloma or EBV-transformed B-lymphoblastoid cell lines with antigen-primed human B lymphocytes to yield human–human hybridomas secreting monoclonal antibodies of predefined antigenic specificity (Olsson and Kaplan, 1980; Croce *et al.*, 1980; Sikora *et al.*, 1982; Olsson *et al.*, 1984; Edwards *et al.*, 1982; Eisenbarth *et al.*, 1982; Chiorazzi *et al.*, 1982; Glassy *et al.*, 1983; Larrick *et al.*, 1983). Only a few human myeloma cell lines have been permanently established in culture. Detailed comparisons of these different cell lines for production of viable hybridomas and stability of human monoclonal antibody production has not resulted in a consensus as to the best fusion partners to use. Comparisons have been made even more difficult because antigen-primed human B lymphocytes from different sources have been fused under different conditions. In this chapter we describe several different constructions of mouse–human hybrid cell lines that appear to have uniquely favorable characteristics as malignant fusion partners for human monoclonal antibody production. In addition, we present strategies for *in vitro* antigen priming of naive B lymphocytes and the molecular cloning of human immunoglobulin genes from hybridoma lines for the purpose of stabilizing and reexpressing the genes.

II. General Properties of Mouse–Human Heteromyeloma and Heteromyelolymphoma Cell Lines

There are only a few permanently established human myeloma cell lines extant (Nilsson *et al.*, 1970; Moore and Kitamura, 1968; Thiele and Mushinski, 1982; Togawa et al., 1982; Miller et al., 1982; Karpas et al., 1982), and none of these to our knowledge has proven to be an efficient malignant fusion partner for the generation of human–human hybridomas. It is noteworthy that all these human myeloma cell lines grow rather slowly, with doubling times in the range of 40–60 hr, and possess chromosome numbers close to the normal diploid human chromosomal complement. Work by others (Harris et al., 1969; Stanbridge, 1976) has indicated that suppression of the malignant phenotype results in the normal senescence and death of hybridomas, and is most likely to occur when the malignant fusion partner grows slowly with a near normal karyotype. Our first experiments involved the generation of human–mouse heteromyeloma cell lines by fusion (Oi and Herzenberg, 1979) of a HAT-sensitive nonproducer mouse myeloma line with a HAT-sensitive human myeloma line (Teng et al., 1983a,b). A subclone of the Nilsson original myeloma cell line U266 was reselected in 6-thioguanine (6TG) after it had been freed of mycoplasma contamination. The HAT sensitivity of the 6TG-resistant cells was verified experimentally; unlike an earlier mutant designated SKO-007, the new mutant cell line had no detectable reversion in HAT medium. Like the parental U266 cell line, the mutant line, designated FU-266, had a modal chromosomal number of 44, secreted IgE(λ), and doubled approximately every 40–45 hr. The capacity of FU-266 cells to act as malignant fusion partners with antigen-primed human B lymphocytes was poor (Table II), but was similar to that of the previously described SKO-007 mutant cell line (Olsson and Kaplan, 1980). The cell line FU-266 was transfected by protoplast fusion (Shaffner, 1980) with a neomycin-resistant gene using a recombinant plasmid vector, pSV-2neo^r (Berg, 1981; Southern and Berg, 1982). The details of somatic cell hybrid selection with a dominant selectable marker were described elsewhere (Calvo Riera, 1984). The fastest growing clone, designated FU-266-E1, was selected for fusion. The P3X63Ag8.653-NP mouse myeloma cell line, which is highly sensitive to the neomycin–kanamycin analogue G418, was irradiated (Schneiderman et al., 1979) with a single sublethal dose (500 rad) before fusion (Pontecorvo, 1971) with FU-266-E1. Because human cells are significantly more sensitive to ouabain than mouse cells, selection of the fused heteromyeloma was carried out in ouabain plus G418. Numerous hybrid clones were obtained (Table I). The properties and fusion characteristics of some of the exemplary fusions are presented in Tables I and II. In general, the fusions carried out with pokeweed mitogen-stimulated peripheral blood lymphocytes (PBL–PWM) gave a lower percentage of viable hybrids and immunoglobulin producers than fusions with Epstein–Barr virus (EBV)-transformed human B lymphocytes (PBL–EBV) or malignant lymphoma cells from patients. Most of our fusions used the heteromyeloma as the malignant fusion partner (Teng et al., 1983a; Bron et al., 1984).

Another approach took advantage of the fact that some of the fusions resulted in unusually stable hybridomas (Östberg and Pursch, 1983). One of these was a fusion between heteromyeloma SHM-D3 and B lymphocytes from a lymph node of a patient with ovarian carcinoma. The resultant hybridoma

TABLE I
Properties of Heteromyelomas and Heteromyelolymphomas[a]

Cell line	Derivation	Drug resistance markers	Ig secreted	Karyotype	
				Human	Mouse
Parental					
SKO-007[b]	Human myeloma	8AG	IgE(λ)	44	0
FU-266-E1	Human myeloma	6TG,G418	IgE(λ)	44	0
X63Ag8.653-NP[c]	Mouse myeloma	8AGOUA	0	0	57
SHM hybrid clones	Human–mouse myeloma	6TGOUA,G418			
A6			0	2	95
A10			0	1–2	55
D33			0	5	78
D36			0	6	103
D3			0	12	112
HML hybrid clones	Human lymphoma–mouse myeloma	6TG,OUA			
H10–3			0	4	64
D6–1			0	29	12
D6–2			0	41	13
D6–3			0	35	15
D6–4			0	30	19
D6–6			0	29	17
Triple hybrid clones	Human–mouse myeloma–human B cell	6TG,OUA,G418			
3HL3			IgM(λ)	10	93
3HL3–6			0	11	68
3HL3–8			IgM(λ)	11	69
3HL3–27			0	ND	ND

[a]Selected clones from a total of 120. Abbreviations: 8AG, 8-azaguanine; 6TG, 6-thioguanine; OUA, ouabian; G418, an aminoglycoside antibiotic; ND, not determined.
[b]Faulkner and Zachau (1982).
[c]Kearney et al. (1979).

sustained immunoglobulin production for over 1 year without subcloning. This hybridoma was backselected for HAT sensitivity, and nonproducer clones were designated as the 3HL series. These hybrids had a higher number of human chromosomes than the parent heteromyeloma, grew rapidly, and carried both ouabain and G418 resistance markers. They are excellent fusion partners, with hybrid frequency similar to those of the heteromyelomas. Examples of fusions with various partners are given in Table II.

In contrast to human myelomas, many of the human B-cell or null lymphoma cell lines established in this laboratory grow very rapidly and are highly aneuploid. This suggests the possibility that hybrid cells with significantly more favorable properties for human hybridoma production could be derived from fusing human myeloma cell lines with rapidly growing B- or

TABLE II
Fusion Characteristics[a]

Malignant fusion partner	Growth characteristics	Doubling time (hr)	Donor B lymphocytes	Viable hybrids[b] (% well)	Ig-producing hybrids[c] (%)	Specific hybrid (%)	Specificity	Specific Ig class	Ig production[d]	Stability[e]
SKO-007	Suspension	48	Spleen	0–64	0–36	1.7	DNP[k]	IgG	3–11	NA
			PBL (PWM)	0	0	0	NS	—	—	
FU-266	Suspension	42	PBL (PWM)	1	10	0	NS	IgG	NA	—
HML-D	Suspension	24	PBL (PWM)	0	0	0	—	—	—	
			PBL (EBV)	0	0	0	—	—	—	
3HL-6	Partially adherent	22	PBL (EBV)	42	100	1	LPS (J5)[l]	IgG(λ)	4–5	+
			Lymph node	43	100	16	Idiotype[m]	μ, λ	20	+
3HL-27	Suspension	24	PBL (EBV)	65	100	0	NS	IgG, IgM	NA	+
SHM-D33	Partially adherent	30	Spleen	17	83	5	LPS (J5)	IgM	NA	—
			Spleen (EBV)	34	100	3	LPS (J5)	IgM	10–20	+
			PBL (PWM)	20	40	0	Rh(D)	NA	NA	NA
			PBL (EBV)	100	100	100	Rh(D)[n]	IgG(λ)	1–20	+
			PBL (EBV)[j]	100	100	0.7	ssDNA	IgM(λ)	—	+
						0.5	dsDNA	—	—	+
						1.2	rRNA	IgG	—	
			Lymph node	37	49	45	Idiotype[m]	IgM(λ)	10–20	+
			Lymph node (SAC)[g]	62	94	90	Idiotype	IgM(λ)	10–20	+
			Spleen (in vitro)[h]	22	55	7	DNP	IgM(λ)	10–20	
SHM-D36	Partially adherent	25	Spleen (in vitro)[i]	30	60	8	DNP	IgM	NA	—
			Lymph node	14	0	0	Idiotype[m]	—	—	NA
			Lymph node (SAC)[g]	21	35	35	Idiotype[m]	IgM(κ)	5	
			PBL (EBV)[j]	100	100	52	TT	IgG	1–3	+
			PBL (EBV)	90	100	87	DNP	IgG, IgM	20	+

(continued)

TABLE II (Continued)

Malignant fusion partner	Growth characteristics	Doubling time (hr)	Donor B lymphocytes	Viable hybrids[b] (% well)	Ig-producing hybrids[c] (%)	Specific hybrid (%)	Specificity	Specific Ig class	Ig production[d]	Stability[e]
SHM-A6	Partially adherent	25	PBL (EBV)	40	76	4	TT	IgG	3–10	–
SHM-A6H4	Partially adherent	25	Spleen (EBV)	48	77	7	LPS (J5)	IgM(κ)	10	+
SHM-D3	Partially adherent	30	Lymph node	21	14	0	Ovarian cancer	IgM(λ)	9	+
SHM-A10	Partially adherent	25	PBL (EBV)	56	27	18	TT	IgG	NA	NA
			PBL (EBV)	50	20	0	TT	–	NA	+

[a]Abbreviations: NS, nonspecific; NA, not available; LPS, lipopolysaccharide; TT, tetanus toxoid.
[b]Each microwell was seeded with $(1-2) \times 10^5$ cell.
[c]Expressed as Ig-producers per viable hybrids.
[d]Expressed as μg/10^6 cells per 24 hr; determined by ELISA (Engvall, 1977).
[e]Hybrid clone is considered operationally stable if it maintains growth and Ig production for at least 4–6 months and is indicated by plus, otherwise, by minus.
[f]PBL from patients with systemic lupus erythematosus.
[g]Lymphocytes stimulated with 0.01% Staphylococcus aureus Cowan I (SAC).
[h]Spleenocytes in vitro sensitized to DNP with 50% viability at the time of fusion.
[i]Same as above except 60% viability.
[j]PBL from volunteers vaccinated with tetanus toxoid.
[k]Faulkner and Zachau (1982).
[l]LPS extracted from E. coli 0111:B4 (J5 mutant), which is deficient in the "0" antigenic side chains.
[m]"Rescued" idiotype from patients with various kinds of lymphomas.
[n]Ravetch et al. (1981).

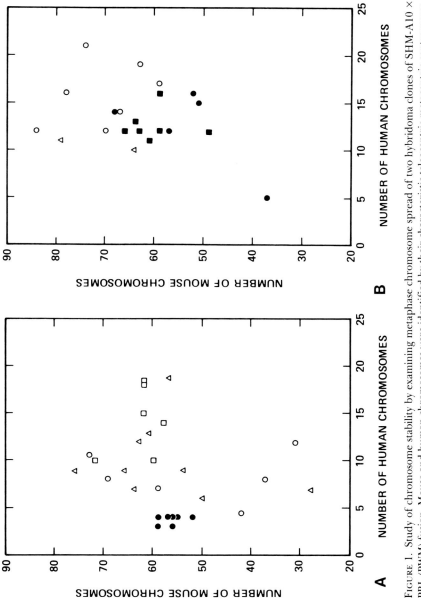

FIGURE 1. Study of chromosome stability by examining metaphase chromosome spread of two hybridoma clones of SHM-A10 × PBL (PWM) fusion. Mouse and human chromosomes were identified by their characteristic teleocentric metacentric centromeres. These hybridoma clones were cultured continuously without subcloning. The modal number of chromosomes and Ig production were determined approximately every 3 weeks (not all data are shown). (A) A general loss of mouse and human chromosomes over a period of 3 months when the clone ceased human Ig production; (○) 1 month after fusion, $T = 4$ weeks; (□) $T = 7$ weeks; (△) $T = 10$ weeks; (●) $T = 14$ weeks. (B) A stable Ig-producer over 8 months; (○) 1 month after fusion, $T = 4$ weeks; (■) $T = 14$ weeks; (△) $T = 25$ weeks; (●) $T = 33$ weeks.

human Ig genes. The molecular cloning of rearranged heavy and light chain genes therefore requires that a library of DNA restriction fragments from a recently subcloned, antigen-specific heterohybridoma be exceptionally representative. An estimated copy number of 0.5 might be considered the upper limit of human Ig representation at the outset, even before passaging and expansion to obtain sufficient material to clone. As a preliminary step toward the cloning of Ig genes, their content and copy number were investigated by Southern hybridization. The rearranged κ chain of two different heterohybridomas was compared with single-copy genomic (unrearranged) controls and the parental fusion partner SHM-D33. As illustrated in Fig. 2, it is readily evident that the Ig loci of both lines are rearranged, but it is also clear that the copy number is much less than one (estimated here to be 0.1 or alternatively one in ten cells containing a complete κ light chain). Similar results regarding copy number are obtained when a heavy-chain-specific probe is used.

These difficulties have caused others to turn to a readily available amplified source of specific Ig material, i.e., mRNA, for the generation of cDNA libraries. An additional advantage of this approach is that the Ig genes, heavy (H) and light (L), are now represented in a processed (spliced) form, which allows for their placement into efficient prokaryotic expression vectors. Two groups have cloned and expressed the various coding domains of human IgE

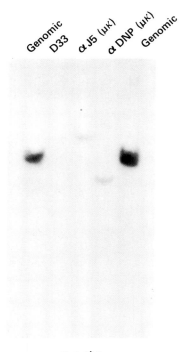

κ **probe**

FIGURE 2. Rearranged human κ chains in heterohybridomas. DNA heteromyeloma from DHL-1 (null cell lymphoma with unrearranged Ig loci) or parental D33 heteromyeloma compared with IgM(κ) anti-J5 (bacterial endotoxin) or IgM(κ)-producing anti-DNP heterohybridomas after cleavage with *Bam*H1, Southern blotting, and hybridization with a κ constant region probe.

from the U266 ND myeloma line (Kurokana *et al.*, 1983; Kenten *et al.*, 1984). Although antigenically active ε peptide was obtained in amounts approaching 18% of total bacterial protein, its binding to cultured basophils as a measure of activity constituted only 20% of the native protein activity (Kenten *et al.*, 1984). This was probably due to the nonglycosylated nature of the peptide produced in bacterial host.

Immunoglobulin proteins produced in *Escherichia coli* are invariably found as inclusion bodies and require solubilization. The very recent production of functional murine anti-CEA (carcinoembryonic antigen) from plasmid constructs placed in *E. coli* required *in vitro* reconstitution of the γ and κ products; *E. coli* coproducing γ and κ chains did not produce active antibody (Cabilly *et al.*, 1984). The only other reported instance of active immunoglobulin production from cDNA clones in *E. coli* (Boss *et al.*, 1984) again required solubilization of the μ and λ chains to obtain antigen binding activity. Plasmids expressing μ and λ when cotransformed into *E. coli* were found to be incompatible with only 5% of *E. coli* expressing antibiotic markers from the different plasmid constructs after 36 hr in culture. Here again, the recovery of active antibody expression after extract dialysis was very poor when compared with the parental hybridoma line.

In addition to the difficulties outlined above regarding specific antibody production from cDNA expression vectors placed in *E. coli*, there has been mounting evidence regarding tissue-specific expression of genes through consensus sequences known as enhancers (Khoury and Gruss, 1983). First discovered in the small DNA papovaviruses SV40 and polyoma, the enhancer elements have been found in the long terminal repeats flanking retrovirus genomes and, more recently, in the immunoglobulin loci. They have been mapped to the large intron of the mouse κ light chain (Queen and Baltimore, 1983; Picard and Schaffner, 1984) and the large intron for the mouse heavy chain (Gillies *et al.*, 1983; Banerji *et al.*, 1983). Through an as yet undefined mechanism, these sequences function (1) in *cis*, at a distance (upward of 10 kb), (2) in an orientation-independent manner to enhance transcriptional activity of genes, and (3) in an apparently cell-type-specific manner (Gillies *et al.*, 1983; Stafford and Queen, 1983). A second canonical sequence located between −90 and −160 base pairs upstream of the κ coding region and different from enhancer elements has recently been discovered that allows for efficient transcription of rearranged κ genes (Faulkner and Zachau, 1984). The so-called pd and dc transcriptional elements are also found upstream of the λ variable chain region and also in the mouse HC enhancer region, and can be characterized as both sufficient and necessary for efficient Ig expression. An additional factor important for Ig expression and secretion not present at any of the Ig loci and apparently active in *trans* has also been described (Faulkner and Zachau, 1982).

Greater success with the introduction and subsequent expression of active Ig molecules has been obtained in eukaryotic systems. Transient expression of functionally rearranged Ig genes was achieved in monkey, mouse, and human fibroblast cultures only after placing the Ig gene in a recombinant plasmid with the SV40 virus promotor (Raison *et al.*, 1982). As noted above, efficient Ig expression in fibroblast cultures requires enhancer elements that are normally active in that cell type (Raison *et al.*, 1982; Stafford and Queen, 1983; Picard and Schaffner, 1983). Transfection and the use of dominant selectable markers has been successful in obtaining correct transcription of active immunoglobulin in myeloma cells as measured by gel electrophoresis and secretion of active antibody (Ochi *et al.*, 1983a; Rice and Baltimore, 1982; Oi *et al.*, 1983). One limiting factor appears to be the very poor transfection efficiency of myeloma cells, ranging from 10^{-4} to 10^{-6} (Ochi *et al.*, 1983a; Oi *et al.*, 1983). Protoplast fusion has been used to introduce cloned heavy and light chains from an antihapten-producing hybridoma when both were present on a plasmid with a dominant selectable marker (Ochi *et al.*, 1983b). This is the only reported instance of the molecular cloning of H and L chains from a hybridoma together with their subsequent reintroduction into cells and a demonstration of reconstitution of antigenic specificity.

These latter points regarding efficient Ig expression only in cells where Ig molecules are normally expressed, together with the difficulties described for prokaryotic expression systems, persuaded us (1) to clone the rearranged Ig chains and/or variable regions directly from hybridoma material, (2) to make use of eukaryotic vector systems for gene delivery into B-lymphocyte cultures, and finally (3) to employ selectable markers to first select and then maintain that population of cells that had stably integrated and expressed the Ig molecules. Of the various strategies currently available to generate representative gene libraries of genetic material, the use of phage vectors provides advantages over that of cosmids principally in terms of screening large numbers of recombinant clones. This is especially important, since the only genes of interest in genomic libraries constructed from hybridoma material would only be the specifically rearranged human Ig molecules.

A genetic complementation system recently described (Seed, 1982) would facilitate the screening procedure by taking advantage of high-frequency homologous recombination between a "probe" sequence inserted into a miniplasmid (πAN7) that carries a synthetic tRNA supressor gene (*sup*F) and the specific recombinant carrying the Ig sequence. A judicious choice of probe sequence isolated from regions known to be shared between rearranged H or L chain genes, once cloned into the miniplasmid, could recombine with infecting phage that carry Ig sequences. The *sup*F gene carried by the π plasmid would then suppress the amber mutated genes located elsewhere in the phage genome and in the process generate phenotypically "wild-type" phage able to productively infect strains of *E. coli* which do not normally allow for replication of amber mutated phage.

The system was tested using a 660-bp fragment isolated from the large first intron of a cloned human IgM gene (Ravetch *et al.*, 1981) and placed in the πAN7 miniplasmid. A major advantage of recombination probe derived from the intron would be that after isolation of the properly rearranged Ig

line that has lost immunoglobulin expression but permits the construction of antibody-secreting hybrid cell lines, *J. Immunol.* **123**:1548–1550.

Kenten, J., Helm, B., Ishizaka, T., Cattini, P., and Gould, H., 1984, Properties of a human immunoglobulin ε-chain fragment synthesized in *Escherichia coli*, *Proc. Natl. Acad. Sci. USA* **81**:2955–2959.

Khoury, G., and Gruss, P., 1983, Enhancer elements, *Cell* **33**:313–314.

Köhler, G., and Milstein, C., 1975, Continuous cultures of fused cells secreting antibody of predefined specificity, *Nature* **256**:495–497.

Kozbor, D., Steinitz, M., Klein, G., Koskimies, S., and Mäkelä, O., 1979, Establishment of anti-TNP antibody-producing human lymphoid lines by preselection for hapten binding followed by EBV transformation, *Scand. J. Immunol.* **10**:187–194.

Kurokana, T., Seno, M., Sasada, R., Ono, Y., Onda, H., Lgarashi, K., Kukuchi, M., Sugino, Y., and Honjo, T., 1983, Expression of human immunoglobulin E ε chain cDNA in *E. coli*, *Nucleic Acids Res.* **11**:3077–3085.

Lane, H. C., Volkman, D. J., Whalen, G., and Fauci, A. S., 1981, *In vitro* antigen-induced, antigen-specific antibody production in man, *J. Exp. Med.* **154**:1043–1057.

Lane, H. C., Shelhamer, J. H., Mostowski, H. S., and Fauci, A. S., 1982, Human monoclonal anti-keyhole limpet hemocyanin antibody-secreting hybridoma produced from peripheral blood B lymphocytes of a keyhole limpet cyanin-immune individual, *J. Exp. Med.* **155**:333–338.

Larrick, J. W., Truitt, K. E., Raubitschek, A. A., Senyk, G., and Wang, J. C. N., 1983, Characterization of human hybridomas secreting antibody to tetanus toxoid, *Proc. Natl. Acad. Sci. USA* **80**:6376–6380.

Levy, R., and Dilley, J., 1978, Rescue of immunoglobulin secretion from human neoplastic lymphoid cells by somatic cell hybridization, *Proc. Natl. Acad. Sci. USA* **75**:2411–2415.

Littlefield, J. W., 1964, Selection of hybrids from matings of fibroblasts *in vitro* and their presumed recombinants, *Science* **145**:709–710.

Miller, C. H., Carbonell, A., Peng, R., Paglieroni, T., and MacKenzie, M. R., 1982, A human plasma cell line—Induction and characterization, *Cancer* **49**:2091–2096.

Misiti, J., and Waldmann, T. A., 1981, *In vitro* generation of antigen specific hemolytic plaque forming cells from human peripheral blood mononuclear cells, *J. Exp. Med.* **154**:1069–1084.

Moore, G. E., and Kitamura, H., 1968, Cell lines derived from patient with myeloma, *N.Y. State J. Med.* **68**:2054–2060.

Morimoto, C., Todd, R. F., Distaso, J., and Schlossman, S. F., 1980, The role of the macrophage in *in vitro* primary anti-DNP antibody in man, *J. Immunol.* **124**:656–661.

Morimoto, C., Reinherz, E. L., and Schlossman, S. F., 1981, Regulation of *in vitro* primary anti-DNP antibody production by functional subsets of T lymphocytes in man, *J. Immunol.* **127**:69–73.

Morimoto, C., Distaso, J., Borel, Y., Schlossman, S. F., and Reinherz, E. L., 1982, Communicative interactions between subpopulations of human T lymphocytes required for generation of suppressor effector function in a primary antibody response, *J. Immunol.* **128**:1645–1649.

Nabholz, M., Miggiano, V., and Bodmer, W., 1969, Genetic analysis with human–mouse somatic cell hybrids, *Nature* **223**:358–363.

Nilsson, K., Bennich, H., Johansson, S. G. O., and Pontén, J., 1970, Established immunoglobulin-producing myeloma (IgE) and lymphoblastoid (IgG) cell lines from an IgE myeloma patient, *Clin. Exp. Immunol.* **7**:477–489.

Ochi, A., Hawley, R. G., Shulman, M. J., and Hozumi, N., 1983a, Transfer of a cloned immunoglobulin light-chain to mutant hybridoma cells restores specific antibody production, *Nature* **302**:340–342.

Ochi, A., Hawley, R. G., Hawley, T., Shulman, M. J., Traunecker, A., Köhler, G., and Hozumi, N., 1983b, Functional immunoglobulin M production after transfection of cloned immunoglobulin heavy and light chain genes into lymphoid cells, *Proc. Natl. Acad. Sci. USA* **80**:6351–6355.

Oi, V. T., and Herzenberg, L. A., 1979, Immunoglobulin-producing hybrid cell lines, in: *Selected*

Methods in Cellular Immunology (B. B. Mishell and S. M. Shiigi, eds.), Freeman, San Francisco, pp. 351–372.

Oi, V. T., Morrison, S. L., Herzenberg, L. A., and Berg, P., 1983, Immunoglobulin gene expression in transformed lymphoid cells, *Proc. Natl. Acad. Sci. USA* **80**:825–829.

Olsson, L., and Kaplan, H. S., 1980, Human–human hybridomas producing monoclonal antibodies of predefined antigenic specificity, *Proc. Natl. Acad. Sci. USA* **77**:5429–5431.

Olsson, L., Andreasen, R. B., Ost, A., Christensen, B., and Biberfeld, P., 1984, Antibody producing human–human hybridomas. II. Derivation and characterization of an antibody specific for human leukemia cells, *J. Exp. Med.* **159**:537–550.

Östberg, L., and Pursch, E., 1983, Human × (mouse × human) hybridomas stably producing human antibodies, *Hybridoma* **2**:361–367.

Paslay, J. W., and Roozen, K. J., 1981, The effect of B-cell stimulation on hybridoma formation, in: *Monoclonal Antibodies and T-Cell Hybridomas: Perspectives and Technical Advances* (G. J. Hämmerling, U. Hämmerling, and J. F. Kearney, eds.), Elsevier/North-Holland, Amsterdam, pp. 551–559.

Picard, D., and Schaffner, W., 1983, Correct transcription of a cloned mouse immunoglobulin gene *in vivo*, *Proc. Natl. Acad. Sci. USA* **80**:417–421.

Picard, D., and Schaffner, W., 1984, A lymphocyte-specific enhancer in the mouse immunoglobulin κ gene, *Nature* **307**:80–82.

Pontecorvo, G., 1971, Induction of directional chromosome elimination in somatic cell hybrids, *Nature* **230**:367–369.

Queen, C., and Baltimore, D., 1983, Immunoglobulin gene transcription is activated by downstream sequence elements, *Cell* **33**:741–748.

Raison, R. L., Walker, K. Z., Halnan, C. R. E., Briscoe, D., and Basten, A., 1982, Loss of secretion in mouse–human hybrids need not be due to the loss of a structural gene, *J. Exp. Med.* **156**:1380–1389.

Ravetch, J. V., Siebenlist, U., Korsmeyer, S., Waldmann, T., and Leder, P., 1981, Structure of the human immunoglobulin μ locus. Characterization of embryonic and rearranged J and D genes, *Cell* **27**:583–591.

Rice, D., and Baltimore, D., 1982, Regulated expression of an immunoglobulin κ gene introduced into a mouse lymphoid cell line, *Proc. Natl. Acad. Sci. USA* **79**:7862–7865.

Rowley, J. D., and Testa, J. R., 1982, Chromosome abnormalities in malignant hematologic diseases, *Adv. Cancer Res.* **36**:103–148.

Saiki, O., and Ralph, P., 1981, Induction of human immunoglobin secretion. I. Synergistic effect of B-cell mitogen Cowan I plus T cell mitogens, *J. Immunol.* **127**:1044–1047.

Schlom, J., Wunderlich, D., and Teramoto, Y. A., 1980, Generation of human monoclonal antibodies reactive with human mammary carcinoma cells, *Proc. Natl. Acad. Sci. USA* **77**:6841–6845.

Schneiderman, S., Farber, J. L., and Baserga, R., 1979, A simple method for decreasing the toxicity of polyethylene glycol in mammalian cell hybridization, *Somat. Cell Genet.* **5**:263–269.

Schwaber, J., 1975, Immunoglobulin production by a human–mouse somatic cell hybrid, *Exp. Cell Res.* **93**:343–354.

Schwaber, J., and Cohen, E. P., 1973, Human × mouse somatic cell hybrid clone secreting immunoglobulins of both parental types, *Nature* **244**:444–447.

Seed, B., 1982, Screening bacteriophage λ libraries for specific DNA sequences by recombination in *E. coli*, in: *Molecular Cloning* (T. Maniatis, E. F. Fritsch, and J. Sambrook, eds.), Cold Spring Harbor Laboratory, Cold Spring Harbor New York, pp. 353–361.

Shaffner, W., 1980, Direct transfer of cloned genes from bacteria to mammalian cells, *Proc. Natl. Acad. Sci. USA* **77**:2163–2167.

Sikora, K., Alderson, T., Phillips, J., and Watson, J. V., 1982, Human hybridomas from malignant gliomas, *Lancet* **1**:11–14.

Southern, P. J., and Berg, P., 1982, Transformation of mammalian cells to antibiotic resistance with a bacterial gene under control of the SV40 early region promoter, *J. Mol. Appl. Genet.* **1**:327–341.

Stafford, J., and Queen, L., 1983, Cell-type specific expression of a transfected immunoglobulin gene, *Nature* **306:**77–79.

Stanbridge, E. J., 1976, Suppression of malignancy in human cells, *Nature* **260:**17–20.

Steinitz, M., Seppälä, I., Eichmann, K., and Klein, G,, 1979, Establishment of a human lymphoblastoid cell line with specific antibody production against group A streptococcal carbohydrate, *Immunobiology* **156:**41–47.

Teng, N. N. H., Lam, K. S., Calvo Riera, F., and Kaplan, H. S., 1983a, Construction and testing of novel mouse–human heteromyelomas for human monoclonal antibody production, *Proc. Natl. Acad. Sci. USA* **88:**7308–7312.

Teng, N. N. H., Calvo Riera, F., Lam, K. S., and Kaplan, H. S., 1983b, Construction of heteromyelomas for human monoclonal antibody production, in: *Monoclonal Antibodies and Cancer* (R. Dulbecco, R. Langman, and I. Trowbridge, eds.), Academic Press, New York, pp. 135–141.

Teng, N. N. H., Kaplan, H. S., Hebert, J. M., Moore, C., Douglas, H., Wunderlich, A., and Braude, A. I., 1985, Protection against Gram-negative bacteremia and endotoxemia with human monoclonal IgM antibodies, *Proc. Natl. Acad. Sci. USA* **82:**1790–1794.

Thiele, C. J., and Mushinski, J. F., 1982, Human myeloma cell line secreting two forms of δ heavy chains, *Fed. Proc.* **41:**835.

Togawa, A., Inone, M., Miyamoto, K., Hyodo, H., and Namba, M., 1982, Establishment and characterization of a human myeloma cell line (KMM-1), *Int. J. Cancer* **29:**495–500.

Tsuchiya, S., Yokoyama, S., Yoshie, O., and Ono, Y., 1980, Production of diphteria antitoxin antibody in Epstein–Barr virus-induced lymphoblastoid cell lines, *J. Immunol.* **124:**1970–1976.

Weiss, M. C., and Green, H., 1967, Human–mouse hybrid cell lines containing partial complements of human chromosomes and functioning human genes, *Proc. Natl. Acad. Sci. USA* **58:**1104–1111.

Yoshie, O., and Ono, Y., 1980, Anti-phosphorylcholine antibody-producing cells in human lymphoblastoid cell lines established by transformation with Epstein–Barr virus, *Cell Immunol.* **56:**305–316.

Zurawski, V. R., Jr., Haber, E., and Black, P. H., 1978, Production of antibody to tetanus toxoid by continuous human lymphoblastoid cell lines, *Science* **199:**1439–1441.

B. Applications to Infectious Diseases

6

Production and Characterization of Human Monoclonal Antibodies against Gram-Negative Bacteria

Warren C. Bogard, Jr., Elizabeth Hornberger, and Patrick C. Kung

I. Introduction

In the last 20 years, Gram-negative bacteria have become the leading agents of fatal bacterial infections in hospital patients. Each year nosocomial bacteremia develops in approximately 194,000 people in the U.S.; of these about 75,000 die (Maki, 1981). This high frequency of mortality occurs despite the aggressive use of potent antibiotics. The shortcomings of antibiotic therapy may be attributed to the relative impermeability of the outer membrane of Gram-negative bacteria to the drugs and to their inability to counteract or neutralize the lethal effects of bacterial endotoxins (Ziegler et al., 1982). Chemically, the toxiphore of endotoxin is lipopolysaccharide (LPS). They have great structural diversity and are unique to Gram-negative bacteria. LPS is usually composed of three structural regions: the O-specific carbohydrate, the core, and the lipid A (Luderitz et al., 1982). The O-specific chain is typically very immunogenic and structurally heterogeneous from strain to strain. The core and lipid A portions of LPS, however, share similar structures among various strains of Gram-negative bacteria. This is particularly true in

Warren C. Bogard, Jr., Elizabeth Hornberger, and Patrick C. Kung • Centocor, Malvern, Pennsylvania 19355. *Present address for* P. C. K.: T cell Sciences, Inc., Lexington, MA 02173.

the core–lipid A junction, which almost always contains phosphate, 2-keto-3-deoxy-D-*manno*-octonate (KDO), and D-glucosamine (Fig. 1).

It was expected that antiserum against LPS could neutralize its lethal effects *in vivo* (Tate *et al.*, 1966) and might also facilitate bacterial clearance by the reticuloendothelial system. In fact, broad-spectrum protection from challenge by viable Gram-negative bacilli or LPS has been demonstrated by several workers (e.g., Braude and Douglas, 1972; McCabe, 1972; Ziegler *et al.*, 1973; McCabe *et al.*, 1977; Braude *et al.*, 1977; Dunn and Ferguson, 1982) using rough mutants of *Escherichia coli* or *Salmonella minnesota* as immunizing agents. These mutants lack the O-specific carbohydrate and on their surface express portions of core which presumably contain antigenic determinants shared by most Gram-negative organisms. Passive immunization of patients with human antiserum raised against the rough mutant *E. coli* J5 has been shown to be efficacious in treating endotoxin shock induced by nosocomial infections (Ziegler *et al.*, 1982). However, the nature, titer, and specificity of the protective antibodies elicited by the whole bacteria have been difficult to establish. These results suggest that monoclonal antibodies may supercede the conventional polyspecific antisera used for the passive immunotherapy.

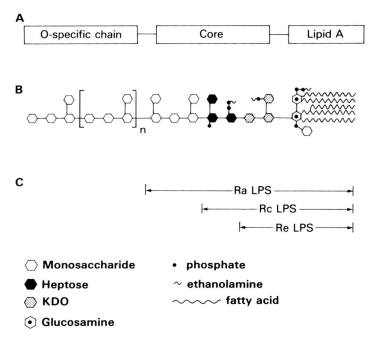

FIGURE 1. Summary of the major structural features of lipopolysaccharide (LPS), the endotoxin of Gram-negative bacteria: (A) schematic diagram of LPS; (B) structure of *Salmonella* LPS; (C) polysaccharide chain termination sites for three representative rough mutant organisms. [Adapted from Luderitz *et al.* (1982).]

tohemagglutinin A-stimulated T-cell supernatant. This resulted in 22% of the well supernatants showing specificity for *E. coli* J5 organisms.

Three hybridomas secreting anti-*E. coli* antibodies were isolated after several serial dilution clonings. The three cloned hybrid lines derived from three separate fusion experiments have continued to secrete the antibodies in culture for over 18 months. These lines were designated by their respective fusion experiment numbers: HM16A, HM22B, and HM28.

Using specific human Ig typing sera, all three hybrids were found to secrete only antigen-specific human IgM antibodies. When the RIA was configured to measure total κ and total λ, HM16A was shown to produce both Ig light chain isotypes (50/50), whereas HM22B and HM28 had predominantly (80/20) and exclusively (100/0) κ, respectively (data not shown). The molecular weight distribution of the total human IgM activity and of the anti-*E. coli* activity were determined by high-performance liquid chromatography. All three antibodies were found to be pentameric IgM. A typical result is shown in Fig. 2.

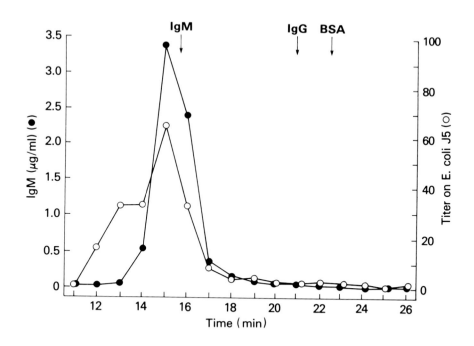

FIGURE 2. Molecular weight distribution of anti-*E. coli* activity in HM16A tissue culture supernatants. Ammonium sulfate-purified ascites containing HM16A was applied to a TSK 4000 SW column (Varian) and 1-min (1-ml) fractions collected. The effluent was monitored for total human IgM and for titer of human IgM on *E. coli* J5 by RIA. The elution time for mouse monoclonal IgM and IgG and for bovine serum albumin are shown.

Growth and secretion rates for the three human hybridomas and for the human lymphoblastoid line were determined (Table II). The cell doubling times for the four cell lines were as follows: 20 hr for HM16A, 16 hr for HM22B, 25 hr for HM28, and 13 hr for WI-L2-729HF2. The total accumulation of IgM specific for *E. coli* J5 was 4.8 μg/ml for HM16A, 0.32 μg/ml for HM22B, and 2.0 μg/ml for HM28. Thus, the lowest Ig-secreting line was the fastest growing line.

Chromosome studies showed that all three hybrid cell lines were nearly tetraploid. Karyotype analysis showed that WI-L2-729HF2 contained an average of 46 chromosomes, including a single X and a single Y chromosome (Fig. 3A). Similar studies on stabilized HM16A hybridoma cells yielded an average of 89 chromosomes. Because the immune lymphocytes were derived from a female donor, three X and one Y chromosomes in the hybrid cell were observed (Fig. 3B) This result confirmed the hybrid nature of HM16A cells.

TABLE II
Summary of Hybrid Growth and Secretion Characteristics

Cell line	Day	Cells $(10^6/\text{ml})$	IgM[a] $(\mu\text{g/ml})$	IgM/24 hr per 10^6 cells[b] $(\mu\text{g/ml})$
HM16A	0	0.10	0	—
	1	0.16	0.07	0.54
	2	0.52	0.60	1.56
	3	1.6	2.93	2.20
	4	1.8	4.00	0.63
	5	2.2	4.80	0.40
	6	4.0	4.00	−0.26
HM22B	0	0.10	0	—
	1	0.24	0.01	0.06
	2	0.74	0.04	0.06
	3	1.7	0.15	0.09
	4	1.4	0.20	0.03
	5	1.5	0.22	0.01
	6	1.3	0.32	0.07
HM28	0	0.10	0	—
	1	0.14	0.20	1.67
	2	0.46	0.53	1.10
	3	1.1	1.10	0.73
	4	1.4	1.60	0.40
	5	1.9	2.00	0.24
	6	1.1	2.00	0.00
729HF2	0	0.10	0	—
	1	0.14	0.00	0.00
	2	0.94	0.01	0.02
	3	2.6	0.08	0.04
	4	3.2	0.08	0.00

[a]Concentration of human IgM as determined by RIA.
[b]Change in IgM concentration per 24 hr normalized to 10^6 cells; calculated as follows: $(M_n - M_{n-1})/[(C_n - C_{n-1})/2]$, where M_n is the IgM concentration at the end of day n and C_n is the number of viable cells per ml at the end of day n.

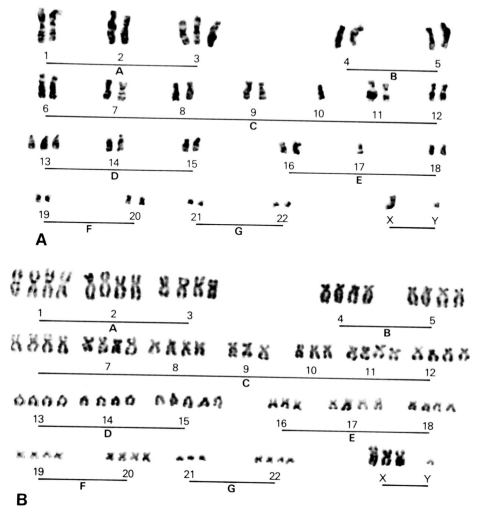

FIGURE 3. Representative chromosome spreads and karyotype of (A) WI-L2-729HF2 and (B) HM16A.

III. Human Monoclonal Antibody Production in Nude Mice

The athymic (nude) mouse has been invaluable as a model for studying the biology of tumor growth and the immune system. Human xenographs and established human carcinoma lines have been sucessfully transplanted into nude mice (Giovanella *et al.*, 1978; Herlyn *et al.*, 1980). Although the potential utility of human antibodies is enormous, the production of milligram (mg) quantities of human monoclonal antibodies of a predefined specificity from human–human hybrids has been limited. Noeman *et al.* (1982) demonstrated that mg quantities of specific monoclonal antibody could be derived from rat–mouse hybridomas in irradiated nude mice.

Numerous attempts to induce ascites production in nude mice with the human hybridoma cell line HM16A by varying priming parameters and cell doses failed. Further efforts focused on subcutaneous solid tumor formation in both irradiated and nonirradiated adults and in neonates. These results were also equivocal. Finally, a schedule utilizing a primed and irradiated nude mouse model system was initiated. Athymic nude mice (outbred; BALB/c background) were obtained at 4 weeks of age (Harlan Sprague-Dawley) and housed under a flexible barrier condition (Sedlacek *et al.*, 1981) and quarantined for 2 weeks. The athymic nude mice were primed with an intraperitoneal injection of 0.2 ml of pristane (Aldrich Chemical Co.). On day 8, the mice were divided into three groups and irradiated with a cesium source (Best Industries) at 300 rad. Previous irradiation experiments determined the LD_{50} to be within the range 500–700 rad. Hybridoma HM16A cells were harvested, washed three times in Hank's Balanced Salt Solution, and adjusted to various cell concentrations and injected ip in 1 ml of saline on day 10. Ascites fluid was collected 39–60 days later. The effects of irradiation levels and cell dose on ascitic tumor formation in pristane-primed nude mice are shown in Table III. None of the five animals irradiated with 300 rad developed ascites when injected with 1×10^6 or 2×10^6 cells, but one mouse of five did become positive at 5×10^6 cells. When the irradiation dose was increased to 350 rad, two of five injected with 1×10^6 cells were positive, while no positives appeared at the 2×10^6 cell level. When the radiation dose was increased to 400 rad, three of five mice (60%) were positive at 1×10^6 and 2×10^6 cells/mouse. The criteria for positivity included volume of ascites tapped and titer (see Table IV). Chromosome analysis confirmed that recovered cells from the ascites fluid were human in origin and had the same number of chromosomes as the *in vitro*-passaged cells (data not shown).

In order to ascertain whether these results might have general utility, the two other human antibody-producing hybridomas were tested in the irradiated and primed nude mouse system. These results are summarized in Table IV. Ascitic tumors formed at an acceptable level for all cell lines tested using a dose of 1×10^6 cells per mouse and an irradiation dose of 400 rad. Moreover, titers of the ascites fluids were 100- to 1000-fold enhanced relative to titers of supernatants of ascites-recovered hybridoma cells collected after 3–5 days in culture. Preliminary data indicate that multiple passaging of the ascites cells improves the positive take rate and volume of ascites collected. Similar results have been obtained with other human–human hybrid lines of different antigen specificities in which 729HF2 cells were used as the fusion partner (A. Quinn, unpublished result). Although large-scale production of human monoclonal antibodies will probably rely on large-scale tissue culture techniques, this system may provide thousandfold amplification of yield so that mg amounts of antibody can be obtained for immediate use or testing.

TABLE III

Production of Antibody-Containing Ascitic Fluid
from Human Hybridoma HM16A in Nude
Mice: The Effect of Cell Dose and Radiation

Cell dose[a]	Number of ascitic tumors/total at given radiation dose		
	300 R	350 R	400 R
1×10^6	0/5	1/5	3/5
2×10^6	0/5	0/5	3/5
5×10^6	1/5	1/5[b]	NT[c]

[a]Groups of five athymic nude females were inoculated with HM16A antibody-producing cells intraperitoneally, 10 days post priming with pristane (0.2 ml/mouse, ip), and 2 days postradiation. Ascites fluid was collected between 4 and 7 weeks.
[b]One additional animal was positive for solid tumor only.
[c]Not tested.

TABLE IV

Human Antibody Production in Irradiated Athymic Nude Mice
from Three Human Hybridomas

Cell line	Specificity	Percent positive[a]	Antibody production (ml/mouse)	Titer	
				Supernatant[b]	Ascites[c]
HM16A	Anti-*E. coli* J5	60 (5)	2.6	2.6×10^2	$(0.2–2) \times 10^5$
HM22B	Anti-*E. coli* J5	87 (15)	2.3	1.6×10^1	$(1.0–2) \times 10^3$
HM28	Anti-*E. coli* 0111:B4	42.8 (21)	2.4	5.1×10^2	$(0.3–5) \times 10^5$

[a]Number of mice per injection in parentheses.
[b]Titer on supernatant from ascites cells grown in tissue culture.
[c]Range of titers for individual ascites taps.

IV. Characterization of Antibody Specificity

Tissue culture supernatants from the three hybrid lines and from the lymphoblastoid line were screened in the RIA against several strains of Gram-negative and Gram-positive bacteria. Positive binding to bacilli was observed by development with ^{125}I-labeled goat anti-human IgM antisera that had been affinity-purified. The results of these experiments are summarized in Table V. HM16A supernatant demonstrated binding activity to all eight Gram-negative bacterial strains. HM22B and HM28 showed binding to four and two stains, respectively. None of the supernatants gave positive results on the two Gram-positive organisms tested. The WI-L2-729HF2 supernatants served as negative control. Curiously, in this experiment, HM28 was negative on *E. coli* J5, the organisms against which it was originally selected. It was later shown that HM28 bound to old heat-inactivated J5 organisms but only very weakly to freshly prepared organisms.

The cell culture supernatants were also screened in RIA for binding to purified LPS from the Gram-negative strains shown in Table V. It was found that HM16 bound very weakly to several of the LPS samples (i.e., at low titer); in contrast, HM22 showed no reactivity to any LPS tested. The results for HM28 in the RIA were unusual. HM28 bound strongly (maximum counts and titer) to *E. coli* 055:B5 LPS and *S. minnesota* LPS, but not to *E. coli* 0111:B4 LPS. This was in contrast to the whole-cell assay (Table V), where HM28 bound to *E. coli* 0111:B4 and *E. coli* 055:B5 organisms but not to *S. minnesota* organisms.

We have previously shown that murine monoclonal antibodies that cross-react with many genera of Gram-negative bacteria were of anti-LPS specificity (more specifically, anti-lipid A). Moreover, by sodium dodecyl sulfate–poly-acrylamide gel electrophoresis (SDS–PAGE) and immunoblotting, these cross-reacting murine antibodies were shown to interact predominantly to LPS components that lack O-specific carbohydrate (i.e., the fast-migrating silver-stained bands in Fig. 4A). This same system was utilized to analyze the human antibodies for LPS binding. Preliminary results showed that HM16A behaved as the cross-reacting murine antibodies did; that is, it bound only to

TABLE V

Binding of Three Human Monoclonal Antibodies to Heat-Inactivated Bacteria by RIA

Bacteria[a]	Counts per minute[b] for given cell culture supernatant[c]			
	HM16A	HM22B	HM28	WI-L2-729HF2
Gram-negative				
Escherichia coli J5	9482	1154	304	389
E. coli 0111:B4	4188	228	11900	363
E. coli 055:B5	6906	369	13849	285
Salmonella minnesota	10973	2723	284	241
S. minnesota Re595	10644	4641	480	314
Klebsiella pneumoniae	4958	213	261	217
Serratia marcescens	11270	600	227	263
Pseudomonas aeruginosa	4903	1368	283	295
Gram-positive				
Staphylococcus aureus	330	174	300	126
Streptococcus faecalis	348	162	200	126

[a]Coated onto polyvinylchloride plates of 5×10^6 in 50 µl of 0.9% (w/v) sodium chloride.
[b]^{125}I-Labeled goat anti-human IgM used as probe (5×10^4 cpm/50 µl).
[c]Incubated (50 µl) for 2 hr at 37°C.

the fast-migrating bands. However, the intensity of the immuno-staining was weak for HM16A. HM22 was completely negative for LPS specificity by this technique. The results for HM28 are shown in Fig. 4. In agreement with the RIA, HM28 recognized components of *E. coli* 055:B5 LPS and *S. minnesota* LPS, but not *E. coli* J5 LPS or *E. coli* 0111:B4 LPS. Surprisingly, however, HM28 interacted with most of the silver-stained components for *S. minnesota*

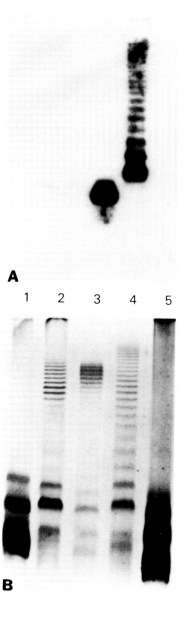

FIGURE 4. Analysis of the binding of human monoclonal antibody HM28 to LPS components by polyacrylamide gel electrophoresis and immunoblotting techniques. (1) *E. coli* J5; (2) *E. coli* 0111:B4; (3) *E. coli* 055:B5; (4) *S. minnesota;* (5) *S. minnesota* Re595. (A) Immunoblot with HM28; (B) gel stained with silver by the method of Tsai and Frasch (1982).

LPS, but only a fast-migrating component of *E. coli* 055:B5 LPS. Thus, HM28 appeared to recognize LPS, but the unusual specificity remains unexplained.

Notwithstanding the unusual specificity of HM28, the most perplexing problem was that HM16A had high titer activity against heat-inactivated organisms by RIA, but only weak anti-LPS activity (by RIA and SDS–PAGE immunoblotting). This was in contrast to our experience with murine anti-Gram negative bacteria, where high titer cross-reactivity correlated well with anti-LPS activity in both the RIA and blotting assays. It may well be that HM16A recognized LPS structure or conformation that exists on the bacterial outer membrane but not in purified antigen. Similar arguments may apply to HM22. The lack of any activity could simply reflect the tenfold lower specific antibody concentration in the cell culture supernatants.

V. Discussion

During the past few years many laboratories have engaged in the advancement of producing human monoclonal antibodies (e.g., Olsson and Kaplan, 1980; Croce *et al.*, 1980; Hoffman, 1980; Kozbor and Roder, 1981; Crawford *et al.*, 1983; Larrik., *et al.*, 1983; Strike *et al.*, 1984). These efforts are related to (1) the development of B-cell lines as optimal fusion partners, (2) methods of *in vitro* immunization, and (C) the techniques of mass production of human monoclonal antibodies. Significant progress has been made in each of these areas of investigation [for review see Kozbor and Roder (1983)].

Our laboratory has been interested in developing human monoclonal antibodies that are effective in protecting patients from Gram-negative bacteria-induced shock. Using 729HF2 as a fusion partner, we have been successful in obtaining several stable human hybridomas secreting anti-Gram-negative bacteria monoclonals. In the course of performing these experiments we have confirmed the high fusion frequency between the peripheral and splenic mononuclear cells and the 729HF2 cells (Strike *et al.*, 1984). However, we noticed that the resulting hybridomas were relatively unstable in the first few months postfusion. It required close attention and extensive labor to derive a stable hybridoma. To date, several human B- and myeloma cell lines have been tested as fusion partners. The resultant hybridomas derived from these partners may suffer from either stability problems in the first few months postfusion or from low fusion frequency (Abrams *et al.*, 1983).

Since programmable *in vivo* immunization is generally unavailable, the source of immune B lymphocytes usually presents a serious obstacle in producing desirable human monoclonal antibodies. In our fusion experiments designed to isolate human monoclonal antibodies specific for hepatitis B surface antigen, we often observed culture wells containing hybridomas that secreted anti-Gram-negative bacteria antibodies; the results suggested the prevalent exposure of the population to the bacteria. In a recent systematic

7

Human Monoclonal Antibodies to Defined Antigens

Toward Clinical Applications

Karen G. Burnett, Julia P. Leung, and Joanne Martinis

I. Production of Monoclonal Antibodies for Diagnostic and Therapeutic Use

In recent years there has been an increasing number of reports detailing techniques for producing human monoclonal antibodies. Most of these human antibodies are derived from primary human lymphocytes by Epstein–Barr virus (EBV) transformation or by hybridization with lymphoid tumor lines. In addition, *in vitro* culture of primary human B cells promises to become yet another approach to making monoclonal antibodies. We have chosen to immortalize human lymphocytes using hybridoma technology rather than EBV transformation for several reasons. First, gram quantities of mouse monoclonal antibodies made by this technique already have been produced and safely used for *in vivo* diagnosis and immunotherapy in human patients. Second, using hybridoma technology, it is possible to produce human monoclonal antibodies without the complication of possible Epstein–Barr virus contamination. Third, while there have been many reports of success producing human antibodies by hybridoma technology, most workers will admit that they have very little control over the production of antigen-

Karen G. Burnett, Julia P. Leung, and Joanne Martinis • Hybritech, San Diego, California 92121

specific human monoclonal antibodies. Consequently, our goal has been and continues to be to develop procedures for routinely making specific human antibodies that can perform defined functions.

One can begin to appreciate the difficulty in developing useful human antibodies by looking at the current state of mouse hybridoma technology. It is relatively easy to produce mouse monoclonal antibodies to large protein antigens. However, making monoclonal antibodies to other antigens such as carbohydrates and small or highly conserved proteins can pose many problems. An antigen may be poorly immunogenic; it may be immunogenic but not clonogenic (not yield antigen-specific hybridomas) or it may yield monoclonal antibodies with undesirable characteristics such as low affinity, high cross-reactivity, or unwanted isotype. Such difficulties may be solved by using various immunization strategies, such as employing high or low doses of immunogen, conjugating the antigen to large protein carriers, varying routes of injection or changing adjuvants, or simply screening enough hybridomas or designing special assays to find the "right" monoclonal antibody. Therefore, even in the easily manipulated mouse system it can be very difficult to "tailor-make" useful mouse monoclonal antibodies to specific applications.

Making human monoclonal antibodies by hybridoma technology presents even greater difficulties. There are two basic problems. First, the ability to immortalize human lymphocytes is still a technical feat. Much experimental effort has gone into finding the ideal lymphoid fusion partner for human lymphocytes. Instability and poor fusibility are still commonly encountered problems. Therefore, the number of human monoclonal antibodies that have been produced and studied is still very limited by comparison to the mouse system. Second, the human antibodies that have been described to date generally have poor specificity and low affinity, properties that prevent any useful diagnostic or therapeutic application. This poor quality reflects our general reliance on *in vivo* immunization to provide antibodies of high affinity and good specificity. *In vivo* antigen-primed lymphocytes can be derived routinely in only a few model systems. Some examples are standard vaccinations for antigens such as hepatitis B and tetanus toxin, autoimmune disease for DNA and nuclear protein antigens, and diagnosed carcinoma for tumor-associated antigens. *In vitro* immunization techniques are still poorly defined for human lymphocytes, yielding primarily low level, IgM responses. In addition, we do not have regular access to the most activated, lymphocyte-rich tissues of the reticuloendothelial system, such as the spleen and lymph nodes. Therefore we must learn to adapt our procedures to use peripheral blood lymphocytes (PBLs).

Given the constraints and unique problems of the human system, we are developing procedures to increase hybridoma production in general and to produce and select for human antibodies with clinically useful qualities. In this chapter we discuss the use of normal human PBLs to generate routinely large numbers of mouse–human and human–human hybridomas. Hepatitis B surface antigen (HBsAg) and tetanus toxin have been used as model systems; the implications for other antigen systems are very broad. These studies demonstrate that if appropriately selected and handled, myeloma cell lines are now available that can immortalize human lymphocytes and realistically can be expected to generate stable hybridomas producing antigen-specific human monoclonal antibodies.

II. Peripheral Blood as a Source of Antigen-Primed Lymphocytes

Human lymphocytes can be obtained from many tissue sources. Spleen, lymph nodes, tonsils, and peripheral blood are particularly rich in lymphocytes. Lymphocytes can also be isolated in relatively low numbers from other normal and neoplastic nonlymphoid tissues. To minimize our reliance on lymphocytes stimulated by disease and obtained by major surgery, we have optimized our procedures to use PBLs from normal donors specifically immunized with the target antigen. Peripheral blood is certainly not an optimal source of activated, antigen-primed lymphocytes. A unit of blood yields approximately 500 million lymphocytes, of which only 20% are B cells. It has been estimated that following specific vaccination, at most only 1% circulating B cells bear surface immunoglobulin capable of binding the immunogen. Therefore, assuming all PBLs fuse equally well, only one in 500 hybridomas should produce specific antibody. Furthermore, following specific immunization, antigen-specific B cells appear only transitorily in the peripheral circulation. The kinetics of their appearance and disappearance is dictated by the individual donor immune response, the immunization history, and the nature of the antigen and genetic reportoire of that individual. Although for some antigens the genetically heterogeneous human population responds fairly uniformly, response to others may be extremely diverse. This means that for each antigen it is necessary to determine when peripheral blood contains the greatest number of lymphocytes producing specific antibody,

We initially chose to work with tetanus toxin as a model antigen because booster-immunized donors are easily available. This selection was fortunate for two more reasons. First, individual responses to this protein antigen were quite uniform across our survey population. Second, most volunteers exhibited a secondary, predominantly IgG response to antigen stimulation. In our survey group we first measured serum antitetanus IgG and IgM by ELISA at a 1:1000 dilution. Over a group of 14 donors we could correlate antitetanus IgG ELISA signal with time lapse since last booster immunization. By comparison, antitetanus IgM ELISA values were relatively low over the survey population even at 1:100 dilution and were difficult to measure over nonspecific background serum binding to the antigen. Next, serum titer response of six individuals to tetanus immunization was monitored (Table I). Serum titer was taken as that dilution giving 25% of an arbitrary positive control

TABLE I
Antitetanus Serum Responses Following Booster Immunization

Donor	Time since last tetanus immunization (months)	IgM titer[a] at given number of days following booster immunization			IgG titer[a] at given number of days following booster immunization		
		0	6	14	0	6	14
B141	2	31	40	28	1300	1250	1200
B14	3	10	10	10	500	600	500
B35	8	160	150	160	960	1100	1200
B100	17	58	45	96	480	940	1400
B72	18	38	35	40	340	600	900
B103	60	20	40	ND	100	1100	ND

[a]Titer: reciprocal value of that serum dilution giving 25% of an arbitrary positive control reference in specific antitetanus ELISA (OD_{495}) on toxoid antigen. ND, Not determined.

serum sample. Antitetanus IgM measured preboost and at days 6 and 14 following immunization remained unchanged or increased less than twofold in all donors. Preboost antitetanus IgG titers varied by only tenfold, from 1:100 to 1:1300, among these six individuals, who ranged from 2 months to 5 years since their last tetanus vaccination. After booster immunization, circulating antitetanus IgG titer in five out of six donors ranged from only 1:900 to 1:1400. Two donors, both immunized less than 3 months prior to this new round of immunizations, did not respond to the vaccine. One donor, who had not been vaccinated for 5 years, showed the most marked response, from 1:100 preboost to 1:1100 at day 6 postboost. These data demonstrate that immune response to tetanus toxin is reasonably predictable.

Our next step was to determine when lymphocytes producing antitetanus antibodies were present in the peripheral circulation. In this assay we assumed that antigen-primed B lymphocytes would be capable of producing specific antibody during *in vitro* culture. Donors were immunized with 5 Lf units of tetanus toxoid vaccine (Wyeth) and whole blood was drawn at day 0 and subsequently at 3-day intervals over 3 weeks after vaccination. Lymphocytes were isolated by Ficoll density gradient centrifugation and cultured *in vitro* with and without the polyclonal activator pokeweed mitogen (PWM). Supernatants were sampled at days 3 and 7 of culture and assayed for specific antibody content by ELISA. As diagrammed in Fig. 1 for one good responder, lymphocytes obtained at day 6 following immunization and cultured without PWM stimulation produced the highest amount of antigen-specific IgG. This antibody was secreted during the first 3 days of culture. When stimulated with 1% (v/v) PWM, lymphocytes obtained at day 9 and as long as 2 months after immunization secreted antitetanus IgG. This antibody production occurred later between days 4 and 7 of *in vitro* culture, as a result of indirect T-cell-mediated B-cell activation by PWM. Based upon this and sim-

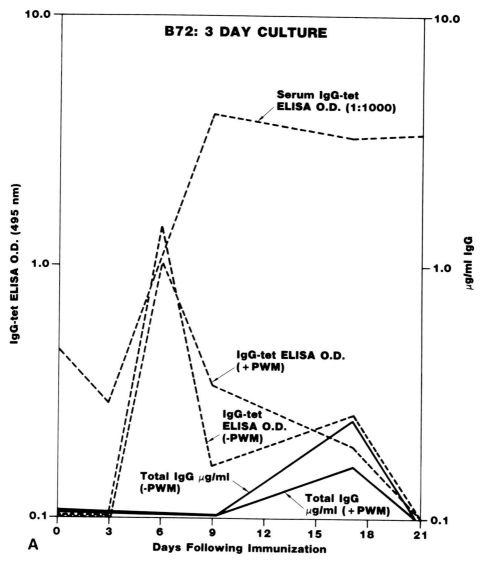

FIGURE 1. Total IgG and specific antitetanus IgG produced *in vitro* by human PBL (donor B72) obtained at various time points after tetanus booster immunization. (A) Antibody in PBL supernatants produced during the first 3 days of *in vitro* culture with or without PWM. (B) Antibody in PBL supernatants produced during 7 days of *in vitro* culture with or without PWM.

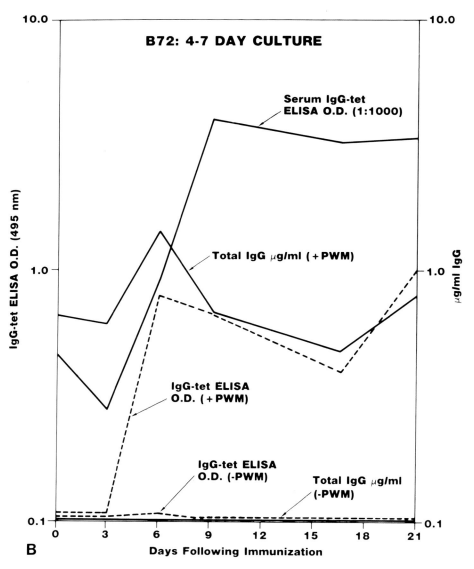

FIGURE 1. (*Continued*)

ilar data from several other donors, we have pinpointed day 6 peripheral blood as the richest source of specific antibody-producing lymphocytes following tetanus secondary immunization. Furthermore, the response pattern indicates that lymphocytes taken at later times (9 days to 2 months) contain B cells that can be secondarily activated *in vitro* to produce specific antibody. These also may be good sources for lymphocytes to be immortalized in producing antigen-specific monoclonal antibodies.

While they are the most routinely available lymphocytes, PBLs have few activated B cells and are the most poorly fusible human lymphocyte population. Table II compares the fusibility of human lymphocytes from three major tissue sources: spleen, lymph node, and peripheral blood. As might be expected, these lymphocyte pools have very different abilities to form hybrids. The variation is due to the diverse medical histories, genetic backgrounds, and environmental stimuli encountered by the individual donors, to the health of the tissue upon removal (particularly spleen and lymph node), and in large part to the nature and function of that component of the reticuloendothelial system. In these comparisons, myelomas and lymphocytes were carefully and routinely handled in order to minimize variations that can arise from other sources, for example, fusion and plating conditions. Lymphocytes were not deliberately stimulated *in vitro* and no feeder or filler cells were added. Data in Table II were generated using lymphocytes from many different donors, in order to demonstrate the realistic variability encountered when working with human lymphocytes. Almost without exception, spleen and lymph node lymphocytes fuse more efficiently than PBLs, regardless of fusion partner. In order for two cells to fuse and produce a viable hybrid, not only must the plasma membrane fuse, but in the heterokaryon both nuclei must be drawn into mitosis simultaneously, so that a single nuclear membrane will be constructed to contain chromosomes from both parents. A lymphoid tumor line is an actively dividing cell population. Lymphocytes in peripheral blood are largely T cells and resting or memory B cells, and therefore should not produce large numbers of Ig-secreting hybrids relative to lymph node, tonsil, or spleen lymphocytes.

Because PBLs have relatively poor fusion efficiency, many investigators routinely culture these cells in the presence of polyclonal activators for several days prior to fusion in order to increase lymphocyte fusibility. Two problems are often encountered when assessing the effects of PWM on hybridoma production: (1) T-cell clones proliferating in response to PWM can easily be mistaken for true hybridomas; (2) PWM indirectly stimulates B-cell Ig secretion, causing high levels of background (residual) Ig production in fusion wells. Therefore, all presumptive hybridomas obtained from PWM stimulation experiments are maintained in culture at least 2 months to ensure continued growth and Ig production. In our hands, PWM stimulation has had extremely variable success and we are continuing to collect data to explain this variability.For these experiments, PBLs isolated on Ficoll density gradients

TABLE II

Comparative Fusibility of Human Lymphocytes from Three Primary Lymphoid Tissue Sources[a]

Lymphoid cell	Primary lymphocyte tissue source	Number of fusions	Total number of lymphocytes ($\times 10^6$)	Number of donors	Total number of clones	Range of fusion frequency ($\times 10^{-6}$)	Number of clones/10^6 lymphocytes ($\bar{x}$)
729/HT[b]	Peripheral blood	50	1010	14	22	<0.02–0.5	0.02
	Lymph node	21	240	11	249	<0.1–6.0	1.0
	Spleen	14	210	5	133	<0.03–3.0	0.6
P3/HT[c]	Peripheral blood	90	1800	38	5126	<0.2–12.0	2.8
	Lymph node	69	940	27	4060	<0.05–18.0	4.3
	Spleen	25	430	5	3108	<0.02–20	7.2

[a]For each fusion, $(1–3) \times 10^7$ human lymphocytes were fused to $(1–3) \times 10^7$ P3/HT or 729/HT. Cells were fused by the method of Gerhard (1980) using 35% PEG 1000 + 7.5% DMSO and diluted into the appropriate HAT-selective medium (Littlefield, 1964). Fused cells were plated into 96-well microtiter dishes at 10^5 cells/well without feeder layers. Growth medium for 729/HT hybrids was RPMI 1640 plus 10% fetal calf serum; for P3/HT hybrids growth medium was autoclavable MEM with 8% horse and 2% fetal calf serum.
[b]729/HT is derived from 729-6 (Lever et al., 1974).
[c]P3/HT is a subline of P3X63Ag8.653 (Kearney et al., 1979).

are either fused immediately or cultured *in vitro* with or without 1% PWM up to 9 days. Periodically during *in vitro* culture, PWM-stimulated and unstimulated lymphocytes are fused to a human or mouse lymphoid tumor cell line. In nine experiments, *in vitro* stimulation had no effect or decreased clone production. In one experiment, PWM stimulation dramatically enhanced clone production, but yield of Ig-producing clones remained low. Based upon our experiments to date, we feel that PWM does not reliably increase the yield of clones or specific human monoclonal antibodies from PBL fusions.

III. A Comparison of Mouse and Human Lymphoid Fusion Partners

Myeloma and lymphoblastoid lines also vary widely in their fusion efficiencies. Because PBLs fuse relatively poorly, and because antigen-specific lymphocytes are present in very low frequency in this lymphocyte population, it is particularly important to select the best fusion partner. The optimal lymphoid fusion partner will fuse reliably and with high frequency; it will support high levels of human Ig secretion and not produce its own non-specific immunoglobulin. Furthermore, the resulting hybridomas must be stable, that is, they must continue to grow rapidly and produce human immunoglobulin for many months without constant subcloning. A pervasive assumption in the recent scientific literature has been that for a human hybridoma to be stable it must be produced from an established human lymphoid cell line. Early experimental work in the area of somatic cell hybridization with fibroblast lines suggested that intraspecific hybrids would be more stable than interspecific hybrids. However, in our experience hybrid stability appears to be a function of the particular cell lines involved. Interspecific hybrids can be stable when constructed with an appropriately selected fusion partner.

In initial experiments to select the optimal fusion partner for human lymphocytes we surveyed the fusion efficiency of human PBLs with four human and three mouse lymphoid lines. Pertinent details regarding the tested cell lines are provided in Table III. Fusion results are presented in Table IV. In our hands the most fusible human cell line was 729/HT, a derivative of 729-6 originally described by Lever *et al.* (1974). All three of the mouse myelomas NS-1, SP2/0, and P3/HT fused well with human lymphocytes. However, it was noted that hybridomas produced with P3/HT continued to secrete human immunoglobulin for many months in culture, while at least 50% of all hybridomas with NS-1 or SP2/0 lost human Ig production very rapidly. Clearly the only two acceptable candidates for fusion partners with human PBLs were 729/HT, a human lymphoblastoid cell line, or P3/HT, a mouse myeloma line.

TABLE III
Lymphoid Lines Surveyed

Name	Species origin	Parent line	Ig production	Cell type	Reference
729-6/HT	Human	729-6	IgM(κ)	EBNA+, lymphoblastoid	Lever *et al.* (1974)
ARH077 Az	Human	ARH077	IgG1(κ)	EBNA+, lymphoblastoid	I. Royston, personal communication
GM607.11	Human	GM607	IgM(κ)	EBNA+, lymphoblastoid	Hybritech
GM4672	Human	GM1500	IgG2(κ)	EBNA+, lymphoblastoid	Croce *et al.* (1980)
NS-1	Mouse	P3X63Ag.8	κ	EBNA−, plasmacytoma	Köhler and Milstein (1975)
SP2/0	Mouse	NS-1	None	EBNA−, hybridoma	Shulman *et al.* (1978)
P3/HT	Mouse	P3X63Ag.8	None	EBNA−, plasmacytoma	Kearney *et al.* (1979)

TABLE IV

Comparative Fusibility of Human PBLs with Established Human and Mouse Lymphoid Tumor Cells[a]

	Number of fusions	Total number of lymphocytes ($\times 10^6$)	Number of donors	Total number of clones	Range of fusion frequency ($\times 10^{-6}$)	Number of clones/10^6 lymphocytes ($\bar{\Sigma}$)
Human						
729/HT	50	1010	14	22	<0.02–0.5	0.02
ARH077 Az	9	200	4	0	<0.01	0
GM607.11	19	650	8	6	<0.01–0.2	0.01
GM4672	3	30	1	1	<0.03–0.1	0.03
Mouse						
NS-1	9	150	4	98	<0.2–3.0	0.7
SP2/0	69	850	20	2143	<0.02–20.0	2.5
P3/HT	90	1800	38	5126	$<0.02–12.0 \times 10^{-7}$	2.8

[a]Fusions were performed and cells cultured as described in Table II.

Subsequently, P3/HT and 729/HT were directly compared to assess those characteristics that are most important to production of human monoclonal antibodies. These tests included: fusibility, yield of human Ig-producing hybridomas, levels of Ig secretion, and stability of specific antibody production. First, data were accumulated on clone production from fusions of P3/HT and 729/HT with spleen, lymph node, and peripheral blood lymphocytes. As shown in Tables II and IV, fusions of human PBLs with P3/HT produced 100 times more clones than with 729/HT. However, this difference in fusibility was much less marked when using spleen or lymph node lymphocytes.

Second, the relative yields of human Ig-secreting hybridomas from the two lymphoid fusion partners were compared by fusing 729/HT and P3/HT at the same time to the same pools of human lymphocytes. Table V summarizes the Ig-production data from those fusions with clone growth in less than 33% of seeded wells, to ensure that each hybridoma tested represented a single fusion event. From these results it is evident that not only did P3/HT yield more Ig-secreting clones, but also that a greater number of these hybrids produced IgG.

Next, we compared the amount of immunoglobulin produced by these mouse–human and human–human hybridomas. Both 729/HT and P3/HT hybridomas in mass cultures routinely secrete as much as 5–20 μg/ml of human Ig as measured by ELISA against a standard of polyclonal human Ig. Sometimes clone supernatants will initially contain greater than 20 μg/ml human Ig, but these levels drop to the expected range with subsequent passage. Based on data from spleen, lymph node, tonsil, and PBL fusions (data not shown), P3/HT and 729/HT produce roughly comparable amounts of human Ig.

Last and most significant, human Ig-secreting hybridomas made with P3/HT are even more stable than hybridomas made with 729/HT. Figure 2 presents stability data compiled during fusion efficiency comparisons of the human and mouse lymphoid tumor lines. These data also summarize observa-

TABLE V

Immunoglobulin Production by Human–Human and Mouse–Human Hybrids[a]

Cell line	PBL		Lymph node		Spleen	
	% IgM	% IgG	% IgM	% IgG	% IgM	% IgG
729/HT	ND	ND	23	13	20	6.7
P3/HT	28	2.3	68	23	55	31

[a]After three feedings, clone supernatants were assayed for the presence of human IgG or IgM by ELISA. The Ig levels were determined by comparison to a polyclonal IgG or IgM standard curve. Positive clones secreted greater than 0.1 μg/ml of human Ig. ND, Not determined (inadequate data).

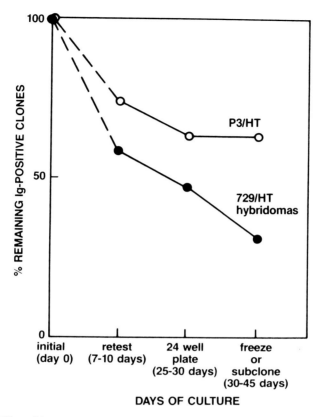

FIGURE 2. Stability of human Ig-secreting hybridomas made with P3/HT or 729/HT. Clones secreting greater than 0.1 μg/ml human IgG or IgM were identified by ELISA on culture supernatants 3–5 weeks after fusion or when microtiter wells were approximately one-third confluent. Positive clones were transferred to a second or "retest" microtiter well and refed. Clones that were still positive at this stage were transferred to 24-well plate wells and were assayed again. Clones remaining positive were transferred to T-25 flasks and were reassayed for Ig production prior to freezing or subcloning.

tions from fusions with growth in fewer than 33% of seeded microtiter wells, thus ensuring that each hybridoma is monoclonal, and minimizing the complication of overgrowth by nonproducer hybridomas. Figure 2 traces the stability of P3/HT and 729/HT hybridomas after initial detection of human IgG or IgM (greater than 0.1 μg/ml by ELISA) in clone supernatants. When retested approximately 2 weeks after the initial screen many P3/HT and 729/HT hybrids have lost Ig production. This instability may be due to residual lymphocyte Ig secretion or to early chromosome segregation that can be seen with any hybrid carrying greater than the normal diploid chromosome complement. In subsequent passages, however, the mouse–human hybridomas are remarkably stable, even more so than the human–human hybridomas. Since these initial observations, we have confirmed stable production (longer than 6 months) of antigen-specific human monoclonal antibodies by 11 P3/HT–human lymphocyte hybrids after a single round of subcloning.

There are, in addition, two major advantages to the P3/HT line. This mouse plasmacytoma is EBNA-negative; in contrast, 729/HT is an EBNA-positive lymphoblastoid cell line. Also, P3/HT does not produce mouse heavy or light Ig chains that can be detected in culture supernatant, on the cell surface, or in the cytoplasm by standard fluorescence staining techniques. However, 729/HT produces its own IgM(κ) human Ig molecules, which can be detected by ELISA in cell culture supernatants and on the cell surface and in the cytoplasm by fluorescence staining. It is quite possible that 729/HT hybridomas will secrete the parental Ig heavy or light chains (for which we have indirect evidence) and/or EBV components. Either possibility would considerably complicate the use of resulting human monoclonal antibodies as pharmaceuticals.

In summary, P3/HT–human lymphocyte hybridomas are more easily produced, yield greater numbers of human Ig-secreting hybridomas, and are more stable than 729/HT hybridomas. Furthermore, P3/HT is an EBNA-negative, non-Ig-producing lymphoid tumor line. Therefore, we have concentrated on the use of this mouse fusion partner to produce antigen-specific human monoclonal antibodies.

IV. Human Antibodies to Specific Antigens

A. Tetanus Toxin

To obtain human monoclonal antibodies to tetanus toxin, five volunteers were vaccinated with 5 Lf units of tetanus toxoid and 30–90 ml whole blood obtained from each person 6 days after immunization. Lymphocytes were purified by Ficoll–Hypaque density gradient centrifugation, washed two times in phosphate-buffered saline (PBS), and fused with P3/HT. These fusions produced 1365 clones, of which 611 secreted >0.1 μg/ml human IgG or IgM. The Ig-positive clones were assayed in a specific ELISA for tetanus toxoid as described above. By this assay five clones were identified that produced antibodies to tetanus toxoid and the purified exotoxin (Calbiochem). Four of the antitetanus hybridomas were successfully subcloned and these subclones were passaged for 6 months in culture until they were arbitrarily terminated. The four mouse–human hybridomas also produced ascites in nude mice with injection of 2×10^6 cells per animal. Two of the four clones gave ascites with greater than 1 mg/ml human IgM. However, in subsequent animal-to-animal passages, IgM content declined. A summary of antibody

TABLE VI
Human Monoclonal Antibodies to Tetanus Toxin

Clone	Culture supernatant			Ascites	
	IgM[a](μg/ml)	Titer[b]	Inhibition[c] (%)	IgM[a](μg/ml)	Titer[b]
YTJ083	8.1	1:2	78	0.03	ND
YTJ088	12.8	1:10	95	1.11	1:1000
YTJ139	10.2	1:16	96	0.13	ND
YTK019	9.6	1:4	77	1.12	1:400

[a]ELISA
[b]ELISA: antibody dilution giving 25% positive control reference OD$_{495}$ on B fragment (10μg/ml). ND, Not determined due to low human IgM content.
[c]Percent inhibition of binding to B fragment at 40 μg/ml tetanus toxin.

production and reactivity data for the four human antitetanus antibodies is provided in Table VI. It should be noted that these antibodies do not bind ^{125}I-exotoxin in a liquid RIA system, suggesting that they have relatively low affinity for the antigen ($<10^9$ liters/mole).

We are now beginning to collect data in the tetanus model system to determine if yield of specific antibody-producing hybridomas from PBLs can be correlated with the time interval between booster immunizations or the serum titer response. Just as immunization protocols are critical to the design of mouse monoclonal antibodies, it is expected that the spectrum of human monoclonal antibodies produced from human PBLs will reflect to some extent individual immunization history and serum vaccine response.

B. Hepatitis B Surface Antigen

In contrast to the remarkably uniform human response to the tetanus toxoid vaccine, response to HBsAg as presented in the Heptavax-B vaccine (Merck, Sharp and Dohme) is much less uniform. The standard series calls for initial immunization, with two boosters given 1 and 6 months afterward. Among the donor population certain individuals respond to the vaccine with dramatic increases in the serum of antigen-specific IgG. In the HBsAg liquid-phase RIA serum assay, serum drawn 2 weeks after the first Heptavax booster vaccine and titrated by quadrupling dilutions from 1:30 to 1:1920 is incubated with ^{125}I-labeled HBsAg (Abbott) and with Sepharose beads conjugated with monoclonal anti-human IgG or IgM antibodies. Three of 13 individuals tested showed strong serum response to the vaccine. PBLs of two such good responders were fused with P3/HT to yield 1092 clones, of which 569 produced human IgG or IgM. Antibody-producing hybridomas were then screened for HBsAg-specific antibody in the RIA described above. One

Table VII

Epitope Definition of Human Monoclonal Antibody YHA002 to HBsAg with Various Murine Monoclonal Antibodies

Inhibiting murine antibody	Primary specificity	Percent inhibition of human Ab, at 50% titer point (cpm)
HYB410	*a* (epitope 1)	48 (741)
HBA259	*a* (epitope 2)	0 (1517)
HBI456	*a* (epitope 2)	11 (1279)
HYB449	*ay*	3 (1395)
GDJ352	Gardnerella	0 (1459)
Culture media	—	0 (1434)

human IgG1(λ) anti-HBsAg antibody, YHA002, was identified. Following two subclonings, YHA002.2.3 was produced in cell culture in liter quantities for more than 8 months. In defined medium (HB102) from Hanna Biologicals) this mouse–human hybridoma produced 1–3 µg/ml human IgG. As nude mouse ascites, YHA002.2.3 yielded a maximum of 108 µg/ml human IgG. Initial characterizations of this human anti-HBsAg antibody were performed using this ascites-derived antibody.

Inhibition assays with three HBsAg subtypes, *adr*, *adw*, and *ayr* (kindly provided by G. Dreesman), suggested that YHA002 recognizes the *a* determinant. Subsequently, competition assays with a panel of mouse monoclonal antibodies of known epitope specificity have confirmed that YHA002 binds the *a* determinant of HBsAg (Table VII). Even more striking, by Scatchard analysis as shown in Fig. 3, YHA002 has an apparent affinity of 2×10^9 liters/mole. This affinity is comparable to the best of our mouse anti-HBsAg monoclonal antibodies, HYB410. YHA002 demonstrates that given the proper source of antigen-primed lymphocytes, hybridoma technology can yield human monoclonal antibodies of high affinity and defined specificity.

V. Clinical Applications

Human monoclonal antibodies ultimately may be extremely useful for *in vivo* diagnosis and therapy of cancer and infectious diseases. Thus, it is now becoming necessary to perform assays to demonstrate clinical utility of these human antibodies. In the area of immunotherapy, prototype animal models already exist in which to test human γ globulin preparations for treatment of such illnesses as rabies, vaccinia, Rh disease, and tetanus.

As a preliminary screen for the therapeutic efficacy, each of the human antibodies to tetanus toxin has been tested for its ability to confer *in vivo* protection in a mouse model system (Table VIII). For each experiment 0.4 ml

lent technical assistance, to Sandi Peever for typing this manuscript, and to our many colleagues at Hybritech for their suggestions and encouragement.

References

Croce, M., Linnenbach, A., Hall, W., Steplewski, Z., and Koprowski, H., 1980, Production of human hybridomas secreting antibodies to measles virus, *Nature* **288**:488–489.

Gerhard, W., 1980, Fusion of cells in suspension and outgrowth of hybrids in conditioned medium, in: *Monoclonal Antibodies* (R. Kennett, T. J. McKearn, and K. G. Bechtol, eds.), Plenum Press, New York, pp. 370–371.

Kearney, J. F., Radbruch, A., Liesegang, B., and Rajewsky, K., 1979, A new mouse myeloma cell line that has lost immunoglobulin expression but permits the construction of antibody-secreting hybrid cell lines, *J. Immunol.* **123**:1548–1550.

Köhler, G., and Milstein, C., 1975, Continuous cultures of fused cells secreting antibody of predefined specificity, *Nature* **256**:495–497.

Lever, J. E., Nuki, G., and Seegmiller, J. E., 1974, Expression of purine overproduction in a series of 8-azaguanine-resistant diploid human lymphoblast lines, *Proc. Natl. Acad. Sci. USA* **71**:2679–2683.

Littlefield, J. W., 1964, Selection of hybrids from matings of fibroblasts *in vitro* and their presumed recombinants, *Science* **145**:709–710.

Shulman, M., Wilde, C. D., and Köhler, G., 1978, A better cell line for making hybridomas secreting specific antibodies, *Nature* **276**:269–270.

8

Production of Human Monoclonal Antibodies Using a Human–Mouse Fusion Partner

STEVEN K. H. FOUNG, SUSAN PERKINS, ANN ARVIN,
JEFFREY LIFSON, NAHID MOHAGHEGHPOUR,
DIANNE FISHWILD, F. CARL GRUMET,
AND EDGAR G. ENGLEMAN

I. Introduction

In man, the use of antigen-specific antibodies is an important clinical tool for diagnostic testing (e.g., blood typing for transfusion, tissue typing for transplantation) and for therapy (e.g., prophylaxis of Rh hemolytic disease of the newborn and zoster immune plasma) (Yankee *et al.*, 1969; Grumet *et al.*, 1982; Davey and Zipursky, 1979; Ross, 1962; Zaia *et al.*, 1983). The limited availability or specificity of many of these reagents has placed an important restraint on their use. The production of hybrids between myeloma cell lines and lymphocytes from immunized hosts appears to make possible the unlimited production of monoclonal antibodies to predefined antigens (Köhler and Milstein, 1975). Successful application of this technique, primarily with rodents, is of limited clinical use because xenogeneic immunization with human cells mainly yields antibodies against monomorphic, species-specific antigens

STEVEN K. H. FOUNG, SUSAN PERKINS, JEFFREY LIFSON, NAHID MOHAGHEGHPOUR, DIANNE FISHWILD, F. CARL GRUMET, AND EDGAR G. ENGLEMAN • Department of Pathology, Stanford University School of Medicine, Stanford University Medical Center, Stanford, California 94305. ANN ARVIN • Department of Pediatrics, Stanford University School of Medicine, Stanford University Medical Center, Stanford, California 94305.

rather than polymorphic alloantigens. Moreover, rodent hybridomas have a theoretical limitation for therapeutic use because their secreted antibody would be treated by human recipients as a foreign protein with potential for inducing serum sickness.

The production of human monoclonal antibodies has been difficult to achieve. Two approaches that have been explored extensively are transformation of B cells by Epstein–Barr virus (EBV) and hybridization of human B cells with appropriately drug-marked mouse or human myeloma and human lymphoblastoid cell lines (Steinitz *et al.*, 1977; Nowinski *et al.*, 1980; Olsson and Kaplan, 1980; Croce *et al.*, 1980). A major problem with EBV transformation has been the difficulty of establishing stable antibody-secreting clones (Steinitz *et al.*, 1977). In our own experience, antigen-specific EBV clones appear to have a limited life span, while fusions of human lymphocytes with human B-cell lines (EBV lymphoblastoid or ostensible myelomas) have had limited success due to a low frequency of hybrid formation. Fusion of human lymphocytes with mouse myelomas will result in a substantial number of hybrids, but the hybrids have been unstable, presumably due to chromosomal loss (Nowinski *et al.*, 1980). However, many investigators have isolated mouse–human hybrids that continued to secrete Ig for an extended period (Lane *et al.*, 1982; Schlom *et al.*, 1980).

II. Generation of a Human–Mouse Fusion Partner

To overcome the problems of poor fusion efficiency and rapid loss of immunoglobulin secretion, we developed a human mouse cell line, SBC-H20, that fuses efficiently to stimulated normal human donor B lymphocytes and produces stable human Ig-secreting hybridomas (Foung *et al.*, 1984). The SBC-H20 cell line was derived from a fusion between a mouse myeloma line, SP2/08AZ, and human peripheral B lymphocytes isolated from a normal donor. A hybrid clone that had secreted human Ig for more than 6 months was placed in medium containing 2×10^{-6} M 6-thioguanine (see Appendix, Chapter 8, for complete description of protocol for generating HAT-sensitive lines). Over the following month, the concentration of 6-thioguanine was progressively increased to 2×10^{-5} M. After the establishment of 6-thioguanine resistance, a non-Ig-secreting subclone was selected, SBC-H20, which serves as our fusion partner. This human–mouse-derived line is sensitive to medium containing hypoxanthine–aminopterin–thymidine (HAT) or azaserine–hypoxanthine (Foung *et al.*, 1982). Furthermore, SBC-H20 is relatively ouabain-resistant and will grow at 10^{-6} M ouabain. This is important for the purpose of using EBV activation to initially expand human B cells secreting antigen-specific Ig and then fusing these cells to the SBC-H20 for stabilization and amplification of Ig synthesis. EBV-transformed cells are relatively ouabain-sensitive and generally will not survive at $(1-2) \times 10^{-7}$ M

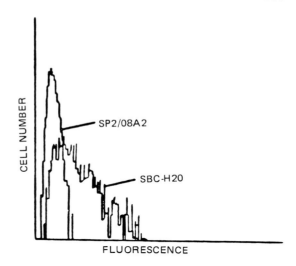

FIGURE 1. Confirmation of retention of human genes encoding cell surface antigens; 10⁶ cells of SP2/08AZ and SBC-H20 were stained with W6/32 antibody and examined by cytofluorography. The majority of SBC-H20 are brightly stained by this anti-human HLA antibody.

ouabain. The SBC-H20 cell line has been maintained in continuous culture for over 2 years with stable expression of human MHC class I antigens as defined by indirect immunofluorescence binding of W6/32 monoclonal antibody (Fig. 1). This antibody recognizes a framework determinant on all HLA-A, -B, -C antigens (Brodsky *et al.*, 1979).

III. Human Anti-A Red Blood Cell Antibody

One of the antigen-specific human monoclonal antibodies we have produced is an anti-A red blood cell antibody of the IgM class. In these experiments we compared the level and stability of antigen-specific Ig synthesis between a cloned EBV-transformed cell line and hybrids produced by fusion of this line with SBC-H20 or a mouse line (SP2/08AZ). First, EBV transformation was used to activate B lymphocytes isolated from splenocytes of a type O individual requiring splenectomy because of severe hemolytic disease (for details see Larrick et al., this volume, Chapter 9). B lymphocytes were transformed by EBV-containing supernatant from the B-958 marmoset lymphoblastoid line (Sly *et al.*, 1976). Cells were plated at 10⁵/well in microtiter trays and cultured 14 days prior to initial assay. Positive wells were expanded in liquid medium culture.

The EBV-activated cells were then fused to the SBC-H20 or SP2/08AZ cells (see Appendix, Chapter 8 for greater details on fusion protocol). Cultures were grown in a selection medium that included 100 μM hypoxanthine, 800 nM aminopterin, and 15 μM thymidine (HAT) and 0.1 μM ouabain at 37°C in a humidified 6% CO_2 incubator. By day 10, 100% of unfused parental cells were dead. Ouabain selection was used for 10 days and HAT selection was used for 14 days. Monoclonality was assured by sequential soft agar and limiting dilution cloning.

Specific antibody determination was accomplished by the following procedure (Parker *et al.*, 1978). Supernatants from wells containing growing hybrids were tested against type A_1 and B red blood cells by an agglutination assay using V-bottom microtiter trays (Falcon Lab). Reactivity was read after centrifugation of the trays at $250 \times g$ for 5 min and addition of anti-human IgM globulin. Titrations were performed with doubling dilutions of 3% bovine serum albumin in normal saline and the endpoint was recorded at the highest dilution with macroscopic red cell agglutination.

Quantitation of Ig antibody in hybridoma supernatants was determined by an enzyme-linked immunoassay using affinity-purified, class-specific goat anti-human Ig. The tests were specific for each Ig class over a range of 500 ng/ml to 10 µg/ml. Fusions with both the SBC-H20 and the SP2/08AZ cell lines resulted in greater than 90% of the parent wells secreting anti-A antibodies with identical heavy and light immunoglobulin chains to those of the parent EBV line (Table I). Attempts at cloning by limiting dilution resulted in rare SP2-derived hybrids producing the anti-A antibody (Table I). Of 23 colonies of SP2-derived hybrids isolated, none contained cells that secreted anti-A antibody. Cloning of the SBC-H20-derived hybrids resulted in greater than 50% of clones secreting the antibody and, more importantly, the isolation of a number of clones with antibody titers substantially greater than that of the original EBV anti-A clone (Table I). The titer of antibody against an A cell from one such SBC-H20-derived hybrid was 16,384, compared to 2000 from the EBV line. These SBC-H20-derived hybrid clones have continued to produce antigen-specific immunoglobulin for over 24 months. The growth

TABLE I

Frequency and Titer of Hybridomas Secreting Human Anti-A Antibody[a]

Secreting line	Number of wells with anti-A activity	Titer[b]
EBV line	—	2,000
SP2 hybrids		
Parents	19/22	32
Clones	0/23	0
SBC-H20 hybrids		
Parents	29/31	8,192
Clones	13/21	16,384
Subclones	36/53	32,768

[a]All antigen-specific IgM with κ light chain.
[b]Maximum titer detected.

TABLE II

Reactivity of Human Monoclonal Anti-A Antibody against
Random Donor Cells

Red cell phenotype	Number tested	Percent positive
A_1	59	100
A_2	13	100
A_1B	4	100
A_2B	1	100
A_{int}	2	100
$A_{int}B$	7	100
B	16	0
O	71	0

rate and quantity of Ig produced (greater than 10 μg/10^6 cells per 24 hr) approximate the level of production by typical murine hybridomas.

The antigen specificity of the human monoclonal anti-A red blood cell antibody was confirmed by testing the supernatant from a hybrid clone against a random panel of human red blood cells using direct hemagglutination. In tests of the supernatant against 133 red blood cells of groups A_1, A_2, A_{int}, A_1B, A_2B, O, and B, positive reactions were observed with all type A groups but no other groups (Table II); the monoclonal anti-A antibody reacted as well as or better than commercial antisera. Against a panel of phenotyped red blood cells that includes all known antigenic systems of red blood cells, no other specificity was detected.

IV. Human Monoclonal Antibodies to Varicella Zoster Virus

Varicella zoster virus (VZV) infections remain one of the major problems in recipients of allografts and other patients (oncology patients and premature infants) who are immunocompromised (Atkinson et al., 1980; Meyers et al., 1980; Feldman et al., 1975). Of the five herpes viruses that affect humans, cytomegalovirus and VZV cause significant mortality and morbidity (Watson, 1983). After organ or bone marrow transplantation (BMT), approximately 40% of patients develop VZV infections (Watson, 1983). Of those who develop VZV infections, 20–40% have disseminated disease, with a 12% mortality rate among all infected patients. Administration of human plasma with high anti-VZV antibody titers has been effective in prevention or modification of primary VZV infection. While initial clinical trials with attenuated, live

VZV vaccines have had favorable results, efficacy and consequences of immunization in the immunocompromised host remain relatively unknown. More importantly, problems of latency and potential oncogenic effects of live virus still exist with this mode of vaccination (Weller, 1983; Takahashi *et al.*, 1974). Because of these observations, the ability to produce human monoclonal antibodies to VZV should provide a potentially unlimited and safe source of antigen-specific antibodies that can be used to explore their roles in the immune response of normal and diseased individuals and ultimately to diagnose and treat VZV infections.

B lymphocytes were isolated from a patient recovering from an acute varicella infection and were fused with SBC-H20 as outlined above. Hybridoma growth was observed in 37 of 58 seeded wells. Supernatants were tested by a solid-phase radioimmunoassay for human anti-VZV IgG activity (Arvin and Koropchak, 1980). Specific antibody binding was considered present if the ratio of the mean counts per minute (cpm) of wells containing supernatant and VZV antigen to wells containing control antigen was greater than or equal to 2.5. Antibodies produced by two subclones that had consistent anti-VZV IgG secretion for 8 months (1-A2 and 2-1D5) were selected for further characterization. As shown in Table III, the titers of VZV IgG in the supernatants from subclones of the two hybridomas were consistently high, with a range of 256–16,384.

Antibody 1-A2 was characterized as IgG1(κ) and 2-1D5 as IgG1(λ). Immunoglobulin was present in supernatants at a concentration greater than 10 μg/10^6 cells after 24-hr culture of both subclones, as determined by an enzyme-linked immunoassay. The specific reactivity of each of the two antibodies with VZV-infected human fibroblasts was further demonstrated by indirect immunofluorescence (Fig. 2). VZV-infected and uninfected human fibroblasts were air-dried on microscope slides and acetone-fixed. Human

TABLE III
Neutralizing Activity of Human Monoclonal Antibodies to VZV[a]

Antibody	Virus	Inoculum (pfu/ml)	Ig neutralizing activity (μg/ml)
1-A2	VZV-32	196	1.0
	VZV-BB	160	5.0
	VZV-CH	88	4.0
	HSV-1	180	>1000
2-1D5	VZV-BB	160	5.0
	VZV-CH	88	2.0
	HSV-1	180	>1000

[a]Neutralizing activity of human monoclonal antibodies to VZV against laboratory (VZV-32) and clinical isolates (VZV-BB and VZV-CH) of VZV and herpes simplex virus-1. Neutralization is defined as greater than 50% reduction in plaque-forming units (pfu) of the original inoculum. Amount of Ig is the lowest concentration resulting in neutralization.

with the monoclonal antibody. The BJAB cell line was also negative with the monoclonal. Staining is consistently and reproducibly observed, however, with Raji and P3HR1. The staining pattern is predominantly cytoplasmic, with some nuclear staining; both methanol- and acetone-fixed cells are stained. With acetone fixation, there appears to be some "leakage" of reactivity just outside the cell membrane. Following sodium butyrate induction, the percentage of stained cells increases to 8–10% for both Raji and P3HR1. Studies with TPA-induced cells are in progress. These data suggest that the monoclonal antibody reacts with a component of the EA(D) complex.

VI. Human Monoclonal Antibodies to Mycobacterium leprae

One other group of antigen-specific human monoclonal antibodies we have produced is against *Mycobacterium leprae*. Non-rosette-forming (NR) lymphocytes were isolated from the peripheral blood of a patient with lepromatous leprosy as outlined above, and cultured in the presence of supernatants from the B-958 marmoset lymphoblastoid line. Cells were plated at 10^5/well in microtiter plates for 6 days, after which initial screening for antibody production was carried out with an enzyme-linked immunoabsorbent assay using affinity-purified, isotype-specific goat anti-human Ig, and armadillo-derived *M. leprae* sonicate (prepared by Dr. P. Brennan, Colorado State University, Fort Collins, Colorado) as antigen (Hunter *et al.*, 1982). Controls used in each assay included diluent alone, culture medium used for propagation of hybrids, known positive human sera from lepromatous patients, human monoclonal anti-A antigen (of the A, B, O red blood cell system), and anti-VZV antibodies. EBV-transformed B cells from positive wells were plated at ten cells/well in liquid medium over irradiated human red blood cells as feeders. Aliquots of the growing polyclones secreting antibody were fused with SBC-H20 cell lines at a ratio of 1:5 and plated in 96-well, flat-bottom plates at 5×10^4 cells/well. Fourteen days after fusion initial screening was carried out and hybrids from positive wells were cloned and subcloned by limiting dilution at 0.5 cell/well. In addition, non-rosette-forming cells from a second lepromatous patient were fused with SBC-H20 cell lines without EBV transformation and preselection.

Three of 75 hybrids derived from the hybridization of EBV-transformed B cells were found to secrete IgM with anti-*M. leprae* activity (Tables IV and V). In comparison, only 0.3% of hybrids screened during the second fusion secreted antibody reactive with *M. leprae* sonicate (Tables IV and V). Cloning of the SBC-H20-derived hybrids resulted in about 38% of clones secreting anti-*M. leprae* antibody. Antibody production by hybrid clones was stable in more than 80% of the clones grown in continuous culture for 4 months, and

TABLE IV
Hybridoma Screening

	OD$_{410}$	
Hybrid	Ig	Anti-M. *leprae*
1.1G7	1.839	1.833
1.1D11	1.260	1.746
1.2F11	1.302	1.685
2.2D11	1.483	1.542
2.6E5	1.785	0.896
Serum from LL patient	1.982	1.734
Anti-A red blood cell antibody[a]	1.964	0.078
Anti-varicella zoster antibody[a]	1.671	0.110

[a]Human monoclonal antibody.

quantities of at least 10 μg/24 hr per 10^6 cells were produced. The anti-*M. leprae* reactivity of the human monoclonal antibodies produced by these hybrids was confirmed by testing the supernatants from the subclones against three antigen preparations: a soluble antigen, sonicated *M. leprae,* and a phenolic glycolipid antigen (provided by Dr. P. Brennan).

VII. Concluding Comments

We have described the production of human monoclonal antibodies to a variety of antigens. Depending on the target antigen, two approaches have been successful: (1) isolation of B lymphocytes, a significant proportion of which are probably activated *in vivo* from patients during acute infection, and fusion to the SBC-H20 cell line; (2) use of EBV to stimulate and transform, *in vitro,* B lymphocytes isolated from individuals recently challenged with anti-

TABLE V
Frequency of Hybrids Secreting Human Anti-M. leprae Antibody

Cells fused	Number of wells with hybrid	Number of hybrids secreting Ig	Number of hybrids secreting antibody
EBV/NR[a]	21/75 (28%)	8 (11%)	3[b] (4%)
NR	274/660 (41%)	44 (7%)	2 (0.3%)

[a]Polyclones of EBV-transformed non-rosette-forming lymphocytes.
[b]All antigen-specific IgM.

gen, followed by cloning of EBV-activated cells to isolate relevant Ig-secreting clones for subsequent fusion to the SBC-H20 cell line to preserve Ig-secreting cells. These results substantiate the feasibility of obtaining human monoclonal antibodies from stable B-lymphocyte-derived hybridomas. The use of SBC-H20 proved advantageous in the generation of these human monoclonal antibodies since the derived hybrids appeared to be produced at a higher frequency and with superior stability than by alternate methods; e.g., EBV transformation alone, fusion with mouse myeloma lines, or fusion with human lymphoblastoid lines. The production of human monoclonal antibodies should provide an important new approach to the study of the host response to these agents and form the basis of a potentially unlimited source of relevant human monoclonal antibodies for prophylactic therapy of patients at high risk for developing life-threatening infection.

ACKNOWLEDGMENTS

The authors would like to thank the following individuals, who participated in the characterization of the above human monoclonal antibodies: Drs. J. Larrick, E. Lennette, A. Raubitschek, and in particular G. Lizak for her superb technical assistance. We thank Charlotte Morrison, who typed this chapter. The work was supported in part by grants HL29572, A32075, and CA24607 from the National Institutes of Health and a grant from the Cetus Corporation, Berkeley, California.

References

Arvin, A. M., and Koropchak, C. M., 1980, Immunoglobulins M and G to varicella-zoster virus measured by solid-phase radioimmunoassay: Antibody responses to varicella and herpes zoster infections, *J. Clin. Microbiol.* **12**:367.

Atkinson, K., Meyers J. D., Storb, R., Prentice, L., and Thomas, E. D., 1980, Varicella-zoster virus infection after marrow transplantation for aplastic anemia or leukemia, *Transplantation* **29**:47.

Brodsky, F. M., Parham, P., Barnstable, C. J., Crumpton, M. J., and Bodmer, W. F., 1979, Monoclonal antibodies for analysis of the HLA system, *Immunol. Rev.* **47**:3.

Croce, C. M., Linnenbach, A., Hall, W., Steplewski, Z., and Koprowski, H., 1980, Production of human hybridomas secreting antibodies to measles virus, *Nature* **288**:488.

Davey, M. G., and Zipursky, A., 1979, McMaster Conference in Prevention of Rh Immunization, *Vox Sang.* **36**:50.

De-The, G., 1982, Epidemiology of Epstein–Barr virus and associated diseases in man, in: *The Herpesviruses*, Volume 1 (B. Roizman, ed.), Plenum Press, New York, p. 25.

Feldman, S., Hughes, W. T., and Daniel, C. B., 1975, Varicella in children with cancer: Seventy-seven cases, *Pediatrics* **56**:388.

Foung, S. K. H., Sasaki, D., Grumet, F. C., and Engleman, E. G., 1982, Production of functional human T–T hybridomas in selection medium lacking aminopterin and thymidine, *Proc. Natl. Acad. Sci. USA* **79**:7484.

Foung, S. K. H., Perkins, S., Raubitschek, A., Larrick, J., Lizak, G., Fishwild, D., Engleman, E. G., and Grumet, F. C. 1984, Rescue of human monoclonal antibody production from an EBV-transformed B cell line by fusion to a human–mouse hybridoma, *J. Immunol. Meth.* **70:**83.

Grose, C., Edmond, B. J., and Brunell, P. A., 1979, Complement enhanced neutralizing antibody response to varicella-zoster virus, *J. Infect. Dis.* **139:**432.

Grose, C., Edwards, D. P., Friedrichs, W. E., Weigle, K. A., and McGuire, W. L., 1983, Monoclonal antibodies against three major glycoproteins of varicella-zoster virus, *Infect. Immunol.* **40:**381.

Grose, C., Edwards, D. P., Weigle, K. A., Friedrichs, W. E., and McGuire, W. L., 1984, Varicella-zoster virus-specific gp 140: A highly immunogenic and disulfide-linked structural glycoprotein, *Virology* **132:**138.

Grumet, F. C., Fendly, B. M., Fish, L., Foung, S., and Engleman, E. G., 1982, A monoclonal antibody (B27M2) subdividing HLA-B27, *Hum. Immunol.* **5:**61.

Henle, W., and Henle, G., 1982, Immunology of Epstein–Barr virus, in: *The Herpesviruses*, Volume 1 (B. Roizman, ed.), Plenum Press, New York, p. 209.

Hunter, S. W., Fujiwara, T., and Brennan, P. J., 1982, Structure and antigenicity of the major specific glycolipid antigen of *Mycobacterium leprae*, *J. Biol. Chem.* **257:**15072.

Köhler, G., and Milstein, C., 1975, Continuous cultures of fused cells secreting antibody of predefined specificity, *Nature* **256:**495.

Lane, H. C., Shelhomer, J. H., Mostowski, H. S., and Fauci, A. S., 1982, Human monoclonal anti-keyhole limpet hemocyanin antibody-secreting hybridoma produced from peripheral blood B lymphocytes of a keyhole limpet hemocyanin-immune individual, *J. Exp. Med.* **155:**333.

Meyers, J. D., Flournoy, N., and Thomas, E. D., 1980, Cell-mediated immunity to varicella-zoster virus after allogeneic marrow transplant, *J. Infect. Dis.* **141:**479.

Nowinski, R., Boglund, C., Lane, J., Lastrum, M., Bernstein, I., Young, W., Hakomori, S., Hall, L., and Cooney, M., 1980, Production of antibody to tetanus toxoid by continuous human lymphoblastoid cell lines, *Science* **199:**1439.

Olsson, L., and Kaplan, H. S., 1980, Human–human hybrids producing monoclonal antibodies of predefined antigenic specificity, *Proc. Natl. Acad. Sci. USA* **77:**5429.

Parker, J., Marcoux, D. A., Hafleigh, E. B., and Grumet, F. C., 1978, Modified microtiter tray method for blood typing, *Transfusion* **18:**417.

Ross, A. H., 1962, Modification of chickenpox in family contacts by administration of gamma globulin, *N. Engl. J. Med.* **267:**369.

Schlom, J., Wunderlich, D., and Teramoto, Y. A., 1980, Generation of human monoclonal antibodies reactive with human mammary carcinoma cells, *Proc. Natl. Acad. Sci. USA* **77:**6841.

Sly, W. S., Sekhon, G. S., Kennett, R., Bodmer, W. F., and Bodmer, J., 1976, Permanent lymphoid lines from genetically marked lymphocytes: Success with lymphocytes recovered from frozen storage, *Tiss. Antigens* **7:**165.

Steinitz, M., Klein, G., Koskimies, S., and Makela, O., 1977, EB virus-induced B lymphocyte cell lines producing specific antibodies, *Nature* **269:**420.

Takahashi, M., Otsuka, T., Okuno, Y., Asano, Y., Yazaki, T., and Isomura, S., 1974, Live vaccine used to prevent the spread of varicella in children in hospital, *Lancet* **2:**1288.

Tamura, G. S., Dailey, M. O., Gallatin, W, M., McGrath, M. S., Weissman, I. L., and Pillemer, E. A., 1984, Isolation of molecules recognized by monoclonal antibodies and antisera: The solid phase immunoisolation technique, *Anal. Biochem.* **136:**458.

Watson, J. G., 1983, Problems of infection after bone marrow transplantation, *J. Clin. Pathol.* **36:**683.

Weller, T. H., 1983, Varicella and herpes zoster, *N. Engl. J. Med.* **309:**1362.

Yankee, R. A., Grumet, F. C., and Rogentine, G. N., 1969. The selection of compatible platelet donors for refractory patients by lymphocyte HLA typing, *N. Engl. J. Med.* **281:**1208.

Zaia, J. A., Levin, M. J., Preblud, S. R., Leszczynski, J., Wright, G. G., Ellis, R. J., Curtis, A. C., Valerio, M. A., and LeGore, J., 1983, Evaluation of varicella-zoster immune globulin: Protection of immunosuppressed children after household exposure to varicella, *J. Infect. Dis.* **147:**737.

Those most successful have been able to preselect the population of B cells to be transformed or to postselect the antigen-specific transformed population by panning or rosetting techniques (Kozbor *et al.*, 1979; Steinitz *et al.*, 1978). More recently we and others have used EBV transformation combined with cell fusion to generate human monoclonal antibodies (Kozbor and Roder, 1983a, 1984; Teng *et al.*, 1983). Several observations have prompted this approach: (1) instability of immunoglobulin secretion by the EBV-transformed lines, (2) increased immunoglobulin secretion by these hybridomas when compared to EBV lymphoblastoid cell lines, and (3) higher frequencies of "rescue" of the antigen-specific populations.

Table I demonstrates the use of EBV transformation and subsequent cell fusion for the generation of human monoclonal anti-*Pseudomonas* exotoxin A antibodies. To begin, we chose high-titer cystic fibrosis patients: patients had serum anti-exotoxin A titers (IgM, IgG, and IgA) all greater than 1:2000 (Moss *et al.*, 1984). When peripheral B cells from the patients were fused directly *ex vivo* or after pokewood mitogen stimulation to a human fusion partner developed in our laboratory (Larrick *et al.*, 1983) or to a mouse–human fusion partner, no stable lines survived. However, using EBV transformation, subculturing, and cell fusion, it was possible to generate several clones with anti-exotoxin A binding. Figure 1 gives the ELISA results of these anti-exotoxin A hybridomas during various stages of cloning corresponding to the protocol described in Table I. At day 20, 22 out of 480 wells were highly positive by exotoxin A ELISA screen (Fig. 1a). Six of these wells were subcultured at 500 cells/well; a second screen revealed that many wells had lost antibody activity (Fig. 1b). Loss of antibody secretion is a common occurrence with EBV infection, reflecting the instability of antibody production in the young EBV transformants and their overgrowth by rapidly dividing nonproducers. After the second subculture, two clones were selected, subcultured

TABLE I

EBV-Cell Fusion Protocol. Anti-Exotoxin A Human Monoclonal Antibodies

Day   1: Draw 50 ml citrated blood from cystic fibrosis patient with high exo A titer.
       a. 5.2×10^6 cells after AET-rosetting to remove T cells (Madsen and Johnson, 1979)
       b EBV transformation with B-958 Supe
       c. Plate at 1×10^4/well in five 96-well plates
Day 20: Twenty-two of 480 wells positive by specific exo A ELISA
Day 24: Six high-titer wells subcultivated at 500 cells/well
Day 37: All wells of #20 positive; further subcultured
Day 48: Highest titer wells of #14 expanded and further subcultured
Day 51: Highest titer EBV culture #20 fused to F3B6 mouse–human cell line
Day 58: Highest titer EBV culture #14 fused to F3B6
Day 69: Two of 15 growing wells from fusion with #20 positive by specific exo A ELISA
Day 70: Two positive hybridomas from #20 fusion cloned by limiting dilution
Day 78: Two highest titer clones from day 70 picked for expansion and antibody production
Day 79: Four of 27 growing wells from fusion with #14 positive by specific exo A ELISA
Day 80: Two positive hybridomas from #14 fusion cloned by limiting dilution

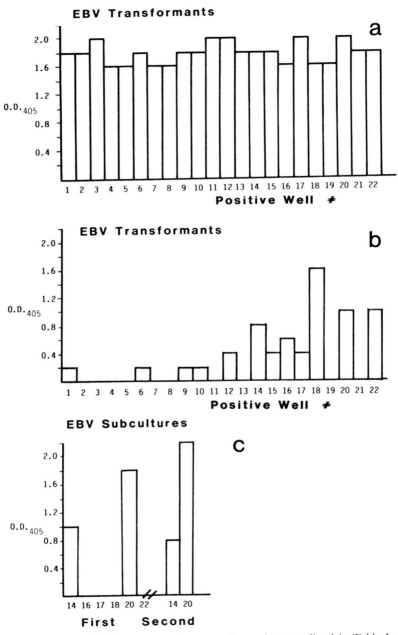

FIGURE 1. Exotoxin A ELISA corresponding to wells or clones outlined in Table I. (a) EBV transformants. (b) Subcultures of the initial transformants. (c) Subculture of the two highest titered EBV transformants. (d) Hybridomas of EBV well #20 fused to mouse–human cell line F3B6. (e) Hybridomas of EBV well #14 fused to mouse–human cell line F3B6. (f) Clones of one of the hybridomas (#20-15).

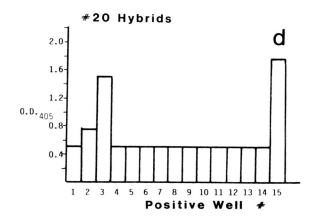

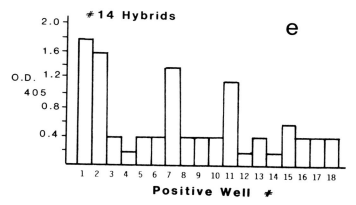

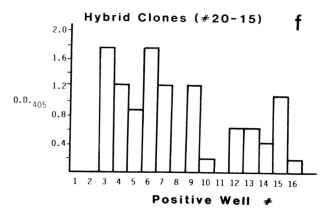

FIGURE 1 (*continued*)

further (Fig. 1c), and eventually fused to the 6TG-resistant mouse–human cell line F3B6. Because this cell line contains predominantly mouse chromosomes, it is also ouabain-resistant. Ouabain (5×10^{-7} M) was used in the selection medium to kill unfused EBV transformants. Unfused F3B6 cells were killed by the addition of hypoxanthine (100 μM) and azaserine (5 μg/ml) (Buttin *et al.*, 1978) to the medium. Growing hybrids usually appear within 2–3 weeks, and, as Figs. 1d and 1e show, both parent EBV cell lines yielded positive anti-exotoxin A-secreting progeny. Figure 1f shows that most of the clones of well #20-15 make appreciable amounts of specific antibody. All of these initial antibodies were of the IgM class. Many, but not all, of the antibodies generated by the EBV fusion technique have been of the IgM class. EBV most frequently infects and transforms IgM-bearing B cells, but B cells secreting other classes of immunoglobulin can also be made into long-term lines using this technique (Brown and Miller, 1982).

Two of the IgM antibodies generated above were used to immunoblot exotoxin A. They recognize the single-chain 66-dalton exotoxin A protein (Fig. 2). A mixture of these antibodies gives a threefold increase in the LD_{50} of exotoxin A activity in a fibroblast proliferation assay (Fig. 3).

B. Anti-Blood Group A Monoclonal Antibodies Generated by in Vitro Stimulation and EBV Fusion

Using the EBV fusion approach, we have generated anti-blood group A human monoclonal antibodies. Ficoll–Hypaque-separated splenocytes from a group O donor were cultured at 2×10^6/ml in Iscove's DME medium with 15% heat-inactivated fetal calf serum and 0.3% group A red blood cells. After 3 days, T cells were removed by AET–SRBC rosetting (Madsen and Johnsen, 1979) and residual cells were transformed by EBV-containing B958 cell supernatant. Cells were plated at 10^5/well and screened by direct group A red cell hemagglutination after 14 days. Positive wells were expanded and cloned in soft agar. An EBV-transformed cell line with IgM anti-A activity was selected for characterization. This line was fused to three different parent cell lines: (1) a mouse plasmacytoma (SP2/0Ag14); (2) a drug-marked mouse–human heterohybrid, and (3) a human lymphoblastoid cell line known to produce human hybrids successfully (Larrick *et al.*, 1983).

Table II gives the anti-A titers of clones of these fusions. The cell line with a mouse parent produced more specific immunoglobulin than the hybrids constructed with either of the cell lines possessing human chromosomes. The reasons for this are unclear. The mouse cells may (1) have more protein synthetic machinery required for high levels of antibody production, (2) have more "efficient" *trans*-acting regulatory DNA sequences, or (3) have a more mature "plasmacytoid" differentiation state. It is also possible that the human hybrid lines produce enough immunoglobulin themselves to interfere with efficient production of the anti-A antibody (i.e., hybrid antibody molecules). To clone successfully the highest producing clones, anti-A secreting

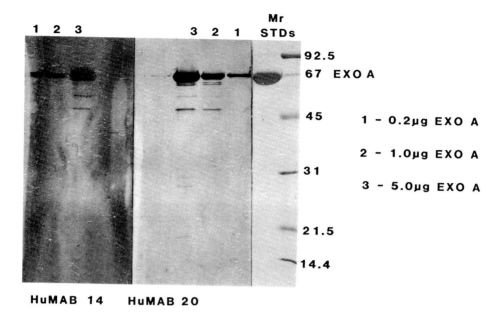

FIGURE 2. Exotoxin A immunoblot. Two human monoclonal anti-exotoxin A antibodies (HuMAB 14, HuMAB 20) recognize electrophoresed and transblotted exotoxin A.

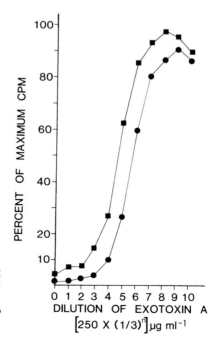

FIGURE 3. Partial neutralization of exotoxin A killing of fibroblasts by a mixture of anti-exotoxin A human monoclonal antibodies. (●) Exotoxin A alone (■) exotoxin A with monoclonals (HuMABs were mixed to give a final concentration of 5 μg/ml).

TABLE II

Comparison of Anti-Blood Group A Agglutination Titers of Human Hybridomas

	Titer[a] at given day					
	Day 1	2	3	4	5	6
Mouse plasmacytoma parent	128	256	1024	2048	2048	—
Mouse–human parent	4	16	32	64	64	—
Human lymphoblastoid parent	8	32	128	128	256	256

[a]Reciprocal of highest positive dilution of supernatant yielding agglutination of human A red cells.

hybridomas were adapted to soft agar culture, and antibody production was measured *in situ* by a direct plaque assay. This technique permits one to not only eliminate nonsecreting clones, but also to select for high-secreting clones by comparing the size of the zone of lysis. Figure 4 shows the anti-blood group A plaques produced by a high-producing clone derived from the mouse parent.

A synthetic group A polysaccharide matrix, Synsor-A (Chembiomed, Edmonton, Canada), was used to affinity-purify the human anti-A IgM anti-

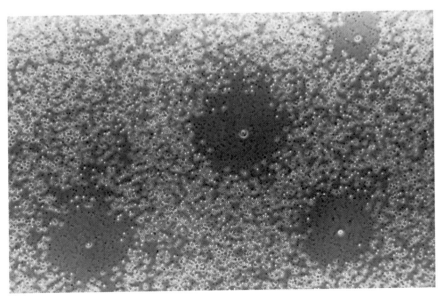

FIGURE 4. Anti-blood group A plaque-forming cells. Mouse–human hybridoma cells were cultured in soft agar with papain-treated human group A red cells. After 4 hr, rabbit complement absorbed with group A red cells and was added to develop the plaques.

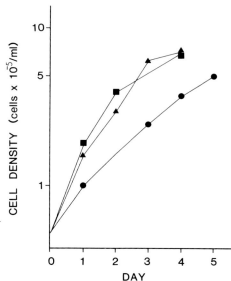

FIGURE 5. Comparative growth rates of hybridomas made with (■) mouse plasmacytoma, (▲) a 6TG-resistant mouse–human heterohybridoma, and (●) a human lymphoblastoid parent cell line.

body. The antibody recognizes a single determinant shared by blood group A subgroups A_1, A_2, A_{int}, A_3, A_x, and A_5 (Raubitschek *et al.*, 1985).

Figure 5 graphically depicts the comparative growth rates of the hybrid lines constructed with the three different parent cell lines. The mouse hybrids not only produce more antibody (Table II), but they also grow faster than the all-human hybrids.

With frequent cloning and plaque selection we have been able to expand the anti-A human hybridomas without loss of antibody secretion. Because it was reported that chromosomal loss frequently destroyed the antibody-secreting capacity of heterohybridomas, we measured DNA histograms on the cell lines making anti-A antibodies after 1 year in culture. Figure 6 shows the parent cell lines compared to each hybrid clone. The all-human hybridomas have segregated very few chromosomes. In contrast, many heterohybrid cell lines we have examined have had less than a tetraploid amount of DNA. Despite the decreased chromosome numbers, the two chromosomes required for antibody manufacture have still been retained (chromosome 14 for μ heavy chain; chromosome 2 for κ light chain), since both of these hybrids continue to secrete anti-A antibody. Some workers have suggested that chromosome 14, carrying the heavy chain genes, and chromosome 22, carrying the light chain genes, may be preferentially retained, whereas chromosome 2, carrying the κ chain genes, may be preferentially lost (Croce *et al.*, 1980; Erickson *et al.*, 1981). To maintain high-secreting heterohybrids, we have routinely recloned our cell lines every few months using the antigen-specific plaque technique or a nonspecific reverse plaque technique.

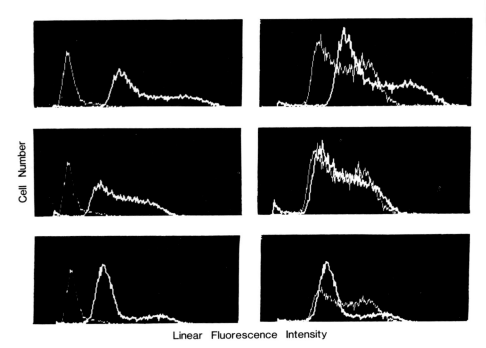

Linear Fluorescence Intensity

FIGURE 6. DNA histograms comparing hybridomas made with mouse, mouse–human, and human parent cell lines. An EBV cell line with a diploid number of chromosomes is used for comparison on the left (light histogram). Cell line SP2/0Ag14 is used for comparison on the right (light histogram). The top histograms compare the mouse/human × EBV anti-group A hybrids (heavy). The middle histograms compare the mouse (SP2/0Ag14) × EBV anti-group A hybrids (heavy). The lower histograms compare the human lymphoblastoid × EBV anti-group A hybrids (heavy). The human hybrids are tetraploid and have approximately as much DNA as the fused and backselected mouse parent cell line SP2/0Ag14 (Shulman et al., 1978). The two mouse hybridomas have much less than a tetraploid complement of DNA when compared to the SP2/0Ag14 parent.

IV. Class Switching of Human Hybridomas

Obviously one of the limitations of the EBV fusion technique has been the predominance of IgM class antibodies. IgG antibodies have longer *in vivo* half-lives, are easier to handle biochemically, and may mediate more desirable effector functions via their Fc regions. For these reasons we have attempted to class switch several of our IgM-secreting human hybridomas.

We have tried positive selection (i.e., fluorescein-labeled anti-IgG positive cell sorting or anti-IgG panning), as well as negative selection (anti-IgM and complement) techniques. Work from other laboratories (Dangl et al., 1982) has suggested that spontaneous isotype switching is not uncommon (10^{-7}), but that class switching is much less frequent. Figure 7 shows a cell sorter histogram of parent IgM-producing cells compared to cells that had been

Steinitz, M., Klein, G., Koskimies, S., and Makela, O., 1977, EB virus-induced B lymphocyte cell lines producing specific antibody, *Nature* **269:**420–422.

Steinitz, M., Koskimies, S., Klein, G., and Makela, O., 1978, Establishment of specific antibody producing human lines by antigen preselection and Epstein–Barr virus (EBV) transformation, *Curr. Top. Microbiol. Immunol.* **81:** 156–163.

Teng, N. N. H., Lam, K. S., Riera, F. C., and Kaplan, H. S., 1983, Construction and testing of mouse/human heteromyelomas for human monoclonal antibody production, *Proc. Natl. Acad. Sci. USA* **80:**7308–7312.

Truitt, K. E., Larrick, J. W., and Raubitschek, A., 1984, Fusion of nonadherent human cell lines, in: *Monoclonal Antibodies and Functional Cell Lines* (R. H. Kennett, K. B. Bechtol, and T. J. McKean, eds.), Plenum Press, New York, pp. 371–373.

Tsuchiya, S., Yokoyama, S., Yoshie, O., and Ono, Y., 1980, Production of diphtheria antitoxin antibody in Epstein–Barr virus induced lymphoblastoid cell lines, *J. Immunol.* **124:**1970–1976.

Winger, L., Winger, C., Shastry, P., Russell, A., and Longenecker, M., 1983, Efficient generation *in vitro*, from human peripheral blood cells, of monoclonal Epstein–Barr virus transformants producing specific antibody to a variety of antigens without prior deliberate immunization, *Proc. Natl. Acad. Sci. USA* **80:**4484–4488.

10
Cell-Driven Viral Transformation

Anthony W. Siadak and Mark E. Lostrom

I. Introduction

Since the advent of hybridoma technology, one of the most provocative applications for monoclonal antibodies has been immunotherapy. Early reports of experiments performed in mice suggested that monoclonal antibody therapy was beneficial against murine T-cell lymphoma (Bernstein *et al.*, 1980) and that it might be useful to deliver potent toxins to undesirable cells *in vivo* [reviewed in Moller (1982)]. Murine monoclonals have more recently been administered without major adverse reactions to immunocompromised human patients with leukemia or lymphoma (Levy and Miller, 1983). Results from these studies have shown, however, that the therapeutic effects of these reagents were difficult to maintain, due in large part to a host response to mouse immunoglobulin (Ig) which resulted in accelerated clearance of successive doses (Levy and Miller, 1983). This observation together with the goal of prophylactically and therapeutically treating a broader group of human patients have provided incentive to develop human monoclonal technology.

Cell lines producing human monoclonal antibodies to a variety of antigens have been reported over the past 10 years. Early cell lines were produced by Epstein–Barr virus (EBV) transformation of human B lymphocytes (Steinitz *et al.*, 1977; Koskimies, 1980). More recently, human–human and human–mouse hybridomas have also been described [for a review see Kozbor and Roder (1983); Larrick and Buck (1984)]. However, due to a myriad of unresolved technical issues, human hybridoma technology has not yet achieved the productivity and reproducibility of its murine counterpart. Although con-

Anthony W. Siadak and Mark E. Lostrom • Genetic Systems, Seattle, Washington 98121.

tinued refinement of these methods may lead to more widespread utility, it is of interest to explore alternate means of generating human monoclonal antibodies. This chapter describes in detail a process termed cell-driven viral transformation, which is a convenient, reproducible method for the preparation of large numbers of EBV-transformed human lymphoblastoid cell lines, each secreting human monoclonal antibody. Further, this process has been applied to the development of *in vivo* protective human monoclonals to *Pseudomonas aeruginosa* whose features are also described.

II. Derivation of the Driving Cell Line

The Epstein–Barr nuclear antigen (EBNA)-positive human lymphoblastoid cell line GM 1500 (Genetic Mutant Cell Repository, Camden, New Jersey) was cultured for 24 hr in growth medium [RPMI 1640 containing 15% (v/v) fetal calf serum (FCS), 2 mM L-glutamine, 1 mM sodium pyruvate, penicillin (100 IU/ml), and streptomycin (100 μg/ml)] supplemented with 300 μg/ml of the mutagen ethylmethane sulfonate (EMS; Sigma Chemical Co., St. Louis, Missouri). Following mutagenesis, the surviving cells were subcultured in growth medium containing gradually increasing concentrations of the purine analogue 6-thioguanine (6TG; Sigma) to render the cells deficient in the purine salvage enzyme hypoxanthine-guanine phosphoribosyltranferase (HGPRT). After several months, a vigorously proliferating cell line resistant to 30 μg/ml 6TG was established. This cell line, termed DS-300, died when introduced into hypoxanthine–aminopterin–thymidine (HAT)-supplemented growth medium (Littlefield, 1964).

DS-300 was investigated as a potential fusion partner for the development of human–human hybridomas. Initial attempts to prepare hybrids between these cells and peripheral blood lymphocytes (PBLs) via the polyethylene glycol (PEG) fusion method of Kennett (1979) resulted in pronounced mixed lymphocyte reactions due to activation and proliferation of donor T cells in response to the DS-300 cells. Because these mixed lymphocyte reactions appeared detrimental to the outgrowth of hybrid cells, subsequent fusions were performed with donor PBLs depleted of T cells by sheep red blood cell (SRBC) rosetting (E⁻PBLs) (Madsen and Johnson, 1979). When T-depleted lymphocytes were combined with DS-300 in a PEG fusion experiment, 75% of the wells in 96-well microtiter plates contained proliferating cell lines by day 14. Microscopic examination of proliferating cells showed them to be morphologically heterogeneous. Although round and elongated cells were present, the majority of cells were pear-shaped, with one or several slender pseudopodia located at one end. Most cells appeared to favor growth in clusters of various size and shape, although single cells were often present.

Analysis of several clones derived from the above fusion, to verify that the cells were true hybrids, resulted in some very interesting observations.

With the exception of one clone, all cells were found (1) to be diploid, (2) to display the HLA type of the lymphocyte donor only, (3) to lack a Y chromosome (GM 1500 is of male origin and all fusions were performed with lymphocytes from female donors), (4) to secrete monoclonal human Ig composed of only one type of heavy and light chain, and (5) to express EBNA. The one exception displayed a near-tetraploid karyotype, but otherwise possessed the characteristics just described. It was readily apparent from these findings that fusion between DS-300 and donor lymphocytes was not responsible for the generation of Ig-producing cell lines. Instead, the observed properties of these lines were uniquely consistent with those of lymphoblastoid cell lines (LCLs) generated by EBV transformation of human B lymphocytes (Nilsson and Klein, 1982). It has since been noted that PEG is nonessential to the development of the Ig-producing cell lines by the above method. Thus, DS-300 cells, when mixed and cocultivated with donor B lymphocytes in the presence of HAT-supplemented growth medium, appeared to effectively facilitate the EBV-mediated transformation of susceptible B cells. This process has been given the name cell-driven viral transformation and is summarized in Fig. 1.

In order to determine if a subpopulation of cells in the uncloned DS-300 cell line was responsible for the above phenomenon, the DS-300 line was subsequently cloned by limiting dilution techniques and the clones assayed for

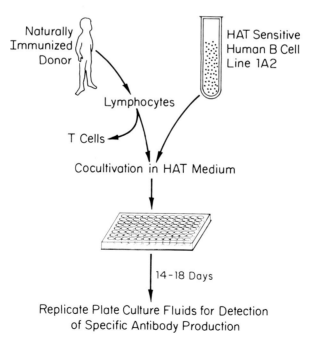

FIGURE 1. Schematic representation of the cell-driven viral transformation process.

their ability to promote transformation. As shown in Table I, clone 1A2 was markedly superior to the parental DS-300 cell line in its ability to facilitate transformation and subsequent outgrowth of LCLs. Of the remaining clones tested, only one other clone (1A1) demonstrated any transforming capacity, albeit quite low. From these data it was concluded that a subpopulation of the DS-300 cells represented by the 1A2 clone was responsible for the generation of antibody-secreting LCLs.

One suspected reason for the superior transforming ability of the 1A2 clone as compared to its sister clones was that it produced far more transforming virus than the other clones. To test this possibility, the 1A1 and 1A2 clones were compared with the EBV-producing B95-8 cell line (Miller and Lipman, 1973) and the GM 1500 cell line for the presence of EBV membrane antigens (MA). These antigens are expressed on the viral envelope and the cell surface of virus-producing but not virus-nonproducing cell lines (Ernberg and Klein, 1979). Analysis was performed on a fluorescence-activated cell sorter (FACS IV; Becton-Dickinson, Mountain View, California) using an indirect immunofluorescence assay on live cells with a monoclonal antibody specific for a 250,000-dalton EBV MA (Hoffman *et al.*, 1980). Results indicated that approximately 5% of the 1A2 and B95-8 cells were positively stained for MA, whereas the 1A1 and GM 1500 cells displayed a barely detectable (0.2–0.5%) level of fluorescence. Surprisingly, when cell-free 4-day culture supernatants from the 1A1 and 1A2 clones were tested for the ability to transform E⁻ PBLs (under conditions where B95-8 supernatant generated proliferating cells in 100% of the plated wells), no induction of continuously growing cell lines was observed. We have seen, however, that a sonicate of 1A2 cells, free of live cells, was quite efficient at promoting LCL outgrowth under the same condi-

TABLE I

*Comparison of the DS-300 Cell Line and Four Clonal
Derivatives for the Ability to Generate LCLs[a]*

Cell line	Percentage of wells containing proliferating cells
DS-300 (uncloned)	62.5
DS-300 clone 1A1	2.1
DS-300 clone 1A2	88.6
DS-300 clone 1B3	0
DS-300 clone 1B4	0

[a]Aliquots of E⁻PBLs from the same donor were combined with each of the different cell lines at a 1:2 ratio in HAT medium and plated at 1.2×10^5 cells/200 µl per well into half of a 96-well flat-bottom microtiter plate. Cultures were fed every third day by replacement of half the supernatant with fresh HAT medium and scored for proliferating cell lines on day 15.

tions. It thus appeared that although the 1A2 clone was a substantial producer of EBV, the virus was not released from intact cells in appreciable quantities.

A precise calculation of the efficiency with which the 1A2 cell line can promote the transformation of adult human B lymphocytes into continuously proliferating cell lines awaits investigation by limiting dilution analysis. Nevertheless, it has been noted that wells seeded with as few as 2000 B cells routinely give rise to vigorously growing cell lines in all wells plated. Application of Poisson distribution analysis to this observation suggests that, at the very least, one in every 300–400 adult B cells can be immortalized by the cell-driven viral transformation process. This is far superior to immortalization frequencies engendered by fusion techniques, $1-10 \times 10^{-7}$ [reviewed in Kozbor and Roder (1983)] and compares quite favorably with those observed in conventional EBV transformation systems under the most optimal conditions (Brown and Miller, 1982; Stein and Sigal, 1983; Yarchoan et al., 1983; Martinez-Maza and Britton, 1983).

Isotype analysis of the immunoglobulins secreted by cell-driven viral transformants has demonstrated that all three major classes of human Ig are produced. As shown in Fig. 2, IgG and IgM constitute the predominant isotypes, and the percentage of cells that produce each appear to be comparable. IgA-secretors were also encountered, but at a lower frequency. This pattern of isotype commitment contrasts with that observed by other investigators, who have reported that IgM-secretors make up the majority of LCLs generated by conventional EBV transformation (Brown and Miller, 1982; Stein et al., 1983; Yarchoan et al., 1983) Whether the observed differences reflect variation in the immune status of lymphocyte donors, the timing of isotype analysis (Stein and Sigal, 1983), use of dissimilar culture systems, or more fundamental disparities with respect to the transforming viruses themselves is at present unknown.

III. Application of the Cell-Driven Viral Transformation Process to the Generation of Specific Human Monoclonal Antibodies

We have most recently used the process of cell-driven viral transformation to produce specific and protective human monoclonal antibodies against the Gram-negative organism *Pseudomonas aeruginosa*. Normally of low virulence in healthy individuals, this bacterium continues to be rather problematic in the hospital environment and particularly in those patients with marginal or defective host immunity. Because of its inherent insensitivity to many antibiotics, infections with this organism have in the past been associated with significant morbidity and mortality (Andriole, 1978). Whereas treatment with ever more potent and specific antibiotics has greatly improved the

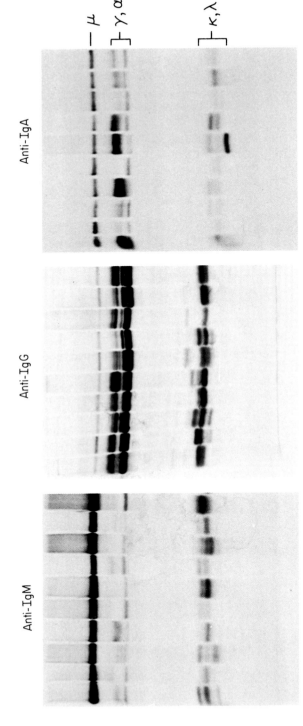

FIGURE 2. SDS–polyacrylamide gel electrophoresis of [³⁵S]methionine immunoglobulins. Ten random wells were selected from a cell-driven viral transformation of adult E⁻PBL. One million cells from each well were cultured for 18 hr in the presence of [³⁵S]methionine, after which cell-free supernatants were harvested and frozen at −70°C. Rabbit anti-human colostrum IgA-, rabbit anti-human IgG-, and rabbit anti-human IgM-coated beads (Biorad, Richmond, California) were individually mixed and incubated (60 min on ice) with 250 μl of antibody-containing supernatants from each of the wells. Following four washes in RIP buffer (Siadak and Nowinski, 1981) at 4°C to remove unbound constituents, the beads were resuspended in 15 μl of sample buffer (Siadak and Nowinski, 1981) and heated to 95°C for 5 min. Ten microliters of each sample, after centrifugation, was run on a 10% bis-acrylamide discontinuous minigel (Laemmli, 1970) for 70 min at 125 V. Gels were dried and bands visualized by autoradiography on NS-2T film (Kodak). It should be noted that each of the antiserum-coated beads exhibited a minor cross-reaction to the other immunoglobulin classes in this assay.

outcome of these often fatal infections, it is generally recognized that prevention of infection in individuals at risk and therapy of already infected patients are still far from optimal (Andriole, 1978). This has prompted the search for alternative prevention and treatment modalities. Given the availability of an improved methodology for making human monoclonal antibodies, we have recently considered passive immunotherapy with antibodies specific for *P. aeruginosa* as one such alternative.

A. B-Lymphocyte Source for Cell-Driven Viral Transformation

Human B lymphocytes were derived from the spleen of a deceased individual known to have had previous infections with *Pseudomonas aeruginosa*. The spleen, obtained at autopsy, was cut into slices approximately 15 mm thick. Cells were liberated from the capsule and connective matrix into a large petri dish by gently perfusing each slice with calcium–magnesium-free phosphate-buffered saline (PBS) delivered through an 18 gauge needle attached to a syringe. Mononuclear cells were separated from the splenic cell preparation by standard centrifugation techniques on Ficoll–Hypaque (Boyum, 1968) and washed twice in calcium–magnesium-free PBS.

The mononuclear cells were depleted of T cells using a modified E-rosetting procedure. Briefly, the cells were first resuspended to a concentration of 1×10^7 cells/ml in PBS containing 20% (v/v) FCS at 4°C. One milliliter of this suspension was then placed in a 17×100 mm polystyrene round-bottom tube to which was added 1×10^9 2-amino-ethyl-isothiouronium bromide-treated sheep red blood cells (AET–SRBC) from a 10% (v/v) solution in RPMI 1640 medium (Madsen and Johnson, 1979). The suspension was very gently mixed for 5–10 min at 4°C and the E-rosetted cells then removed by centrifugation on Ficoll–Hypaque for 8 min at $2500 \times g$ and 4°C. The E-rosette-negative splenic mononuclear cells (E⁻Spl) banding at the interface were washed once in RPMI 1640 medium and resuspended in the same containing 15% (v/v) FCS, 2 mM L-glutamine, 1 mM sodium pyruvate, penicillin (100 U/ml), streptomycin (100 μg/ml), hypoxanthine (1×10^{-4} M), aminopterin (4×10^{-7} M), and thymidine (1.6×10^{-5} M). This medium is referred to as HAT medium.

B. Cell-Driven Viral Transformation of Cells

1A2 cells in logarithmic growth phase were suspended in HAT medium and combined with the E⁻Spl cells at a ratio of 30 1A2 cells per E⁻Spl cell. The cell mixture was plated into ten flat-bottom 96-well microtiter plates at a concentration of 155,000 cells/well in a volume of 200 μl per well, and the cultures were incubated at 37°C in a humidified atmosphere containing 6% CO_2. Cultures were fed every 3–4 days by replacement of half the supernatant with fresh HAT medium. The wells were observed every other day on an inverted microscope for signs of cell proliferation. Two weeks after plating the cells, subsequent feeding of the wells was accomplished with a new medium formulation identical to HAT medium except that it lacked the aminopterin component. Eighteen days postplating it was observed that approximately 70% of the wells contained proliferating cells and that in most of the wells, the cells were of sufficient density for removal and testing of supernatants for anti-*P. aeruginosa* antibody.

C. Detection of Specific Antibody-Secreting Cells

Supernatants were screened for the presence of anti-*P. aeruginosa* antibodies using an enzyme-linked immunosorbent assay (ELISA) technique (Engvall, 1977). The antigen plates consisted of flat-bottom 96-well microtiter plates (Nunc), the wells of which contained whole bacterial cells that had been ethanol-fixed to the bottom of the well. Plates were prepared by addition of 50 μl of a washed bacterial suspension (OD_{660} = 0.2) in PBS into the wells, centrifugation of the plates for 20 min at $1500 \times g$, aspiration of PBS, addition of 75 μl of 95% ethanol, fixation for 10 min, removal of ethanol, and finally air drying. The antigen plates used in the screening included: (1) a pool of *P. aeruginosa* Fisher immunotypes 1 (ATCC 27312), 2 (ATCC 27313), and 3 (ATCC 27314); (2) a pool of *P. aeruginosa* Fisher immunotypes 4 (ATCC 27315), 5 (ATCC 27316), 6 (ATCC 27317), and 7 (ATCC 27318); (3) a clinical isolate of *Escherichia coli;* (4) *Klebsiella pneumoniae* (ATCC 8047); and (5) a microtiter plate with no bacteria.

Prior to assay, the wells of the plates were blocked against further protein adsorption by a 1-hr incubation with 100 μl of 5% bovine serum albumin (BSA) in PBS, pH 7.2. The ELISA assay was performed in four steps:

1. Supernatants from wells of the culture plates were replica plated into the corresponding wells of the antigen plates (50 μl/well) and incubated for 30 min at 37°C. Nonbound antibodies were then removed by washing the wells three times with PBS containing 1% BSA (1% BSA–PBS).

2. Fifty microliters of biotinylated goat anti-human Ig (Tago, Burlingame, California; diluted 1:1000 in 1% BSA–PBS) was added to each well and the plates incubated for 30 min at 37°C. Nonbound reagent was then removed by washing three times with 1% BSA–PBS.

3. Fifty microliters of a preformed avidin–biotinylated horseradish peroxidase complex (Vectastain ABC Kit, Vector Laboratories, Burlingame, California) was added to each well and the plates incubated

for 30 min at 25°C. Nonbound complex was then removed by washing three times with 1% BSA–PBS.

4. One hundred microliters of enzyme substrate (0.8 mg/ml *ortho*-phenylenediamine dihydrochloride in 100 mM citrate buffer, pH 5.0, plus 0.03% H_2O_2 in deionized H_2O, mixed in equal volumes just before plating) was added to each well and the plates incubated for 30 min at 25°C in the dark. Then 50 μl of 3 N H_2SO_4 was added to each well to terminate reactions. Culture supernatants containing antibodies corresponding to the plate's antigen were detected by positive color development in the corresponding wells and the strength of the reaction quantitated by measuring the absorbance at 490 nm on a Dynatech MR 580 micro ELISA reader.

Approximately 20% of the culture supernatants contained antibody that bound to the *P. aeruginosa* antigen plates. Many of these, however, were also positive on the other bacterial antigen plates and the plate that contained no antigen. We have found this result to be due to the presence of "sticky" antibodies in these supernatants and have since shown that the majority of such antibodies are of the IgM class. Three supernatants (4G9, 6F11, and 10B2) did, however, demonstrate a more restricted reactivity pattern with specificity for the *P. aeruginosa* Fisher immunotypes 1–3 plate but not the *P. aeruginosa* Fisher immunotypes 4–7 plate or any of the control plates. It was subsequently determined in a similar ELISA assay on the individual Fisher immunotypes that each of these three culture supernatants contained antibody specific to the Fisher 2 immunotype. Furthermore, when biotinylated goat anti-human Ig subclass reagents [i.e., anti-IgG, anti-IgM, and anti-IgA (Tago; diluted 1:500 in 1% BSA–PBS)] were used instead of the more broadly reactive anti-Ig reagent, positive reaction of the three culture supernatants with Fisher immunotype 2 bacteria was observed only with the anti-IgM reagent, thus demonstrating an IgM isotype for the relevant antibody in each of these supernatants.

D. *Cloning of Specific Antibody-Producing Cells*

The cells in wells 4G9, 6F11, and 10B2 were cloned by limiting dilution on a semiconfluent layer of human foreskin fibroblasts in flat-bottom 96-well plates. Media consisted of RPMI 1640 containing 15% (v/v) FCS, 2 mM L-glutamine, 1 mM sodium pyruvate, penicillin (100 IU/ml), and streptomycin (100 μg/ml). Cultures were fed every third day by replacement of half the supernatant with fresh media. In general, wells were of sufficient lymphoblastoid cell density between 2 and 3 weeks postplating for analysis of antibody specificity as described above. In this manner, the cells in wells 4G9, 6F11, and 10B2 that were secreting anti-Fisher immunotype 2 antibody were cloned after two and in some cases (4G9 and 10B2) three successive rounds of cloning. Clonality in this system was defined as specific antibody activity present in 100% of examined clonal supernatants.

E. Characterization of the Molecular Target Recognized by Monoclonal Antibodies

The observation that the monoclonal antibodies from each of the above clones reacted exclusively with a single (in this case Fisher 2) immunotype and that the Fisher immunotyping system (Fisher *et al.*, 1969) is based on diversity of the lipopolysaccharide (LPS) molecules on *P. aeruginosa* (Hanessian *et al.*, 1971) suggested that the antibodies were directed against LPS antigens. To examine this further, additional ELISA assays were performed with the 4G9, 6F11, and 10B2 clonal supernatants on plates containing whole, fixed bacteria of each of the 17 International Antigenic Typing Scheme (IATS) strains (Brokopp and Farmer, 1979) of *P. aeruginosa*, *Pseudomonas aureofaciens*, the J5 mutant of *E. coli* 0111:B4, and a clinical isolate of *Providencia stuartii*. In complete agreement with a comparison of the Fisher immunotypes and their corresponding LPS-based serotypes in the IATS (Brokopp and Farmer, 1979), each of the anti-Fisher immunotype 2 clonal supernatants was reactive with only IATS strain 11. No reactions were observed on any of the non-*P. aeruginosa* bacteria. Furthermore, consistent with the known outer membrane location of LPS molecules on Gram-negative bacteria, all three monoclonal antibodies demonstrated a very bright and complete surface staining of live Fisher immunotype 2 bacteria in an indirect immunofluorescence assay. Based on stronger reactivity of the antibody in ELISAs and better growth properties of the respective cell line, the 6F11 monoclonal was chosen for further study.

Biochemical characterization of the molecular species recognized by the 6F11 antibody was accomplished by immunoblot analysis. As shown in Fig. 3, 6F11 reacted only with crude Fisher immunotype 2 LPS and outer membrane preparation of Fisher immunotype 2 bacteria (also known to contain LPS). In both instances, the 6F11 antibody appeared to recognize a series of regularly spaced molecular entities, giving rise to a "ladder-like" pattern on the immunoblot. This profile was entirely consistent with that seen in polyacrylamide gel electrophoretic analysis of LPS in the presence of SDS, where it has been demonstrated that the heterogeneous size profile exhibited by such a banding pattern is due to a population of LPS molecules differing by weight increments equivalent to the number of O-antigenic oligosaccharide side chain units present per molecule (Pavla and Makela, 1980; Goldman and Leive, 1980). Since serologic specificity of LPS molecules is based on the structure of

1 2 3 4 5 6 7 8 9 10

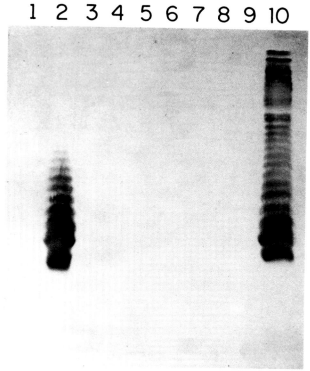

FIGURE 3. Immunoblot analysis of human monoclonal antibody 6F11. Twenty micrograms of crude LPS [prepared by the hot phenol–water method of Westphal *et al.* (1952)] from Fisher immunotypes 1 (lane 1), 2 (lane 2), 3 (lane 3), 4 (lane 4), 5 (lane 5), 6 (lane 6), and 7 (lane 7), 20 μg of chromatographically purified LPS (List Laboratories, Campbell, California) from *E. coli* 0111:B4 (lane 8), and *Klebsiella pneumoniae* (lane 9), and 50 μg of an outer membrane preparation (Tam *et al.*, 1982) of Fisher immunotype 2 bacteria (lane 10) were each subjected to SDS–PAGE (Hancock and Carey, 1977). Separated molecular species were transferred from the gel to a nitrocellulose membrane (NCM) (Towbin *et al.*, 1979) and the NCM blot blocked for 1 hr in PBS–Tween (Batteiger *et al.*, 1982). The blot was then incubated for 1 hr at 25°C in 30 ml PBS–Tween containing 3 ml of spent culture supernatant from the 6F11 line. Following four 5-min rinses in PBS–Tween, the blot was incubated in a 1:5000 dilution (in PBS–Tween) of rabbit anti-human Ig for 1 hr at 25°C. The blot was rinsed four times in PBS–Tween and then placed in 30 ml of a solution containing a 1:2000 dilution (in PBS–Tween) of protein A–horseradish peroxidase (Zymed Laboratories, San Francisco, California). After a 1-hr incubation at 25°C the blot was rinsed four times in PBS–Tween and then submerged in 60 ml of substrate prepared as follows: 120 mg of horseradish peroxidase–color development reagent (Bio-Rad Laboratories, Richmond, California) was dissolved in 40 ml cold methanol; 120 μl of 30% H_2O_2 was added to 200 ml Tris-buffered saline (20 mM Tris, pH 7.4, 0.5 M NaCl); the two solutions were mixed just prior to addition to the blot. After appropriate color development (usually 15–45 min after addition of substrate) the reaction was quenched by rinsing the blot several times in deionized water.

the repeating oligosaccharide units and/or their glycosidic linkages (Westphal *et al.*, 1983), the specificity and immunoblot data clearly suggested that monoclonal antibody 6F11 was specific for some part of the oligosaccharide unit or the linkage between such units rather than the more serologically conserved structures of LPS represented by the core region and lipid A.

F. In Vitro Functional Activity of the 6F11 Monoclonal Antibody

In humans, the primary mechanism of immunity to *P. aeruginosa* appears to be a combination of opsonization of the bacteria by specific antibodies followed by their phagocytosis by polymorphonuclear leukocytes (neutrophils) (Pollack, 1979). To determine if the 6F11 human monoclonal antibody could mimic this activity, it was examined in an *in vitro* opsonophagocytic assay, which compared the uptake of radiolabeled bacteria by human neutrophils in the presence of complement (C′) when the 6F11 monoclonal was present and not present.

Radiolabeled bacteria in the assay were prepared by inoculating 5 ml of *Pseudomonas* in minimal medium with 100 μl (1 μCi) of [^{3}H]leucine (146.5 Ci/mmole; New England Nuclear, Boston, Massachusetts) and 30 μl of an overnight bacterial suspension cultured in trypticase soy broth. The tube was incubated at 37°C on a shaker for 4–6 hr, after which the excess [^{3}H]leucine was removed by four washes in Hank's Buffered Saline Solution containing 0.1% gelatin and 5 mM HEPES (HBSS/gel, pH 7.2) and the bacteria resuspended in the same to a final concentration of 6.67×10^6/ml. Human neutrophils were isolated according to van Furth and van Zwet (1973) with several modifications. Buffy coat from 10 ml of heparinized blood was underlayed with Ficoll–Hypaque and centrifuged. The RBC pellet was washed once in RPMI 1640 medium and resuspended in an equal volume of 37°C PBS. Three milliliters of this suspension was then added to 6 ml of 2% dextran (in 37°C PBS) and the contents gently but thoroughly mixed end over end. After a 20-min incubation at 37°C to allow the RBCs to sediment, the supernatant (containing neutrophils) was removed and washed two times in 4°C PBS. Cells were washed once more in 4°C HBSS–HEPES (pH 7.2) and resuspended in same to 5×10^7 neutrophils/ml. Lyophilized normal rabbit serum (NRS) reconstituted in 0.01 M EDTA (pH 7.2) and twice absorbed with live bacteria (Bjornson and Michael, 1974) representing the seven Fisher immunotypes served as a source of C′.

As indicated in Fig. 4A, the 6F11 monoclonal antibody was capable of opsonizing Fisher immunotype 2 bacteria and promoting their ingestion by human neutrophils. When the experiment was repeated using Fisher immunotype 1 bacteria (Fig. 4B), this activity was not observed, thus corroborating the functional specificity of the 6F11 monoclonal antibody with its specificity as determined by ELISA. It is interesting to note that for the IgM 6F11 monoclonal antibody to act as an opsonin, it had the same obligatory require-

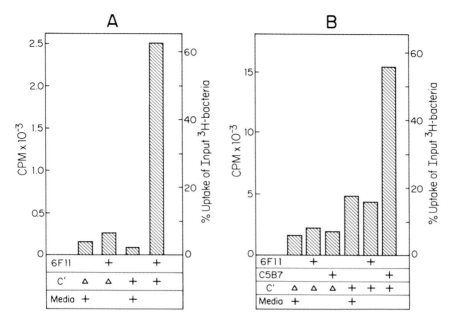

FIGURE 4. Opsonophagocytosis of *P. aeruginosa* by the 6F11 human monoclonal antibody and human neutrophils. (A) Input bacteria: [³H]-Fisher immunotype 2. (B) Input bacteria: [³H]-Fisher immunotype 1. Plus sign indicates the presence of reagent and △ indicates heat inactivation. C5B7 is a human monoclonal antibody specific for Fisher immunotype 1 LPS. In each experiment 300 μl of [³H]-bacterial suspension was added to 100 μl of antibody-containing culture supernatant (diluted 1:1 with △FCS) in a 1.5-ml Eppendorf tube and incubated 20 min on a rotator at 37°C. This was followed by the sequential addition of 50 μl of C′ (or △C′) and then 50 μl of neutrophil suspension with 30- and 45-min incubation periods on a rotator at 37°C after each of the respective additions. Neutrophils were freed of uningested bacteria (as confirmed by microscopic examination) by two washes with cold PBS. Neutrophils were then lysed by incubation in 250 μl of 0.1 N NaOH for 30 min with occasional vortexing. Two hundred fifty microliters of the tube's contents was solubilized in 3 ml of scintillation fluid (Dimilume 30, United Technologies, Packard) and counted. Results are expressed as percent uptake of input radiolabeled bacteria. The cpm associated with input radiolabeled bacteria was determined by counting 250 μl of a control tube's contents that had been subjected to the above procedures except for the addition of △NRS for antibody and no washes to remove uningested bacteria.

ment for complement as has been observed for IgM opsonizing antibodies to *Pseudomonas* in human serum (Young, 1974).

G. *In Vivo Activity of the 6F11 Monoclonal Antibody*

The above data suggested that monoclonal antibody 6F11 would, under appropriate administration, provide specific protection *in vivo* against a lethal challenge of Fisher immunotype 2 bacteria. To test this hypothesis, animal

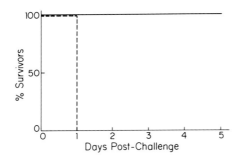

FIGURE 5. Monoclonal antibody therapy of mice challenged with a lethal dose of *P. aeruginosa*. Female BALB/c mice between 21 and 22 g body weight were divided into two groups of ten mice each. (—) Group inoculated ip with 0.5 ml of 6F11 antibody (containing approximately 50 μg antibody as determined by radioimmunoassay) $(NH_4)_2SO_4$-concentrated from spent culture supernatant; (– – –) group receiving ip 0.5 ml of similarly concentrated fresh culture medium. Six hours later, all animals were challenged ip with 0.3 ml of a live bacterial suspension containing five times the LD_{50} of Fisher immunotype 2 *P. aeruginosa*. The bacterial suspension had been prepared from a broth culture in logarithmic-phase growth, from which the bacteria were centrifuged, washed two times in PBS, and resuspended to the appropriate density in PBS. The bacterial challenge represented 1.2×10^8 live organisms.

protection studies were performed with the 6F11 antibody and several Fisher immunotypes of *P. aeruginosa*. In one experiment (Fig. 5) mice were inoculated ip with 6F11 antibody that had been $(NH_4)_2SO_4$-concentrated from spent culture supernatant. An equal number of animals were similarly inoculated with salt-concentrated fresh culture medium as negative controls. Six hours later, all animals were challenged ip with five times the LD_{50} of Fisher immunotype 2 bacteria. Animals were observed for a period of 5 days. Twenty-four hours postchallenge, all the animals that had received concentrated culture media were dead. In contrast, those animals that had received the 6F11 monoclonal antibody were all alive. The latter group appeared quite healthy, with only minor symptoms of bacterial infection (i.e., a slight ruffling of the fur). These symptoms disappeared by 48 hr postchallenge, with no further evidence of bacterial disease during the remainder of the observation period. Similar experiments performed using a challenge of five times the LD_{50} of other Fisher immunotypes of *P. aeruginosa* resulted in no protection by the 6F11 antibody. These data demonstrated that passively transferred 6F11 antibody provided complete and specific protection against a lethal challenge dose of Fisher immunotype 2 *P. aeruginosa*.

IV. Discussion

We have described here a convenient, reproducible, and efficient method for the production of human monoclonal antibodies. The method entails the cocultivation of human B lymphocytes and the HAT-sensitive, transforming, EBV-producing lymphoblastoid cell line 1A2. Two to three weeks after initiation of the culture, continuous cell lines, each producing human monoclonal antibody, can be screened with appropriate assays for desired specificities.

Summarized in Table II are the salient features of the process and the properties of the antibody-producing lymphoblastoid cell lines.

Notable among the features of the process is its simplicity. During the cocultivation in HAT-supplemented growth medium, the death of the 1A2 cells results in the release of transforming EBV into the immediate environment of susceptible B cells. This fresh, high-titered source of virus very efficiently transforms B cells into continuously proliferating LCLs. The ease of mixing the two cell populations, seeding directly into 96-well culture plates, followed by regular feedings has thus obviated the need to prepare and quantitate high-titered stocks of EBV. Further simplifying the protocol, it has been subsequently observed that T-cell depletion is nonessential if cyclosporin A (0.5 μg/ml) is included in the culture medium during the first 2 weeks of the transformation.

Perhaps more important than the simplicity of use is the high efficiency and reproducibility with which antibody-producing cell lines are generated by this process. Any system for the production of human monoclonal antibodies must take into account that the proportion of B cells from native lymphoid populations dedicated to antibody production against a specific antigen is anticipated to be variable and quite small, being on the order of $1-10 \times 10^{-4}$ (Kozbor and Roder, 1983). Given, in most cases, the absence of an ethical means to systematically amplify this small subpopulation by repeated *in vivo*

TABLE II

Properties of Cell-Driven Viral Transformation and Antibody-Producing Lymphoblastoid Cell Lines Generated by the Process

Selective cocultivation system:
    Normal B lymphocytes cultured with HAT-sensitive, EBV-transformed B-cell line
    1A2 in HAT medium; cell fusion not required
Characteristics of 1A2 cells:
    Clonal human lymphoblastoid cell line
    EBNA-positive
    Produces transforming EBV
    Diploid
    IgG$^+$
    HGPRT$^-$: do not survive in HAT
Characteristics of transformed B cells:
    EBNA-positive
    Diploid
    Secrete IgG, IgM, or IgA
    HGPRT$^+$: survive in HAT
Advantages of cell-driven transformation:
    Efficient generation of B-cell lines (frequency $>10^{-3}$)
    Vigorous growth
    High maximum cell density
    Stable antibody production (1–10 μg/ml)

immunization and a poorly developed technology for generating specific human antibody responses *in vitro*, it is advantageous to be able to prepare as many different B-cell lines as possible from a defined number of starting lymphocytes. The cell-driven viral transformation process has reproducibly been shown to immortalize at least one in 300–400 adult B cells from bone marrow, peripheral blood, and spleen into a culturable, clonable, monoclonal antibody-secreting cell line. This process thus appears to be a more effective method for the generation of immortalized human B cells than mouse–human or human–human fusion techniques.

It is apparent from this level of efficiency that the cell-driven viral transformation process should afford the opportunity to examine a broad cross section of the humoral repertoire and to select multiple monoclonal antibodies for therapy or other purposes. In support of this premise, we have isolated and cloned cell lines secreting monoclonal antibody to virtually all of the bacterial antigens thus far included in our experiments. Furthermore, in accordance with our initial studies on isotype commitment, cell lines secreting IgG, IgA, and IgM isotypes of desired specificities have been prepared.

Having devised a means to obtain large numbers of immortalized B cells, we have recently turned our attention to the improvement of the process and, in particular, to our ability to isolate desired clones. The strategy we have adopted to reduce the number of independent cell lines per well and thereby to achieve clonal lines more rapidly has been to utilize a seeding density of $(1–2) \times 10^3$ B cells per well when initiating transformations. Significantly better results have been realized both in transformation and cloning efficiencies from three additional protocol modifications. First, the culture medium now employed is Iscove's Modified Dulbecco's Medium with HEPES buffering. Second, round-bottom culture plates have replaced flat-bottom plates for initiation and cloning of transformants. Third, irradiated human peripheral blood mononuclear cells (1×10^5 cells/well) have replaced primary fibroblasts as feeder layers during cloning procedures. The combination of these changes has resulted in a twofold improvement in the efficiency of transformation and more than a fourfold improvement in the cloning efficiency of desired lymphoblastoid cells. Although variable from one lymphoblastoid cell to another, we have routinely observed that 10–30% of transformed cells can be propagated at the single-cell level using the above culture conditions.

Lymphoblastoid cells derived from cell-driven viral transformations exhibit a range in growth rate and amount of antibody secreted. Once cloned, however, the individuality conferred by these properties appears to be stably maintained. In general, clonal cell lines have demonstrated population doubling times of 24–36 hr. Log-phase cells, cultured at 5×10^5/ml for 3–4 days, typically yield 1–10 μg of antibody per ml. This level is in accordance with the best values reported for LCLs by conventional EBV transformation (Brown and Miller, 1982; Winger *et al.*, 1983) and compares well with production by mouse–human and human–human hybrids (Kozbor and Roder, 1983; Larrick and Buck, 1984).

The simplicity, reproducibility, and efficiency of the cell-driven viral transformation process are perhaps best realized when applied to the development of *in vivo* protective monoclonal antibodies. Well known from previous research and clinical study of *P. aeruginosa* infections are the beneficial therapeutic effects of high-titer antisera. Antibodies reactive with the surface antigens, most notably LPS, of these bacteria appear to cooperate with phagocytic cells and serum complement to remove and render harmless the *P. aeruginosa* organisms and thereby be beneficial to the host (Pollack, 1979). While immune globulin compositions represent a more directed approach compared to γ globulins or broad-spectrum antibiotics, they also contain large amounts of extraneous substances and are relatively low in titer. Human monoclonal antibodies can overcome the problem of low specific titer and, as shown in this chapter, perform as *in vivo* protective immunotherapeutic agents. High-titer, high-purity, and consistent human monoclonal compositions may represent a worthy improvement to the prophylactic and therapeutic treatment of *P. aeruginosa* infections.

Note Added in Proof

Experiments designed to more accurately assess the immortalization frequency of adult B cells using the cell-driven transformation process have recently been initiated in this lab. Results indicate that, one out of every 50 to 100 adult B cells is routinely transformed into a proliferating and antibody secreting cell line when co-cultured with 1A2 cells in HAT-supplemented culture medium.

ACKNOWLEDGMENTS

We would like to express our gratitude to Gary Keizur, Mae Joanne Rosok, Walt Shuford, and Pamela Ansari for their excellent technical assistance in these studies. We also thank Dr. Howard Raff for his help in designing the opsonophagocytic assay and Roxanne Reilley for typing the manuscript.

References

Andriole, V. T., 1978, *Pseudomonas* bacteremia: Can antibiotic therapy improve survival, *J. Lab. Clin. Med.* **94**:196–200.
Batteiger, B., Newhall, W. J., and Jones, R. B., 1982, The use of Tween 20 as a blocking agent in the immunological detection of proteins transferred to nitrocellulose membranes, *J. Immunol. Meth.* **55**:297–307.

Bernstein, I. D., Tam, M. R., and Nowinski, R. C., 1980, Mouse leukemia: Therapy with mono-clonal antibodies against a thymus differentiation antigen, *Science* **207**:68–71.

Bjornson, A. B., and Michael, J. G., 1974, Factors in human serum promoting phagocytosis of *Pseudomonas aeruginosa*. I. Interaction of opsonins with the bacterium, *J. Infect. Dis.* **130**(Suppl):S119–S125.

Boyum, A., 1968, Isolation of mononuclear cells and granulocytes from human blood, *Scand. J. Clin. Lab. Invest.* **21**(Suppl. 97):77–89.

Brokopp, C. D., and Farmer, J. J., III, 1979, Typing methods for *Pseudomonas aeruginosa*, in: *Pseudomonas aeruginosa: Clinical Manifestations of Infection and Current Therapy* (R. G. Doggett, ed.), Academic Press, New York, Chapter 5.

Brown, N. A., and Miller, G., 1982, Immunoglobulin expression by human B lymphocytes clonally transformed by Epstein–Barr virus, *J. Immunol.* **128**:24–29.

Engvall, E., 1977, Quantitative enzyme immunoassay (ELISA) in microbiology, *Med. Biol.* **55**:193–200.

Ernberg, I., and Klein G., 1979, EB virus-induced antigens, in: *The Epstein–Barr Virus* (M. A. Epstein and B. G. Achong, eds.), Springer, New York, Chapter 3.

Fisher, M. W., Devlin, H. B., and Gnabasik, F. J., 1969, New immunotype scheme for *Pseudomonas aeruginosa* based on protective antigens, *J. Bacteriol.* **98**:835–836.

Goldman, R. C., and Leive, L., 1980, Heterogeneity of antigenic-side-chain length in lipopolysac-charide from *Escherichia coli* 0111 and *Salmonella typhimurium* LT2, *Eur. J. Biochem.* **107**:145–153.

Hancock, R. E. W., and Carey, A. M., 1979, Outer membrane of *Pseudomonas aeruginosa:* Heat and 2-mercaptoethanol-modifiable proteins, *J. Bacteriol.* **140**:902–910.

Hanessian, S., Regan, W., Watson, D., and Haskell, T. H., 1971, Isolation and characterization of antigenic components of a new heptavalent *Pseudomonas* vaccine, *Nature New Biol.* **229**:209–210.

Hoffman, G. J., Lazarowitz, S. G., and Hayward, S. D., 1980, Monoclonal antibody against a 250,000-dalton glycoprotein of Epstein–Barr virus identifies a membrane antigen and a neutralizing antigen, *Proc. Natl. Acad. Sci. USA* **77**:2979–2983.

Kennett, R. H., 1979, Cell fusion, *Meth. Enzymol.* **58**:345–359.

Koskimies, S., 1980, Human lymphoblastoid cell line producing specific antibody against Rh antigen D, *Scand. J. Immunol.* **11**:73–77.

Kozbor, D., and Roder, J. C., 1983, The production of monoclonal antibodies from human lymphocytes, *Immunol. Today* **4**:72–79.

Laemmli, U. K., 1970, Cleavage of structural protein during the assembly of the head of bacterio-phage T4, *Nature* **227**:680–685.

Larrick, J. W., and Buck, D. W., 1984, Practical aspects of human monoclonal antibody produc-tion, *Bio Techniques* **2**:6–14.

Levy, R., and Miller, R. A., 1983, Tumor therapy with monoclonal antibodies, *Fed. Proc.* **42**:2650–2656.

Littlefield, J. W., 1964, Selection of hybrids from matings of fibroblasts *in vitro* and their pre-sumed recombinants, *Science* **145**:709–710.

Madsen, M., and Johnson, H. E., 1979, A methodological study of E-rosette formation using AET treated sheep red blood cells, *J. Immunol. Meth.* **27**:61–74.

Martinez-Maza, O., and Britton, S., 1983, Frequencies of the separate human B cell subsets activatable to Ig secretion by Epstein–Barr virus and pokeweed mitogen, *J. Exp. Med.* **157**:1808–1814.

Miller, G., and Lipman, M., 1973, Comparison of the yield of infectious virus from clones of human and simian lymphoblastoid lines transformed by Epstein–Barr virus, *J. Exp. Med.* **138**:1398–1412.

Moller, G. (ed.), 1982, *Antibody Carriers of Drugs and Toxins in Tumor Therapy*, Immunological Reviews, Volume 62, Munksgaard, Copenhagen.

Nilsson, K., and Klein, G., 1982, Phenotypic and cytogenetic characteristics of human B-lymph-oid cell lines and their relevance for the etiology of Burkitt's lymphoma, *Adv. Cancer Res.* **37**:319–380.

Pavla, E. T., and Makela, P. H., 1980, Lipopolysaccharide heterogeneity in *Salmonella typhimurium* analyzed by sodium dodecyl sulfate/polyacrylamide gel electrophoresis, *Eur. J. Biochem.* **107**:137–143.

Pollack, M., 1979, Antibody-mediated immunity in *Pseudomonas* disease and its clinical application, in: *Immunoglobulins: Characteristics and Uses of Intravenous Preparations* (B. M. Alving and J. S. Finlayson, eds.), U.S. Department of Health and Human Services, Washington, D.C., pp. 73–79.

Siadak, A. W., and Nowinski, R. C., 1981, Thy-2: A murine thymocyte-brain alloantigen controlled by a gene linked to the major histocompatibility complex, *Immunogenetics* **12**:45–58.

Stein, L. D., and Sigal, N. H., 1983, Limiting dilution analysis of Epstein–Barr virus-induced immunoglobulin production, *Cell. Immunol.* **79**:309–319.

Stein, L. D., Ledgley, C. J., and Sigal, N. H., 1983, Patterns of isotype commitment in human B cells: Limiting dilution analysis of Epstein–Barr virus-infected cells, *J. Immunol.* **130**:1640–1645.

Steinitz, M., Klein, G., Koskimies, S., and Makel, O., 1977, EB virus-induced B lymphocyte cell lines producing specific antibody, *Nature* **269**:420–422.

Tam, M. R., Buchanan, T. M., Sandstrom, E. G., Holmes, K. K., Knapp, J. S., Siadak, A. W., and Nowinski, R. C., 1982, Serological classification of *Neisseria gonorrhoeae* with monoclonal antibodies, *Infect. Immunol.* **36**:1042–1053.

Towbin, H., Staehelin, T., and Gordon, J., 1979, Electrophoretic transfer of proteins from polyacrylamide gels to nitrocellulose sheets: Procedure and some applications, *Proc. Natl. Acad. Sci. USA* **76**:4350–4354.

Van Furth, R., and van Zwet, T. L., 1973, *In vitro* determination of phagocytosis and intracellular killing by polymorphonuclear and mononuclear phagocytes, in: *Handbook of Experimental Immunology*, Volume 2, 2nd ed. (D. M. Weir, ed.), Blackwell, Oxford, Chapter 36.

Westphal, O., Luderitz, O., and Bister, F., 1952, Über die Extraktion von Bakterien mit Phenol/Wasser, *Z. Naturforsch.* **79**:148–155.

Westphal, O., Jann, K., and Himmelspach, K., 1983, Chemistry and immunochemistry of bacterial lipopolysaccharides as cell wall antigens and endotoxins, *Progr. Allergy* **33**:9–39.

Winger, L., Winger, C., Shastry, P., Russell, A., and Longenecker, M., 1983, Efficient generation *in vitro*, from human peripheral blood cells, of monoclonal Epstein–Barr virus transformants producing specificity antibody to a variety of antigens without prior deliberate immunization, *Proc. Natl. Acad. Sci. USA* **80**:4484–4488.

Yarchoan, R., Tosato, G., Blaese, R. M., Simon, R. M., and Nelson, D. L., 1983, Limiting dilution analysis of Epstein–Barr virus-induced immunoglobulin production by human B cells, *J. Exp. Med.* **157**:1–14.

Young, L. S., 1974, Role of antibody in infections due to *Pseudomonas aeruginosa*, *J. Infect. Dis.* **130**(Suppl.):S111–S118.

C. Applications to Cancer

11

The Generation of Human Monoclonal Antibodies and Their Use in the Analysis of the Humoral Immune Response to Cancer

RICHARD J. COTE AND ALAN N. HOUGHTON

I. Introduction

The discipline of cancer immunology can be defined as having two related but distinct aspects. The first is the search for antigens on tumor cells that might distinguish these cells from their normal counterparts, using immunologic methods. The second is the investigation of the ability of animals and humans to recognize and respond to their own tumors. The discovery that inbred strains of mice are able to recognize antigens expressed by chemically induced sarcomas (Gross, 1943; Foley, 1953; Prehn and Main, 1957) opened up both of these important areas of tumor immunology. Studies of cancer cells with heterologous antibodies, long thought to be the way in which antigens on tumors could best be studied (Bashford, 1913), have not, until quite recently, yielded much useful information. However, the use of mouse monoclonal antibodies as monovalent, heterologous probes has developed into a powerful approach to the serologic analysis of tumors, vastly increasing our knowledge

---

RICHARD J. COTE AND ALAN N. HOUGHTON • Memorial Sloan-Kettering Cancer Center, New York, New York 10021.

about the antigenic phenotypes of cells (Dippold *et al.*, 1980; Ueda *et al.*, 1981; Papsidero *et al.*, 1983). These reagents have already been applied to the histological diagnosis and definition of tumors, and to the localization and treatment of cancer in patients (Epenetos *et al.*, 1982; Miller and Levy, 1981; Osborn and Weber, 1982; Houghton *et al.*, 1985). Although the use of mouse monoclonal antibodies *in vivo* may be limited by their immunogenicity (Houghton *et al.*, 1985; Miller *et al.*, 1982), they have certainly secured a permanent niche in the armamentarium of the basic scientist, pathologist, and clinician interested in cancer.

One area in which mouse monoclonal antibodies (or other heterologous antisera) can give little information is the study of the human immune response to tumors. Evidence from a procedure developed in this laboratory known as autologous typing (Carey *et al.*, 1976), in which serum from a patient with cancer is tested against autologous and allogeneic tumor cell lines for antibody reactivity, has indicated that in at least some cases patients can mount a humoral immune response to antigens present on their cancer cells. This technique has proved to be a versatile and powerful method with which to examine the human immune response to tumors. Using autologous typing, it has been possible to identify and to define serologically antigens that have apparent restriction to tumors (tumor-specific antigens), as well as differentiation antigens (Carey *et al.*, 1976; Garret *et al.*, 1977; Pfreundschuh *et al.*, 1978). However, due to the polyclonal nature of the antibodies in serum (resulting in the presence of multiple antigenic specificities), the ability to detect low-titered reactivities is limited. In addition, the amount of serum available is necessarily finite, severely proscribing efforts to define biochemically those antigens that have been serologically analyzed, and making these reagents unsuitable for diagnostic and therapeutic applications. The generation of human monoclonal antibodies from patients with cancer could, in addition to providing detailed information about the general B-cell repertoire, extend the analysis of the human humoral immune response to cancer and provide reagents for the diagnosis and treatment of cancer.

While the murine hybridoma technology has proved to be a reliable and reproducible method to produce mouse monoclonal antibody (Köhler and Milstein, 1975), methods to generate human monoclonal antibody have been more difficult to develop, despite considerable interest and effort in this area. The two approaches that have been explored most vigorously are transformation of B cells by Epstein–Barr virus (EBV) (Steinitz *et al.*, 1977; Koskimies, 1980; Kozbor and Roder, 1981; Irie *et al.*, 1982; Crawford *et al.*, 1983) and the hybridization of B cells with drug-marked cell lines of mouse or human origin (Nowinski *et al.*, 1980; Schlom *et al.*, 1980; Olsson and Kaplan, 1980; Croce *et al.*, 1980; Sikora *et al.*, 1982; Edwards *et al.*, 1982; Chiorrazzi *et al.*, 1982; Cote *et al.*, 1983; Houghton *et al.*, 1983; Larrick *et al.*, 1983; Glassy *et al.*, 1983). The transformation of human lymphocytes by EBV has yielded cultures of cells that secrete antibody to a variety of well-defined antigens (Steinitz *et al.*, 1977; Kozbor and Roder, 1981; Koskimies, 1980). However, the antibodies have tended to be low-titered, and the cultures are reported to be difficult to clone and unstable for antibody production (Zurawski *et al.*, 1978; Irie *et al.*, 1982). In addition, it appears that not all individuals studied have B cells that are amenable to EBV transformation and subsequent antibody production (Irie *et al.*, 1982), which could severely limit the application of this technique.

The fusion of human lymphocytes with drug-marked mouse myeloma lines results in hybrid cells that secrete human immunoglobulin (Ig) (Nowinski *et al.*, 1980; Schlom *et al.*, 1980; Cote *et al.*, 1983; Houghton *et al.*, 1983). There is, however, a general feeling that these interspecies hybrids tend to lose their ability to secrete human Ig due to the preferential loss of human chromosomes. Nevertheless, several groups have isolated mouse–human hybrids that continued to secrete human Ig over extended periods (Nowinski *et al.*, 1980; Cote *et al.*, 1983; Houghton *et al.*, 1983).

There are an increasing number of reports on the fusion of human lymphocytes with drug-marked cell lines of human origin (Olsson and Kaplan, 1980; Croce *et al.*, 1980; Cote *et al.*, 1983; Houghton *et al.*, 1983; Larrick *et al.*, 1983). However, most studies have indicated that a low frequency of hybrid clones results from these fusions, and this has limited progress with this technology. In addition, most of the cell lines developed for fusions are lymphoblastoid lines, and not myelomas (Croce *et al.*, 1980; Sikora *et al.*, 1982; Edwards *et al.*, 1982; Chiorrazzi *et al.*, 1982; Larrick *et al.*, 1983; Glassy *et al.*, 1983). The experience of this laboratory and others has shown that it is difficult to grow human myelomas in tissue culture. Over the past 3 years only two out of 73 different myeloma specimens have been established as permanent cell lines in this laboratory. Both lines that were established were derived from patients with plasma cell leukemia; one secretes γ heavy chain and κ light chain, while the other only secretes κ light chain. Although one of these lines is relatively vigorous, most myelomas that have been established are slow growing and fastidious (Nilsson *et al.*, 1970; Karpas *et al.*, 1982), which may limit their usefulness as fusing partners.

In an effort to understand further the humoral immune response to cancer in humans, we have investigated the use of mouse and human hypoxanthine-guanine phosphoribosyltransferase (HGPRT)-deficient cell lines as fusing partners in the generation of hybridomas secreting human monoclonal antibody. We have compared five cell lines in fusions with human lymphocytes; the U266-derived SKO-007 human myeloma line (Olsson and Kaplan, 1980), the human lymphoblastoid cell lines LICR-LON-HMy2 (Edwards *et al.*, 1982), GM4672 (Croce *et al.*, 1980), and UC729-6 (Glassy *et al.*, 1983), and the mouse myeloma line NS-1 (Köhler and Milstein, 1976).

II. Properties of Drug-Marked Fusion Partners

Our study includes data from over 234 fusions. Lymphocytes from tumors, lymph node, spleen, and peripheral blood of tumor-bearing patients, as

TABLE I

Characteristics of the Drug-Marked Myeloma and Lymphoblastoid Lines Studied

Cell line	Karyotype	Heavy chain	Light chain	Cell doubling time (hr)	Comments
LICR-2	Human	γ	κ	24	EBNA+
SKO-007	Human	ε	λ	35	Mycoplasma-free
UC729-6	Human	μ	κ	24	EBNA+
GM4672	Human	γ	κ	30	EBNA+
NS-1	Mouse	—	κ	24	—

well as peripheral blood lymphocytes from normal individuals have been used in our fusions. The characteristics of the drug-marked myeloma and lymphoblastoid lines are shown in Table I. LICR-2, GM4672, UC729-6 and NS-1 have approximately the same doubling times, while that for SKO-007 is substantially longer. The LICR-2, GM4672, and UC729-6 lines were found to have the Epstein–Barr virus nuclear antigen (EBNA+) (Edwards et al., 1982; Croce et al., 1980; Glassy et al., 1983). The SKO-007 variant used in these fusions was rendered mycoplasma-free by Dr. Jørgen Fogh (Sloan-Kettering Institute). The cell lines were obtained from the following sources: SKO-007, Becton-Dickinson (Sunnyvale, California); LICR-2, P. Edwards, A. Neville, and M. O'Hare (Ludwig Institute for Cancer Research, London, England); GM4672, Human Genetic Mutant Cell Repository (Camden, New Jersey); UC729-6, M. Glassey, H. Handley, and I. Royston (University of California, San Diego, California); NS-1, U. Hammerling (Sloan-Kettering Institute, New York, New York). The drug-marked cells are maintained in medium consisting of RPMI 1640 supplemented with 7.5% fetal calf serum (FCS), penicillin at 100 U/ml, streptomycin at 100 μg/ml, and 8-azaguanine at 20 μg/ml. The lines are killed in medium containing 0.4 μM aminopterin.

A. Characterization of Fusion Conditions

Prior to fusion, lymphocytes and myeloma/lymphoblastoid lines were washed in RPMI 1640 several times, combined, and pelleted together in the final wash. All excess medium was aspirated away from the pellet, and 0.2 ml of 42% (w/v) polyethylene glycol (PEG) 4000 [in phosphate-buffered saline containing 10% (v/v) dimethylsulfoxide] was slowly added to the cell pellet with gentle mixing for 3 min at 37°C. Ten milliliters of RPMI 1640 with 7.5% FCS was then added drop by drop over 5 min. The resultant cell suspension was gently washed and suspended in postfusion medium (RPMI 1640, 15% FCS, penicillin 100 U/ml, streptomycin 100 μg/ml, 50 μM 2-mercaptoethanol, 0.1 mM hypoxanthine, 16 μM thymidine). The cells were incubated overnight at 37°C, resuspended in postfusion medium containing 0.4 μM aminopterin, and plated in 96-well tissue culture plates (Costar 3596) at a density of no more than 1×10^5 lymphocytes per well (on occasion the plating density was substantially less than this). Feeder layers of BALB/c or C57BL/6 mouse peritoneal cells (1×10^5 cells/well, plated 24–48 hr previously) were used. The medium was changed once a week, and cells were maintained in the presence of 0.4 μM aminopterin for 4–6 weeks.

A number of factors in the fusion procedure were analyzed. The results of fusions were highly variable, even given identical sources of lymphocytes and a given fusion partner. Because of this, a large number of fusions needed to be performed with each drug-marked line in order to compare their efficacy, and firm conclusions regarding optimal conditions were difficult to reach. However, several factors were found to influence results in a generally consistent fashion. These included:

1. Condition of the myeloma/lymphoblastoid lines. The lines were maintained in logarithmic-phase growth at >95% cell viability. Fusions with overgrown cultures resulted in a low frequency of clonal outgrowth.

2. Fusion ratios. Lymphocyte to myeloma/lymphoblastoid cell ratios of 1:1 or 2:1 resulted in 2–8 times greater clonal outgrowth than fusions at 5:1 or 10:1.

3. PEG. PEG used in fusions was maintained at pH 7.5–8.2. PEG at lower pH was found to give poor results.

4. Time of aminopterin addition. A delay in the addition of aminopterin to the fused cells for 24 hr resulted in more vigorous growth of clones and appeared to increase the number of clones obtained.

5. FCS. Significant differences in the frequency of clonal outgrowth were found with different lots of FCS. As initially observed by Edwards *et al.* (1982), some lots of FCS actually inhibited the growth and clonability of the myeloma/lymphoblastoid cell lines and the growth of Ig-secreting clones derived from fusions. Different lots of FCS were therefore prescreened for optimal growth-promoting properties by using these cell types.

6. Other medium supplements. Medium conditioned by several different cell types did not improve the frequency of clonal outgrowth. Supernatant from cultures of peripheral blood T cells (sheep red blood cell rosetting fraction) stimulated 4–6 days with phytohemagglutinin and added to the postfusion medium actually resulted in a marked reduction in resulting clones. No other supplements used appeared to affect clonal outgrowth, although the newly defined B-cell growth and differentiation factors need to be tested.

7. Changes in the fusion partners. The use of NS-1 that has been in continuous culture over long periods of time (6 months to 1 year) appears to result in poorer clonal outgrowth, and hybrids derived from these cells may be less stable for Ig production. We therefore maintain a stock of NS-1 frozen in liquid nitrogen, and keep this cell line in continuous culture for only 3–4 months.

B. Characterization of Fusion Partners

Clones appeared in the wells of the primary fusion plates over a variable period of time, depending on the fusion partner. In general, clones derived from fusion of human lymphocytes with NS-1 appeared 2–4 weeks after fusion, while clones derived from fusions with LICR-2, GM4672, UC729-6 and SKO-007 appeared anywhere from 4 to 7 weeks after fusion. The growth rate of the clones was variable, but in general, clones derived from NS-1 had a doubling time of 24–35 hr, clones derived from LICR-2 and UC729-6 doubled every 35–45 hr, while those from SKO-007 and GM4672 had a doubling time of >40 hr. Because of their earlier appearance and faster rate of growth, NS-1-derived clones could be screened for Ig production and antibody secretion and then subcultured sooner than clones derived from the human fusing partners.

The relative fusion efficiencies of each of the myeloma/lymphoblastoid lines was examined. Since the number of lymphocytes obtained from each specimen was quite variable, we calculated (as a basis for comparison) the number of clones that would have resulted from the fusion of 10^7 lymphocytes. This value was called the frequency of outgrowth. For over a given number of lymphocytes, fusions with NS-1 resulted in an average of four times more clones than fusions with UC729-6, eight times more clones than with LICR-2, and more than 20 times more clones than with GM4672 or SKO-007 (Table II). The fusion efficiency of the human drug-marked cell lines was compared in fusions with lymph node lymphocytes. LICR-2 and UC729-6 give comparable results (nine and 12 clones resulting from fusion with 10^7 lymphocytes, respectively), while fusions with SKO-007 and GM4672 were 5–10 times less efficient (Table II). These results are comparable to those originally published for these lines (Edwards *et al.*, 1982; Olsson and Kaplan, 1980; Croce *et al.*, 1980; Glassy *et al.*, 1983).

LICR-2 and SKO-007 gave the poorest results in fusions with peripheral blood lymphocytes, especially when compared to fusions with lymph node lymphocytes. (Few fusions were performed between peripheral blood lymphocytes and GM4672 or UC729-6, so these results were not included for comparison.) There are several explanations for this observation, including (1) the low percentage of B cells in peripheral blood, (2) suppression of the malignant phenotype of the resultant hybrid by the particular B-cell type in normal blood, resulting in less efficient hybrid outgrowth, (3) the fact that the stage of differentiation or activation of B cells in peripheral blood may not be optimal for hybrid formation or stability, or (4) destruction of hybrid cells by cytotoxic T cells elicited by surface antigens contributed by LICR-2 or SKO-007. If the latter possibility is involved in the low frequency of clonal outgrowth, removal of T cells prior to fusion should increase the frequency of Ig-secreting clones. Initial results indicate that this may be the case (Table II). The fusion frequency of LICR-2 or SKO-007 with T-cell-depleted peripheral

TABLE II
Results of Fusions of Lymphocytes from Different Sources
with Five Myeloma/Lymphoblastoid Lines

Source of lymphocytes	Number of fusions	Clones per 10^7 lymphocytes fused		Percent Ig+ wells[a]	Number of wells with growing clones
		Median	Range		
All fusions					
NS-1	37	50.0	0–250	50	1211
LICR-2	111	7.0	0–100	74	973
SKO-007	68	1.5	0–33	60	230
UC729-6[b]	10	12.1	0–41	51	270
GM4672[b]	8	1.0	0–1	100	8
Lymph node lymphocytes					
NS-1	17	45.0	0–155	53	709
LICR-2	46	9.0	0–100	75	677
SKO-007	30	2.0	0–26	70	88
UC729-6	10	12.1	0–41	51	270
GM4672	8	1.0	0–1	100	8
Peripheral blood lymphocytes					
NS-1	14	53.0	0–240	44	388
LICR-2	44	2.1	0–29	70	102
SKO-007	37	<1.0	0–33	65	86
T-Cell-depleted peripheral blood lymphocytes					
LICR-2	10	6.1	0–25	75	12
SKO-007	5	2.0	0–10	57	14
Splenocytes					
NS-1	1	60.0	—	80	60
LICR-2	4	4.0	1.4–33	70	107
SKO-007	4	1.6	0.67–5.8	20	41
Tumor-associated lymphocytes					
NS-1	5	46.7	0–250	60	54
LICR-2	7	10.1	0–50	80	75
SKO-007	2	<1.0	—	0	1

[a]Percent of wells with growing clones having detectable levels of Ig in the supernatant (>500 ng/ml).
[b]Fused with lymph node lymphocytes only.

blood mononuclear cells is substantially greater than with unseparated peripheral blood lymphocytes, and is comparable to results obtained in fusions with lymph node lymphocytes. Finally, it should be noted that the frequency of outgrowth for fusions of human lymphocytes (from any source) and NS-1 compares favorably with mouse splenocyte–mouse myeloma fusions, where the frequency of outgrowth is 25–100 clones per 10^7 splenocytes fused.

C. Immunoglobulin Production of Hybrid Clones

The composite experience from 234 fusions showed that the percentage of wells with growth that had detectable levels of immunoglobulin (>500 ng of Ig/ml of culture supernatant) was roughly similar for the myeloma/lymphoblastoid lines studied, although clones derived from LICR-2 and GM4672 showed a greater percentage of Ig production (Table II). [The level of γ chain secreted by the LICR-2 line (<100 ng/ml) was generally below the sensitivity of our Ig assay. However, there is some evidence that the production of the LICR-2-derived heavy chain may be increased after fusion (see Fig. 2).] Although all clones derived from GM4672 secreted Ig, too few clones were produced to make any definite statement regarding Ig production. Clones derived from UC729-6 often produced both a γ heavy chain and the parental μ heavy chain, and in cases where only μ heavy chain was detected, the secretion of only the parental heavy chain could not be excluded. (We did not, in general, distinguish Ig secretion of any of the parental lines from Ig secretion of the B cell in our initial screening assays.) Human and mouse light chains and ε heavy chain were not detected in these assays.

Although the mechanisms regulating the level of Ig production are unknown, it does not appear to be a feature conferred on the clone by the myeloma or lymphoblastoid fusion partners, at least not in the case of the cell lines used in this study. The level of Ig secreted was systematically compared for clones derived from NS-1, LICR-2, and SKO-007, where the most data were available (Fig. 1); 70–75% of Ig-secreting clones produced between 1 and 10 μg of Ig/ml and 25–30% produced between 11 and 100 μg/ml. A comparison of the effect of the source of lymphocytes on the level Ig produced did not reveal any consistent differences.

The relative proportion of clones secreting each of the major Ig classes (IgM, IgG, IgA) was independent of the myeloma/lymphoblastoid fusion partner, but appeared to be related to the source of lymphocytes. A higher proportion of clones derived from axillary lymph node lymphocytes of patients with breast cancer secreted IgA than did clones derived from peripheral blood lymphocytes, whereas the proportion of IgM-secreting clones was generally higher in fusions with peripheral blood lymphocytes (Cote et al., 1983). This increase in the IgA/IgM ratio seen in clones derived from axillary lymph node lymphocytes is consistent with work showing an increase in IgA levels and IgA-producing lymphocytes in the lymph nodes and tumors of

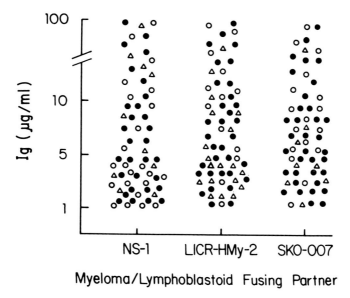

FIGURE 1. Level of Ig secreted by clones derived from fusions of NS-1, L1Cr-2, or SKO-007 with (●) lymph node lymphocytes, (○) peripheral blood lymphocytes, or (△) splenocytes.

breast cancer patients (Eremin *et al.*, 1982; Hsu *et al.*, 1981). It indicates that hybrid clones are derived from representative populations rather than from particular subsets of lymphocytes. This is an important consideration when interpreting these and other data.

D. Stability of Hybrid Clones

There has been a general feeling that clones produced through the fusion of human lymphocytes and mouse myeloma lose their ability to secrete human Ig soon after fusion, primarily due to preferential loss of human chromosomes by these clones. To gain perspective on this question, we have compiled stability data from studies of mouse myeloma–mouse splenocyte hybrids in our laboratory (Table III). Seventeen fusions were studied, from which 67 hybrids secreting antibody (Ab) to cell surface antigens were subcloned. After 1–3 subclonings, 32 of these clones no longer secreted Ab, so that 2–3 months after fusion, 53% of the original cultures retained the ability to secrete mouse monoclonal Ab.

In fusions with human lymphocytes, the percentage of stable Ig-producing clones was compared for fusions with NS-1, LICR-2, or SKO-007 (Table IV). Clones resulting from fusions of human lymphocytes with NS-1 were

TABLE III

Stability of Antibody Production by Hybrids Resulting from Fusions of Mouse Splenocytes with Mouse Myeloma NS-1[a]

Number of fusions studied	Number of Ab+ cultures subcloned	Number of subcloned cultures Ab+ 2–3 months postfusion
17	67	35

[a]Antibody to cell surface antigens detected by red cell rosetting assays.

almost as stable as those derived from fusions with LICR-2 or SKO-007. These results were comparable to those obtained with the mouse hybridomas.

NS-1-derived clones grow rapidly and are easily subcloned, whereas LICR-2- and SKO-007-derived clones grow poorly at limiting dilution, and so are difficult to subclone. Our limited results with clones derived from UC729-6 and GM4672 indicate that these also do not grow well at limiting dilutions. Sixteen percent of LICR-2-derived clones were lost during subcloning because of their inability to grow at low cell densities. The period of greatest loss of human Ig production is the first 2–3 months after fusion. Once the cells are subcloned, Ig-producing mouse–human and human–human hybrids can be selected in 70–80% of cases. So a key factor in maintaining Ig-secreting clones is early and repeated subcloning.

E. Evidence for the Hybrid Nature of the Clones

As the human hybridoma technology developed, it became important to determine whether or not the clones derived were true hybrids, because EBV transformation and B-cell mitogens can give rise to growing cell populations secreting Ig. This determination was particularly pertinent in the cases of the human lymphoblastoid fusing partners (LICR-2, UC729-6, and GM4672), which are EBNA+ and therefore a source of transforming EBV. In theory, the distinction between EBV transformants and hybrids should be straight-

TABLE IV

Stability of Ig Secretion by Clones Resulting from Fusions with NS-1, LICR-2, and SKO-007

Myeloma/lymphoblastoid line	Number of cultures Ig+ 2 months postfusion[a]		Number of cultures Ig+ 3–4 months postfusion[a]	
NS-1	76/126	(60%)	46/104	(44%)
LICR-2	76/102	(75%)	30/54	(56%)
SKO-007	24/34	(70%)	—	

[a]Ig detectable in culture supernatant at levels >500 ng/ml.

forward. EBV-transformed cells tend to be diploid, and secrete only one species of light and heavy chain. It was assumed that hybrid cells would be tetraploid and secrete the Ig product of the myeloma and lymphocyte. However, it is known that some EBV-transformed lines are tetraploid (O'Hare *et al.*, 1982) and we have found that mouse–mouse hybrids are substantially subtetraploid. Because of the problems in interpreting clonal ploidy, the most useful evidence for a human–human hybrid is production of distinct light and heavy Ig chains in addition to those produced by the myeloma or lymphoblastoid line. The secretion products of a series of LICR-2- and SKO-007-derived clones have been studied by sodium dodecyl sulfate–polyacrylamide gel electrophoresis (SDS–PAGE), and the Ig products of the myeloma, as well as new species of Ig heavy and light chains, have been detected (Fig. 2). Note that the production of γ heavy chain by the LICR-2 parent appeared to increase after fusion. In addition, clones derived from fusions with LICR-2 have been studied by immunofluorescent staining for intracytoplasmic κ and λ light chains. Thirty-three percent (3/9) of the clones studied produced λ light chain as well as the κ light chain of the LICR-2 line. The percentage of new λ light-chain-bearing clones corresponds to the percentage of light-chain-bearing lymphocytes in the human. Clones derived from SKO-007 were similarly studied, and it was found that 2/3 were producing a new κ light chain in addition to the λ light chain of the SKO-007 line. These data, along with results from a number of other groups (Olsson and Kaplan, 1980; Sikora *et al.*, 1982; Edwards *et al.*, 1982; Chiorrazzi *et al.*, 1982; Larrick *et al.*, 1983; Glassy *et al.*, 1983), indicate that true hybrids can be obtained from fusions of human lymphocytes with human myeloma or lymphoblastoid cell lines.

The hybrid character of clones derived from NS-1 fusions has clearly been established. Karyotypic analysis of six clones derived from fusions of human lymphocytes with NS-1 and secreting human Ig showed both mouse and human chromosomes. It is of interest that in the six clones studied, the chromosomal number is subtetraploid, although by flow cytometry the stable clones contain a tetraploid complement of DNA. These results suggest that there may be mouse and human chromosomal rearrangements in these hybrids. One possibility for the stability of mouse–human hybrids is translocation of human Ig-coding sequences onto mouse chromosomes, resulting in stable transmission during DNA replication and cell division.

III. Human Monoclonal Antibodies Directed against Cellular Antigens

Now that techniques for the production of human Ig by mouse–human or human–human hybridomas have been sufficiently developed, we have started to define the specificity of the secreted antibody. Because we are

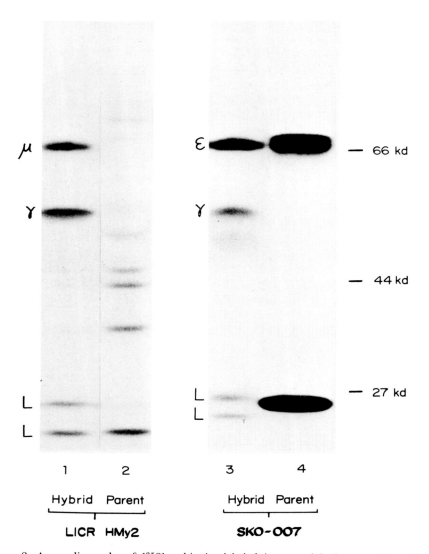

FIGURE 2. Autoradiographs of [^{35}S]methionine-labeled immunoglobulins precipitated from culture supernatants of (1) the Ma4 cell line (2) L1CR-2 human lymphoblastoid line, (3) Be3 cell line, and (4) SKO-007 human myeloma line. Ma4 is derived from a fusion of lymph node lymphocytes with L1CR-2, and Be3 is derived from a fusion of lymph node lymphocytes with SKO-007; both cell lines were subcloned twice at one cell per well. Ma4 produces both μ and γ heavy chains and two distinct light chains (L). One of the two light chains secreted by Ma4 corresponds to the κ light chain secreted by the L1CR-2 parental line. (No γ heavy chain was observed in the L1CR-2 supernatant due to low levels of secretion.) Be3 produces both γ and ε heavy chain and two light chains; one set of heavy and light chains corresponds to the ε and λ products of the SKO-007 parental line.

TABLE V

Immunoglobulin Produced by Cultures Derived from Fusions with Human Lymphocytes Reactive with Cell Surface Antigens[a]

Lymphocyte source	Number of cultures with antibody reactivity/number of Ig+ cultures tested for given fusion partner		
	NS-1	LICR-2	SKO-007
Lymph node	3/297	2/503	0/68
Peripheral blood	1/107	1/66	0/69
Spleen	0/30	0/41	0/4

[a]Reactivity to cell surface antigens was tested on live cells by the PA, IA, and anti-human Ig assays. Panel of human cell lines includes: (1) breast cancer: MCF-7, CAMA, MDA-MB-157, MDA-MB-231, Al Ab; (2) lung cancer: SK-LC-2, SK-LC-5, SK-LC-6, SK-LC-17, SK-LC-21; (3) colon cancer: SW48, SW1222, SK-CO-10; (4) melanoma: SK-MEL-28, SK-MEL-37, SK-MEL-41; (5) astrocytoma: U251 MG, SK-MG-1; (6) renal cancer: SK-RC-2, SK-RC-6, SK-RC-7, SK-RC-9; (7) normal kidney: Pa-An, Qu, Pi

interested in the human immune response to tumors, cultured cancer cells have been the major focus of our analysis of human monoclonal antibodies.

Initial screening of the hybrid supernatants has revealed that seven of 1185 Ig-secreting clones studied, or 0.6%, produce antibody to cell surface antigens present on cultured human tumor cell lines, as detected by the protein A (PA), immune adherence (IA), or anti-human Ig (anti-Ig) red cell rosetting assays (Table V). However, 65 of the 1185 clones studied, or 5.5%, produce antibody to intracellular antigens as detected by indirect immunofluorescence on human tumor cell lines fixed with methanol–acetone (1:1) (Cote *et al.*, 1983; Houghton *et al.*, 1983), 0.08% glutaraldehyde, or 3.7% formaldehyde (5–10 min fixation in each case) (Table VI).

Two general conclusions may be drawn from these results. It appears that a large proportion of the B-cell repertoire in normal individuals and patients with cancer is directed to the production of antibodies to cellular antigens. However, the great majority of these reactivities are directed against intracellular antigens. Antibodies directed against cell surface antigens are rare, possibly due to: (1) a general prohibition against the development of autoantibodies to cell surface antigens due to immunologic tolerance; (2) antigen loss by cultured cells; testing these antibodies against noncultured fresh tissue may demonstrate a greater percentage of cell surface reactivities; (3) greater polymorphism of cell surface vs. intracellular antigens; as a consequence, the appropriate cell lines may not be included in the tissue culture

TABLE VI

Immunoglobulin Produced by Cultures Derived from Fusions
with Human Lymphocytes Reactive
with Intracellular Antigens[a]

Lymphocyte source	Number of cultures with antibody reactivity/number of Ig+ cultures tested for given fusion partner		
	NS-1	LICR-2	SKO-007
Lymph node	14/297	13/503	5/68
Peripheral blood	6/107	4/66	4/69
Spleen	13/30	5/41	1/4

[a]Reactivity to intracellular antigens was tested on fixed cells by indirect immunofluorescence. Panel of human cell lines includes: (1) breast cancer: MCF-7, CAMA, MDA-MB-157; (2) lung cancer: SK-LC-6, SK-LC-17, SK-LC-21; (3) colon cancer: SW48, SW1222; (4) melanoma: SK-MEL-28, SK-MEL-41; (5) astrocytoma: U251 MG, SK-MG-1; (6) renal cancer: SK-RC-6, SK-RC-7, SK-RC-29; (7) normal kidney: Pa-AN, Qu, Pi

panel; and (4) a greater range of determinants within the cell than on the cell surface.

A. Antibody Reactivity with Cell Surface Antigens

Two human monoclonal antibodies directed against cell surface antigens have been tested on a large panel of cells in culture by absorption. In both cases, the antigens being detected show restricted distributions (Table VII).

Ri37 is an IgG antibody derived from a fusion of NS-1 with axillary lymph node lymphocytes of a patient with breast cancer. The hybrid producing this antibody has been subcloned five times and has been stable for antibody production over a 2-year period. It secretes between 2 and 5 μg IgG/ml of culture supernatant and has remained in bulk culture (without further subcloning) for more than 8 months without loss of antibody titer.

The Ri37 antibody is detected by both the PA and anti-Ig assays, but not by IA assays. The antibody titer (reaction with 50% of target cells) on one of the cell lines expressing the antigen (SK-MEL-41) is 1:100,000, and reactivity can be detected at supernatant dilutions of over 1:1,000,000. Absorption tests show that the antigen is expressed by a restricted number of malignant tumors. The only normal cell type that has been found to express the antigen is normal mature B lymphocytes; the antigen is not expressed by any other hematopoietic cell type, including T cells, macrophages, granulocytes, EBV-

TABLE VII
Absorption Analysis of Two Human Monoclonal Antibodies Reactive with Cell Surface Antigens[a,b]

Cell line	Ri37	Ma4
Breast cancer		
MCF-7	—	—
CAMA	—	+
BT-20	—	—
Al Ab	—	+
Colon cancer		
HT-29	—	+
SW680	NT	—
SW1116	—	NT
SW122	—	+
Lung cancer		
SK-LC-6	+	+
SK-LC-8	+	—
SK-LC-13	—	+
SK-LC-LL	+	NT
Renal cancer		
SK-4C-7	—	—
SK-RC-9	—	+
SK-RC-28	—	+
Bladder cancer		
TCC-SUP	+	—
253-J	—	—
Scb	—	+
T-24	—	+
Ovarian cancer		
SK-OV-3	—	—
SK-OV-4	NT	—
OV 2774	—	+
Cervical cancer		
Me-180	—	—
Melanoma		
SK-MEL-19	—	—
SK-MEL-28	—	—
SK-MEL-33	—	+
SK-MEL-41	+	—
Malignant glioma		
SK-MG-1	—	+
SK-MG-4	—	NT
U251 MG	—	—
Hematopoietic tumors		
P-12	—	NT
MOLT-4	—	NT
Raji	—	NT
BALL-1	—	NT
SK-Ly-16	—	—
SK-Ly-18	—	—

(continued)

TABLE VII (*Continued*)

Cell line	Ri37	Ma4
EBV-transformed B cells		
AX, AS, DX, EU	—	—
Adult fibroblasts		
AS, AX, DX, EU	—	—
Normal kidney		
Pa-An, QU, Pi	—	—
Melanocytes		
FS751	NT	—
FS752	NT	—
Hematopoietic Cells		
B cells	+	—
T cells	—	—
Macrophages	—	—
Granulocytes	—	—
Erythrocytes		
A, B, AB, O, Rh+, Rh−	—	—

[a]Equal volumes of packed cells and Ri37 supernatant (diluted 1:1000 to 1:2000) or Ma4 supernatant (diluted 1:64 to 1:256) were mixed and incubated 1 hr at room temperature. After removal of absorbing cells by centrifugation, residual reactivity was tested on SK-MEL-41 in the case of Ri37 or SK-RC-9 in the case of Ma4.
[b]+, Cell line absorbed antibody reactivity; —, cell line did not absorb antibody reactivity; NT, cell line not tested.

transformed B cells, or malignant hematopoietic cells. Thus, in the hematopoietic lineage, Ri37 identifies a B-cell differentiation antigen.

Ma4 is an IgM antibody secreted by a clone derived from a fusion of LICR-2 with regional lymph node lymphocytes of a patient with recurrent melanoma. The line has been subcloned four times and has been stable for antibody production over 2 years. It secretes 5 μg IgM/ml of culture supernatant. This line also secretes IgG (2 μg/ml) presumably derived from the LICR-2 fusion partner (Fig. 2).

The Ma4 antibody is detected by IA and anti-Ig assays, but not by PA assays. The antibody titer on SK-RC-9 is 1:1000. The antigen detected by antibody Ma4 is expressed in a restricted number of malignant tumors and has not been detected on any normal cells tested so far. The antigen has been found to be heat stable and resistant to treatment with trypsin and proteinase K, and it is extractable by treatment with chloroform and methanol. It is, therefore, most likely a lipid antigen, and further characterization is ongoing.

B. Antibody Reactivity with Intracellular Antigens

Human monoclonal antibodies reacting with a wide range of intracellular determinants have been detected, including reactivities with cytoplasmic, cytoskeletal, membrane-associated, and nuclear antigens, as well as Golgi complex and structures consistent with endoplasmic reticulum. The majority of these antibodies (approximately 50%) react with antigens expressed in a wide variety of cell lines. However, a number of human monoclonal antibodies recognize antigens that show tissue specificity or are highly restricted.

The specificity analysis of two human monoclonal antibodies directed against intracellular antigens is shown in Fig. 3. Indirect immunofluorescence assays were perfomed on cells fixed in methanol–acetone (1:1 v/v) for 5 min. M54 detects an antigen found in epithelial cells, and not in cells of neuroectodermal origin (Fig. 3A), while M304 reacts only with cells of neuroectodermal origin, and not with cells of epithelial origin (Fig. 3B).

A series of human monoclonal antibodies have been found that react with cytoskeletal proteins of the intermediate filament family (Thomson *et al.*, 1984). Antibody M307 reacts only with cells of mesodermal origin, and after incubating of these cells with colcemid the reactivity is observed to "collapse" toward the nucleus. By Western blotting, M307 was found to react with a detergent-insoluble protein of molecular weight 57,000. These data indicate that M307 reacts with vimentin. In contrast, several antibodies have been found to react only with cells of epithelial origin (Pa24, C29, Hull, Hu22). Detergent extraction and Western blot analysis indicate that these antibodies react with cytokeratin filaments. We have detected an antibody (De8) that reacts with an epitope common to all classes of intermediate filaments (vimentin, cytokeratins, neurofilaments, glial fibrillary acidic protein, and desmin). These antibodies are able to distinguish the histogenesis of cells and tissues, and are currently used to identify intermediate filament proteins in frozen and paraffin-embedded malignant and normal tissue sections by immunohistochemical analysis (Cote *et al.*, 1984).

These results clearly demonstrate that human monoclonal antibodies that define tumor antigens (e.g., Ma4) and differentiation antigens (e.g., Ri37, M54, M304) can be generated using the techniques described here. Although these data can be interpreted as an indication that patients with cancer may be able to respond in some direct way to their tumor, definitive conclusions are difficult to draw at this time. Our data indicate that hybridomas derived from the lymphocytes of normal individuals can secrete Ab to cellular antigens, and a systematic analysis of the B-cell repertoire in tumor-bearing and normal individuals is now underway. In addition, the significance of antibodies directed against intracellular antigens needs to be determined; do those antibodies play any role in tumor recognition and immunity, or do they simply arise as a result of tumor growth (for example, due to the increased rate of cell

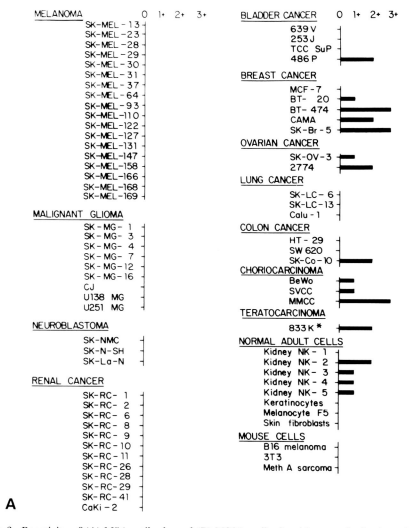

FIGURE 3. Reactivity of (A) M54 antibody and (B) M304 antibody with a panel of cultured cells using indirect immunofluorescence assays. Horizontal bars indicate intensity (0–3+) of immunofluorescence reactions. (*) In the case of 833K teratocarcinoma cell line, only 10% of cultured cells reacted with M54 antibody.

death with subsequent release of intracellular antigens in tumors)? In any event, the ability to produce human monoclonal antibodies is generating detailed information about the B-cell repertoire, and is providing a new class of reagents with which to study tumor antigens, differentiation antigens, and

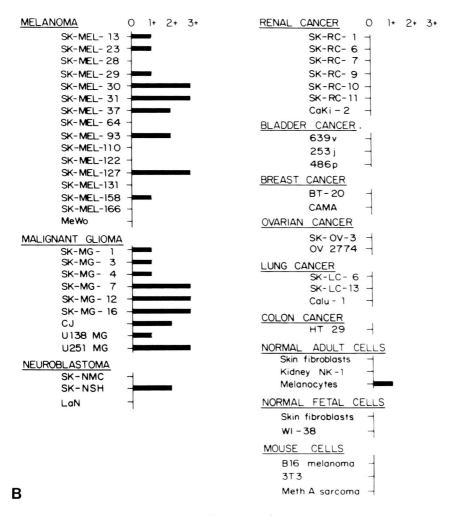

FIGURE 3. (*continued*)

cellular antigens in general. Using this technology, we now have the tools to approach some of the fundamental questions in human tumor immunology.

IV. Summary

Human lymphocytes from peripheral blood, regional lymph nodes, tumor, and spleen from patients with cancer, and from peripheral blood of normal individuals, have been shown to fuse with the human drug-marked cell lines SKO-007, LICR-LON-HMy2, GM4672, and UC729-6, and with the mouse drug-marked cell line NS-1, resulting in hybridomas that secrete human monoclonal Ig. The fusion efficiencies, stability, and percentage of clones that secrete Ig indicate that this technology can now be used to define the B-cell repertoire in normal individuals and patients with cancer. Antibodies that recognize cell surface and intracellular antigens on human tumor (and normal) cell lines have been identified using the technology described here. These include antibodies that distinguish cells of different histogenesis and different stages of differentiation within a given lineage. We can now use these reagents and techniques to extend our analysis of the human immune response to tumors in an effort to determine whether patients with cancer recognize distinctive tumor antigens.

ACKNOWLEDGMENTS

We thank Jannette Rios for her help in the preparation of the manuscript and Dr. Lloyd J. Old for his support and comments. This work was supported in part by grants IM-333 from the American Cancer Society and NCI CA-34079 from the National Cancer Institute, National Institutes of Health. R. J. C. is a recipient of a National Research Service Award (3 F32 CA7325-0151) from the National Cancer Institute.

References

Bashford, E. F., 1913, The constancy and variability of tumor cells during propagation, in: *Transactions of the International Congress of Medicine, London*, Section III, Part 2, p. 59.
Carey, T. E., Takahashi, T., Resnick, L. A., Oettgen, H. F., and Old, L. J., 1976, Cell surface antigens of human malignant melanoma: Mixed hemadsorption assays for humoral immunity to cultured autologous melanoma cells, *Proc. Natl. Acad. Sci. USA* **73**:3278–3282.
Chiorrazzi, N., Wasserman, R. L., and Kunkel, H. G., 1982, Use of Epstein–Barr virus-transformed B cell lines for the generation of immunoglobulin-producing human B cell hybridomas, *J. Exp. Med.* **156**:930–935.
Cote, R. J., Morrissey, D. M., Houghton, A. N., Beattie, E. J., Oettgen, H. F., and Old, L. J., 1983, Generation of human monoclonal antibodies reactive with cellular antigens, *Proc. Natl. Acad. Sci. USA* **80**:2026–2030.
Cote, R. J., Houghton, A. N., Cordon-Cardo, C., Thomson, T. M., Morrissey, D. M., Oettgen, H. F., and Old, L. J., 1984, Immune response of cancer patients: Analysis with human monoclonal antibodies, *Fed. Proc.* **43**:1663 (abstract 1441).
Crawford, D., Callard, R., Muggeridge, M., Mitchell, D., Zanders, E., and Beverley, P. C., 1983, Production of human monoclonal antibody to X31 influenza virus nucleoprotein, *J. Gen. Virol* **64**:697–700.
Croce, C. M., Linnenbach, A., Hall, W., Steplewski, Z., and Koprowski, H., 1980, Production of human hybridomas secreting antibodies to measles virus, *Nature* **288**:488–489.
Dippold, W. G., Lloyd, K. O., Li, L. T. C., Ikeda, H., Oettgen, H. F., and Old, L. J., 1980, Cell surface antigens of human malignant melanoma: Definition of six antigenic systems with mouse monoclonal antibodies, *Proc. Natl. Acad. Sci. USA* **77**:6114–6118.

Edwards, P. A. W., Smith, C. M., Neville, A. M., and O'Hare, M. J., 1982, A human–human hybridoma system based on a fast growing mutant of the ARH-77 plasma cell leukemia-derived line, *Eur J. Immunol.* **12:**641–648.

Epenetos, A. A., Canti, G., Taylor-Papadimitriou, J., Curling, M., and Bodmer, W. F., 1982, Use of two epithelium-specific monoclonal antibodies for diagnosis of malignancy in serous effusions, *Lancet* **ii:**1004–1006.

Eremin, O., Coombs, R. R. A., Prospero, T. D., and Plumb, D., 1982, T-Lymphocyte and B-lymphocyte subpopulations infiltrating human mammary carcinomas, *J. Natl. Cancer Inst.* **69:**1–8.

Foley, E. J., 1953, Antigenic properties of methylcholanthrene-induced tumors in mice of the strain of origin, *Cancer Res.* **13:**835–837.

Garret, T. J., Takahashi, T., Clarkson, B. D., and Old, L. J., 1977, Detection of antibody to autologous human leukemia cells by immune adherence assays, *Proc. Natl. Acad. Sci. USA* **74:**4587–4590.

Glassy, M. C., Handley, H. H., Hagiwara, H., and Royston, I., 1983, UC729-6, a human lympho-blastoid B-cell line useful for generating antibody-secreting human–human hybridomas, *Proc. Natl. Acad. Sci. USA* **80:**6327–6331.

Gross, L., 1943, Intradermal immunization of C3H mice against a sarcoma that originated in an animal of the same line, *Cancer Res.* **3:**326–333.

Houghton, A. N., Brooks, H., Cote, R. J., Taormina, M. C., Oettgen, H. F., and Old, L. J., 1983, Detection of cellular antigens by human monoclonal antibodies, *J. Exp. Med.* **158:**53–65.

Houghton, A. N., Mintzer, D., Cordon-Cardo, C., Welt, S., Fliegel, B., Vadhan, S., Carswell, E., Melamed, M. R., Oettgen, H. F., and Old, L. J., 1985, Mouse monoclonal antibody detecting GD_3 ganglioside: A phase I trial in patients with malignant melanoma, *Proc. Natl. Acad. Sci. USA* **82:** 1242–1246.

Hsu, S.-M., Raine, L., and Nayak, R. N., 1981, Medullary carcinoma of breast: An immu-nohistochemical study of its lymphoid stoma, *Cancer* **48:**1368–1376.

Irie, R. F., Sze, L. L., and Saxton, R. E., 1982, Human antibody to OFA-I, a tumor antigen, produced *in vitro* by Epstein–Barr virus-transformed human B-lymphoid cell lines, *Proc. Natl. Acad. Sci. USA* **79:**5666–5670.

Karpas, A., Fischer, P., and Swirsky, D., 1982, Human plasmacytoma with an unusual karyotype growing *in vitro* and producing light chain immunoglobulin, *Lancet* **i:**931–933.

Köhler, G., and Milstein, C., 1975, Continuous cultures of fused cells secreting antibody of predefined specificity, *Nature* **236:**495–497.

Köhler, G., and Milstein, C., 1976, Derivation of specific antibody-producing tissue culture and tumor cell lines by cell fusion, *Eur. J. Immunol.* **6:** 511–519.

Koskimies, S., 1980, Human lymphoblastoid cell line producing specific antibody against Rh antigen D, *Scand. J. Immunol.* **11:**73–77.

Kozbor, D., and Roder, J. C., 1981, Requirements for the establishment of high-titred human monoclonal antibodies against tetanus toxoid using the Epstein–Barr virus technique, *J. Immunol.* **127:**1275–1280.

Larrick, J. W., Truitt, K. E., Raubitschek, A. A., Senyk, G., and Wang, J. C., 1983, Characteriza-tion of human hybridomas secreting antibody to tetanus toxoid, *Proc. Natl. Acad. Sci. USA* **80:**6376–6380.

Miller, R. A., and Levy, R., 1981, Response of cutaneous T cell lymphoma to therapy with hybridoma monoclonal antibody, *Lancet* **ii:**226–230.

Miller, R. A., Maloney, D., Warnke, R., McDougall, I. R., Wood, G., Kawakami, T., Dilley, J., Goris, M. L., and Levy, R., 1982, Considerations for treatment with hybridoma antibodies, in: *Hybridomas in Cancer Diagnosis and Treatment* (M. S. Mitchell and H. F. Oettgen, eds.), Raven Press, New York, pp. 133–145.

Nilsson, K., Bennich, H., Johansson, S. G. O., and Pontén, J., 1970, Established immunoglobulin producing myeloma (IgE) and lymphoblastoid (IgG) cell lines from an IgE myeloma patient, *Clin. Exp. Immunol.* **7:**477–489.

Nowinski, R. C., Berglund, C., Lane, J., Lostrom, M., Bernstein, I., Young, S., Hill, L., and

Cooney, M., 1980, Human monoclonal antibody against Forssman antigen, *Science* **210**:537–539.

O'Hare, M. J., Smith, C. M., and Edwards, P. A. W., 1982, A new human hybridoma system (LICR-LON-HMy2) and its use in the production of human monoclonal antibodies, in: *Protides of Biological Fluids, Colloquium 30* (H. Peeters, ed.), Pergamon Press, Oxford, pp. 265–268.

Olsson, L., and Kaplan, H. S., 1980, Human–human hybridomas producing monoclonal antibodies of predefined antigenic specificity, *Proc. Natl. Acad., Sci. USA* **77**:5429–5431.

Osborn, M., and Weber, K., 1982, Intermediate filaments: Cell-type specific markers in differentiation and pathology, *Cell* **31**:303–306.

Papsidero, L. D., Croghan, G. A., O'Connell, M. S., Valenzuela, L. A., Nemoto, T., and Chu, T. M., 1983, Monoclonal antibodies (F36/22 and M7/105) to human breast carcinoma, *Cancer Res.* **43**:1741–1747.

Pfreundschuh, M., Shiku, H., Takahashi, T., Ueda, R., Ransohoff, J., Oettgen, H. F., and Old, L. J., 1978, Serological analysis of cell surface antigens of malignant human brain tumors, *Proc. Natl. Acad. Sci. USA* **75**:5122–5126.

Prehn, R. T., and Main, J. M., 1957, Immunity to methylcholanthrene-induced sarcomas, *J. Natl. Cancer Inst.* **18**:769–778.

Schlom, J., Wunderlich, D., and Teramoto, Y. A., 1980, Generation of human monoclonal antibodies reactive with human mammary carcinoma cells, *Proc. Natl. Acad. Sci. USA* **77**:6841–6845.

Sikora, K., Alderson, T., Phillips, J., and Watson, J. V., 1982, Human hybridomas from malignant gliomas, *Lancet* **ii**:11–14.

Steinitz, M., Klein, G., Koskimies, S., and Makel, O., 1977, EB virus-induced B lymphocyte cell lines producing specific antibody, *Nature* **269**:420–422.

Thomson, T. M., Cote, R. J., Houghton, A. N., Oettgen, H. F., and Old, L. J., 1984, Human monoclonal antibodies recognizing intermediate filament (IF) molecules, *Fed. Proc.* **43**:1513 (abstract 564).

Ueda, R., Ogata, S., Morrissey, D. M., Finstad, C. L., Szkudlarek, J., Whitmore, W. F., Oettgen, H. F., Lloyd, K. O., and Old, L. J., 1981, Cell surface antigens of human renal cancer defined by mouse monoclonal antibodies: Identification of tissue specific kidney glycoproteins, *Proc. Natl. Acad. Sci. USA* **78**:5122–5126.

Zurawski, V. R., Haber, E., and Black, P. H., 1978, Continuous human lymphoblastoid cell lines, *Science* **199**:1439–1441.

12
Design and Production of Human Monoclonal Antibodies to Human Cancers

Mark C Glassy, Harold H. Handley,
and Ivor Royston

I. Introduction

Central questions of the tumor immunologist pertain to the type and nature of antigens appearing in the malignant state and methods used to detect them. Monoclonal antibody (MAb) technology (Köhler and Milstein, 1975) provides investigators an opportunity to study virtually any immunogenic molecule with exact precision and has been successful in detecting human tumor antigens (Boss *et al.*, 1983). Recently, hybridoma technology has been extended to the production of human MAbs (Olsson and Kaplan, 1980; Schlom *et al.*, 1980; Croce *et al.*, 1980; Glassy *et al.*, 1981, 1983a; Sikora and Phillips, 1981; Edwards *et al.*, 1982) and is being used to study human tumor antigens.

Tumor patients have been shown to mount both cell-mediated and humoral immune responses to their tumors (Hellstrom and Brown, 1979). Therefore, by immortalizing human B cells producing such antitumor antibodies, a steady supply of antibody will be available not only to study the immune response of the patient, but also to characterize the respective antigens. Schlom *et al.* (1980) demonstrated, and others confirmed (Sikora and

Mark C Glassy, Harold H. Handley, and Ivor Royston • Cancer Center, University of California, San Diego, and Veterans Administration Medical Center, San Diego, California 92103.

Wright, 1981; Glassy *et al.*, 1983a; Lowe *et al.*, 1984), that B lymphocytes in the regional draining lymph nodes of cancer patients are primed to synthesize antibodies against tumor antigens. Therefore, these lymphocytes when immortalized through the now classical hybridoma technique will yield human MAbs reactive with tumor antigens.

The production of human MAbs to human tumor antigens will probably result in an expansion of the library of antitumor MAbs currently available from murine sources and may lead to the development of clinically useful reagents for the detection and therapy of human tumors. Also, a major problem facing the *in vivo* use of murine MAbs is the elicitation of a host immune response to these foreign proteins. The use of human MAbs may obviate this potentially serious problem.

II. Development and Characterization of UC 729-6

To date the production of human MAbs has been hindered by the difficulty of consistently generating stable human Ig-secreting hybridomas, either from interspecies mouse–human hybridomas or intraspecies human–human hybridomas. Mouse–human hybrids preferentially eliminate human chromosomes (Ruddle, 1973; Glassy and Ferrone, 1982) and over time will lose the loci coding for human Ig, a problem encountered by others (Sikora and Wright, 1982). Human–human hybrids have suffered from the lack of a suitable fusion partner. This latter problem has been solved in our laboratory by developing UC 729-6, a diploid 6-thioguanine-resistant human lymphoblastoid B-cell line that, when used as a fusion partner, yields stable human–human hybridomas (Glassy *et al.*, 1981, 1983a; Handley and Royston, 1982). Others (Croce *et al.*, 1980; Chiorazzi *et al.*, 1982) have also demonstrated the feasibility of using 8-azaguanine- or 6-thioguanine-resistant human lymphoblastoid B-cell lines in generating human Ig-secreting human hybridomas. UC 729-6 has reproducibly fused with human lymphocytes isolated from peripheral blood, spleen, tonsils, and lymph nodes. A recent independent report by Abrams *et al.* (1983) compared currently available human cell lines (both B-cell and myeloma) for generating human hybridomas and concluded that UC 729-6 was the optimal cell line to use with respect to the number of Ig-secreting hybridomas generated and their stability over long-term culturing.

UC 729-6, an Epstein–Barr virus (EBV)-positive hypoxanthine phosphoribosyltransferase-negative cell line, was isolated by treating parent WIL-2 cells (Levy *et al.*, 1968, 1971) with 25 μM 6-thioguanine (Lever *et al.*, 1974). Prior to fusions, UC 729-6 cells were incubated with 100 μM 6-thioguanine. Some general characteristics of UC 729-6 are outlined in Table I.

Approximately 95% of the UC 729-6 fusions attempted in our laboratory have resulted in hybrid formation and approximately 85% of those contained

Table I

General Characteristics of UC 729-6

Human lymphoblastoid B-cell line derived from parental WIL-2 cells
6-Thioguanine-resistant and dies in HAT medium within 10 days
F_c-receptor-negative
HLA profile: HLA-A1, A2, B5, B17, DR4, DR7
Diploid, with a $21p^+$ marker chromosome
Secretes ≤ 20–50 ng IgM/10^6 cells per ml per day
Doubles every 17 hr

hybridomas secreting Ig. The fusion frequencies of UC 729-6 with human lymphocytes are shown in Table II. Overall, lymphocytes isolated from lymph nodes and tonsils yielded higher fusion frequencies than those from peripheral blood and spleen. The highest percentage of Ig-secreting hybridomas was obtained with lymph node lymphocytes and IgM-producers were more prevalent than IgG-producers.

UC 729-6 was also fused with malignant B lymphocytes from patients with lymphoma and leukemia. Hybrids formed in approximately 85% of the attempts, with fusion frequencies ranging from 3 to 10 (see note, Table II). All of the resulting hybrids secreted Ig, all of which were either monoclonal κ or λ. Consequently, UC 729-6 is being used in our laboratory to rescue leukemia and lymphoma Ig for the production of anti-idiotypes.

III. Enzyme Immunoassay to Qualitate and Quantitate Human Immunoglobulin

One of the problems associated with generating human MAbs entails the screening of a large number of hybridoma supernatants while searching for

Table II

Fusion Frequencies of UC 729-6[a]

Lymphocyte source	Fusions	Number of hybrid$^+$ wells/10^6 lymphocytes	Percent of hybrids secreting Ig	
			IgG	IgM
Lymph node	12	0.29–3.16 (1.9)	0–24 (11)	0–36 (29)
Peripheral blood lymphocytes	8	0.0–1.31 (0.51)	0	0–66 (41)
Spleen	2	0.27–0.80 (0.54)	0	25–50 (38)
Tonsil	7	0.35–5.34 (2.8)	0–42 (17)	0–37 (20)

[a]After fusion, cells were plated at 1.0×10^5 per well. The means ($\bar{x}$) are shown in parentheses.

antibody specificity. Also, since most human Ig-secreting hybridomas derived from fusions with UC 729-6 grow rapidly (doubling times of about 25–30 hr), questions pertaining to the type, amount, and specificity of these MAbs must be answered quickly to avoid constant culturing. Therefore, an assay that emphasizes speed and simplicity is advantageous. We have developed (Glassy et al., 1983b, 1984) a micro enzyme-linked immunoassay (EIA) utilizing a filtration method that allows the rapid, simple, and sensitive detection of human MAbs that recognize either soluble or cell surface antigens. This assay involves the immobilization of target cells onto a solid support followed by incubation with the test human hybridoma supernatant and subsequent analysis by EIA. This is summarized in Fig. 1. This assay, when read visually, takes no more than 2 hr to complete.

The EIA procedure consists in adding $(1.0–2.0) \times 10^5$ target cells (or the appropriate amount of soluble antigen) suspended in fetal calf serum buffer (FCS buffer; 10% fetal bovine serum, 1% bovine serum albumin, and 0.3% gelatin in PBS with 0.1% thimerosol) per well of a specially designed 96-well plate (Cleveland et al., 1979) that serves as both an incubation chamber and a filtration manifold. Cells and soluble antigens were immobilized onto glass fiber filter disks in these plates by application of 380 mm Hg of vacuum. Fifty microliters of each test human MAb was then added and allowed to incubate 30 min, after which each well of the plate was washed three times with 0.3% gelatin in PBS (gel buffer) by the same vacuum filtration method. After washing, each well received 50 μl of an appropriate dilution of horseradish peroxidase (HRP)-conjugated goat anti-human IgG, IgM, etc. (Tago), incubated 30 min, and again washed three times with gel buffer. All procedures and incubations were carried out at room temperature. The wells were sealed and 250 μl of the substrate for the peroxidase enzyme o-phenylenediamine (400 μg/ml dissolved in 0.05 M citrate buffer, pH 5.0, with 60 ng/ml of H_2O_2) was added to each well and incubated in the dark. The reaction was stopped by adding 50 ul of 2.5 M H_2SO_4 and the plates were either read visually or at 490 nm using a Dynatech micro-EIA reader, model MR 600.

For human MAb concentration determinations, a titration of Ig (e.g., IgG or IgM) of known concentration was added to some wells in lieu of the test MAb and developed as described above to generate a standard curve. The test human MAb concentrations were then obtained from this curve.

IV. Use of Regional Draining Lymph Nodes of Cancer Patients as a Source of Antitumor Antibodies

The immortalization of lymphocytes isolated from regional draining lymph nodes of cancer patients has allowed us to begin a systematic analysis of the immune response generated by these patients to their tumor antigens. A schematic of this process is outlined in Fig. 2. As shown, there are three major

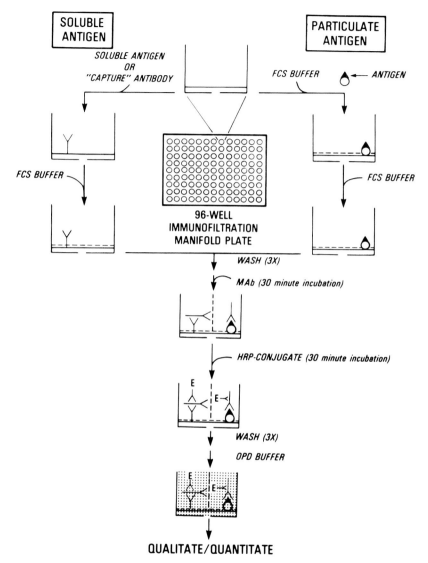

FIGURE 1. Flow chart of the enzyme immunoassay showing separate procedures for both soluble and particulate antigens. Results are either read visually or by an EIA reader.

sources of antigens to which antibodies can be raised, two of which are cancer related. The first consists of shed antigens such as those released, either actively or passively, by tumor cells and filtered out by the lymph node, thereby activating B cells. Second, there are metastatic cells, which embed themselves within the node and generate an antibody response against their tumor antigens. Also included in this diagram are naturally occurring self-

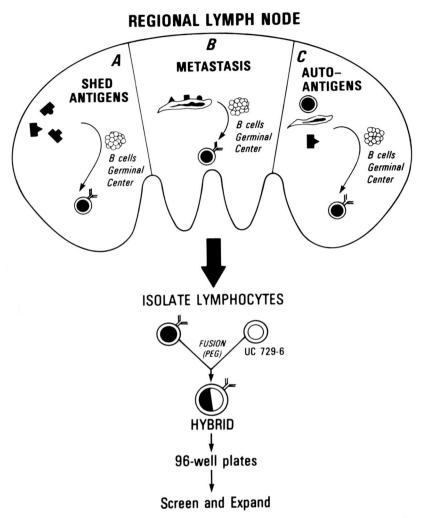

FIGURE 2. Flow diagram illustrating the types of antigens processed by a human lymph node in the generation of anticancer MAbs. (A) Shed antigens (from malignant and/or normal cells) enter the lymph node through the afferent lymphatics and stimulate B-cell proliferation. (B) Metastatic cells, which display both normal and tumor-related antigens, enter the lymph node and stimulate B cells to make antibodies. (C) Though not directly related to cancer, humans may generate antibodies to normal cells and soluble antigens released from these cells. The immunoglobulin-secreting B lymphocytes are isolated (Glassy *et al.*, 1983a) and immortalized by fusion with UC 729-6.

antigens consisting of both shed and cell-bound types, which, under certain conditions, may generate an antibody response possibly giving rise to pathological conditions. In each of these cases, UC 729-6 serves as a suitable vector to immortalize and stablize the Ig-secreting B lymphocyte.

A flow diagram illustrating the sequence of events our laboratory uses in generating anticancer MAbs is shown in Fig. 3. After establishing which human hybridomas are secreting Ig, their supernatants are screened against an appropriate panel of cell types. Although the ideal case would be to first screen the generated human MAbs against autologous tumor tissue, this is difficult to do in practice due to its availability in insufficient amounts or lack of availability altogether. In our approach we utilize cell lines as a first screen since they are readily accessible and easy to grow and manipulate. Subsequent screens, however, do incorporate staining of primary tissue types as frozen sections tested by immunofluoresence and/or immunoperoxidase. Since we postulate that deviations in the relative three-dimensional spatial arrangements of cells may result in altered expression of tumor antigens, we incorporate both established cell lines and tissue sections in screens for anticancer human MAbs.

Both karyotype (Glassy *et al.*, 1983a) and cytofluorographic (Glassy *et al.*, 1983a,c) analyses of our human–human hybrids have shown them to be pseudotetraploid hybridomas and not merely revertants of UC 729-6 or EBV-transformed cells. The presence of genetic elements of both parental cell types, such as a tetraploid DNA content, the $21p^+$ marker chromosome of UC 729-6 (Glassy *et al.*, 1983a), and the rescue of new Ig have shown that the

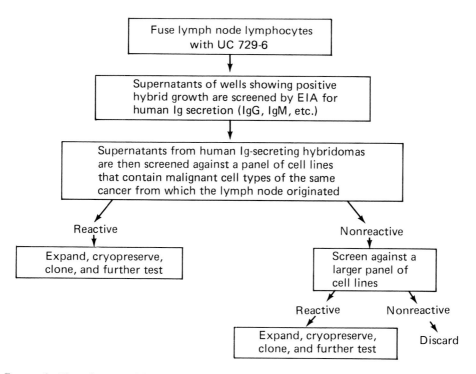

FIGURE 3. Flow chart our laboratory uses in the production and screening of human MAbs to human cancers. See text for further details.

putative hybrids generated from UC 729-6 were true human–human hybridomas. Cytofluorographic analyses of UC 729-6, diploid lymphocytes, the CLNH5 human–human hybridoma (Glassy *et al.*, 1983a), and MHG7, a human IgM-secreting mouse–human hybridoma (Lowe *et al.*, 1984), are shown in Fig. 4. On a scale of 200 units, the relative DNA content of CLNH5 (83 units) is approximately the sum of the peak of UC 729-6 (45 units) plus that of a diploid lymphocyte (42 units). The MHG7 mouse–human hybrid has eliminated several human chromosomes and consists of a mixture of cell types of varying DNA content, indicative of mouse–human hybrids (Ruddle, 1973).

V. Detection of Cell-Bound Antigens

For the most part, the nature of the immune response man generates to his own antigens, including those associated with malignant cells, is unknown. Investigators using sera from cancer patients have successfully demonstrated that these individuals do mount a humoral response to their own tumors (Carey *et al.*, 1976; Ueda *et al.*, 1979). These observations have been confirmed and extended through human hybridoma technology, in that these patients have made antibodies that recognize both cytoplasmic (Cote *et al.*, 1983) and cell surface antigens (Schlom *et al.*, 1980; Sikora and Phillips, 1981; Glassy *et al.*, 1983a,c; Handley *et al.*, 1983; Houghton *et al.*, 1983; Lowe *et al.*, 1984).

We have fused UC 729-6 with human lymphocytes isolated from regional lymph nodes draining cancers of the prostate, cervix, kidney, and vulva. Four human IgM and eight human IgG MAbs producing hybridomas were isolated (Glassy *et al.*, 1983a–c; Handley *et al.*, 1983; Lowe *et al.*, 1984; and M. Glassy, unpublished observations) whose Igs have selectively reacted with human tumor cells by enzyme immunoassay and immunofluorescence. All of these hybridomas have been cloned by limiting dilution without the use of feeder layers. Some of their general characteristics are described in Table III. The reactivity profiles of the MHG7 and CLNH5 IgMs by EIA with a panel of cell lines are shown in Fig. 5. These human IgM-secreting hybridomas showed positive reactivity with cervical (HeLa and CaSki), lung (T293H), and prostate carcinoma cell lines (Ln-Cap and PC-3), but were negative for normal fibroblast cell lines (350Q and WI-38), T-cell lines (CEM, Molt-4, HPB-ALL, and 8402), peripheral blood lymphocytes, red blood cells, and granulocytes (M. C Glassy, unpublished observations). The WLNA6 IgM MAb (Glassy *et al.*, 1983a,c) reacted strongly with the T293H lung cell line, had weak reactivity with the HeLa and CaSki cervical carcinoma cell lines, and was negative with the 350Q and WI-38 normal fibroblasts. Three IgG-secreting hybridomas, termed VLN5C7, VLN3G2, and VLN3F10, were preferentially reactive with a carcinoma of the vulva (A431) and T293H cells in addition to stomach cancer cell lines KATO-III, AGS, and MNK-28. Reactivity by EIA ranged

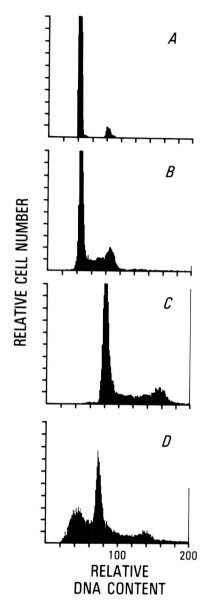

FIGURE 4. Relative DNA content of lymphocytes and human Ig-secreting hybridomas. Cells and hybridomas were stained by the propidium iodide method for the determination of relative cell DNA content and analyzed by cytofluorometry as described by Taylor (1980). Cell number is plotted on the ordinate against relative fluorescent intensity, indicative of DNA content, on the abscissa. (A) Human chronic lymphocytic leukemia cells; (B) UC 729-6 cells; (C) human–human pseudotetraploid hybridoma CLNH5; (D) mouse–human hybridoma MHG7.

from two- to ninefold over backgrounds. Detailed descriptions of our immunoreactive human monoclonal IgGs will be published elsewhere.

Immunofluorescence analysis of the MHG7 IgM MAb demonstrated that it reacted with prostate carcinoma cells but not with normal prostate cells in the same sections of both frozen and paraffin-embedded tissue (Lowe *et al.*,

TABLE III
Characteristics of Selected Human Hybridomas

Cell line/clone	Type	Lymph node source of B cells	Ig secreted	Cell type with highest reactivity by EIA
UC 729-6	Human	—	—	—
MHG-7	Mouse–human	Prostate cancer	IgM	Prostate
CLNH5	Human–human	Cervical cancer	IgM	Cervix
WLNA6	Human–human	Wilm tumor	IgM	Lung
VLN1H12	Human–human	Vulva cancer	IgM	Lung
CLNH11	Human–human	Cervical cancer	IgG	Cervix
VLN3G2	Human–human	Vulva cancer	IgG	Vulva
VLN5C7	Human–human	Vulva cancer	IgG	Stomach
VLN6H2	Human–human	Vulva cancer	IgG	Stomach
VLN2D3	Human–human	Vulva cancer	IgG	Vulva
VLN1F9	Human–human	Vulva cancer	IgG	Stomach
VLN3F10	Human–human	Vulva cancer	IgG	Prostate
VLN2G11	Human–human	Vulva cancer	IgG	Stomach

1984). Table IV summarizes the results of MHG7 reactivity with 28 separate cases. Of the frozen sections, MHG7 reacted with four out of five prostate cancer cases, two out of three benign prostatic hypertrophy (BPH) cases, and zero out of two renal parenchyma cases. Of the formalin-fixed sections, MHG7 reacted with seven out of 12 prostate cancers, four out of six BPH cases, and zero out of three foreskin cases. MHG7 reacted with all grades of sections examined, regardless of whether the tissue was frozen or paraffin-embedded. Of note, both frozen and permanent sections were made from tissues obtained from patients 1–3. MHG7 was reactive with the frozen tissue section of patient 1, while nonreactive with a permanent section of the same tissue. Both the frozen and permanent sections of patient 2 were reactive with MHG7, even though the paraffin sections were much less so. Also, MHG7 reactivity with patient 3 was similar in both types of tissue fixation.

The reactivity of MHG7 with prostate tissue sections has consistently been focal, in that not all of the malignant cells identified were immunoreactive with the MAb. This opens up the possibility that the antigen recognized by MHG7 is a proliferation- or differentiation-dependent macromolecule. The antigen is also subject to degradation or alteration, since a lower percentage of formalin-fixed tissue was reactive with MHG7 than fresh frozen sections. Caution must therefore be exercised when evaluating large panels of formalin-fixed tissues, in that a lack of reactivity may not necessarily mean the lack of antigen.

In addition to the cell lines and malignant prostate tissue sections, we have also demonstrated that the MHG7 MAb reacted with cases diagnosed as BPH in both frozen and formalin-fixed sections. The human humoral re-

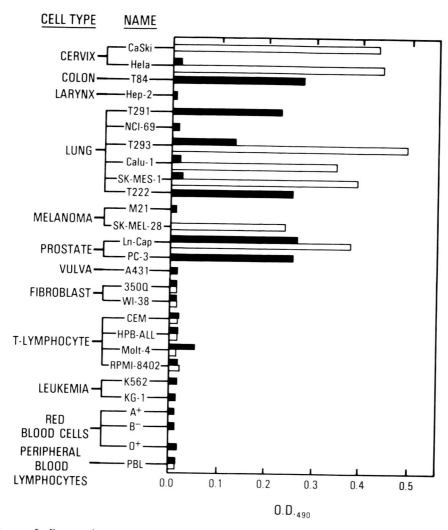

FIGURE 5. Enzyme immunoassay of the human IgM MAbs MHG7 (closed bars) and CLNH5 (open bars) and their reactivity with a panel of normal and malignant human cells. Each well of the immunofiltration manifold plates used in this assay contained 2×10^5 cells. A 1:3000 dilution of HRP-conjugated goat anti-human IgM was used to develop the MAb reactivity with OD_{490} units were obtained on an EIA reader (Dynatech, model MR 600).

sponse to prostate antigens is poorly understood (Webb *et al.*, 1981) and the type of clinically relevant antigens to which the patient may be generating antibodies is unknown. Since MHG7 reacts with both prostate carcinoma cells and BPH but not normal prostate cells, this raises several interesting possibilities about the diagnostic or therapeutic potential of this human MAb. For example, one possibility is that MHG7 may identify an antigen associated with

Table IV

Immunofluorescent Reactivity of MHG7 with Tissue Sections

Patient[a]	Tissue type	Grade[b]	Percent reactivity[c]
Frozen section			
1	Prostate	MW	15–20
2	Prostate	MW	30
3	Prostate	MW	25
4	Prostate	PD	10–15
5	Prostate	MW	—
6	Prostate	BPH	30–35
7	Prostate	BPH	20–25
8	Prostate	BPH	—
9	Kidney	Normal	—
10	Kidney	Normal	—
Permanent section			
1	Prostate	MW	—
2	Prostate	MW	5
3	Prostate	MW	20
11	Prostate	MW	10–15
12	Prostate	MW to PD	25–30
13	Prostate	MW	5
14	Prostate	PD	5
15	Prostate	WD	30
16	Prostate	WD	—
17	Prostate	MW	—
18	Prostate	PD	—
19	Prostate	MW	—
20	Prostate	BPH	30
21	Prostate	BPH	10–15
22	Prostate	BPH	5–10
23	Prostate	BPH	5
24	Prostate	BPH	—
25	Prostate	BPH	—
26	Foreskin	Normal	—
27	Foreskin	Normal	—
28	Foreskin	Normal	—

[a]Twenty-eight separate patients were analyzed in this study, of which patients 1–3 were evaluated by both frozen and permanent sections.
[b]Grade refers to the type of diagnosis. PD, poorly differentiated; MW, moderately well-differentiated; WD, well-differentiated; BPH, benign prostatic hypertrophy.
[c]Percent of tumor ducts reactive with MHG7. A dash refers to samples that showed no demonstrable reactivity.

prostate cancer that is also expressed on a "premalignant" form of BPH. In considering these possibilities, it is important to keep in mind that the human B lymphocytes immortalized in this study were derived from a regional draining lymph node of a patient with prostate carcinoma. Therefore, the patient has mounted a humoral response to his prostate-associated antigens. Since

BPH cells reacted with MHG7, further work will be necessary before we can correlate antigen expression with the malignant state.

VI. Concluding Remarks

Since our laboratory is interested in the human immune response to autologous tumor antigens and the eventual clinical use of human MAbs, we have developed a human–human hybridoma system to achieve this goal. We have developed and characterized UC 729-6, a 6-thioguanine-resistant human lymphoblastoid B-cell line, useful in generating stable Ig-secreting human–human hybridomas. UC 729-6 is diploid, with a $21p^+$ chromosomal marker, and doubles every 17 hr. Resulting human–human hybridomas were pseudotetraploid, containing the $21p^+$ marker, doubled every 20–30 hr, and have secreted up to 9 μg of human Ig/ml per 10^6 cells for over 9 months in continuous culture. In addition, we have developed an EIA that offers many advantages over other conventional antibody–antigen reactions in that this assay is rapid, simple, and sensitive in determining human MAb class, concentration, and specificity to soluble, particulate, or cellular antigens.

We have also exploited the use of regional draining lymph nodes of cancer patients, which we have shown contain B lymphocytes sensitized to their own tumor antigens. These lymphocytes were immortalized by poly-ethylene glycol-mediated somatic cell hybridization with UC 729-6, resulting in a continuous supply of the anticancer MAb. Of the human MAbs generated in our laboratory thus far, none have reacted with hematopoietic cells such as normal peripheral blood lymphocytes, myelomas, lymphomas, leukemias, and erythrocytes. These human MAbs have reacted with a broad range of adherent malignant cell types, and therefore are not specific to one cell type. For example, the MHG7 IgM MAb reacts with a diverse cell population of adherent cell lines of malignant origin in addition to prostate carcinoma cells, and therefore is not prostate-specific. However, since normal prostate cells (except for hyperplastic) were unreactive, MHG7 may recognize a putative tumor-associated antigen.

Human MAbs reactive with human cancers may have advantages over MAbs of other species, particularly those of murine origin. First, murine MAbs are xenogeneic foreign proteins, and, when used clinically, patients have encountered some difficulties, ranging from minor allergic reactions to anaphylaxis (Dillman, 1984). MAb inhibition has also occurred due to an endogenous anti-mouse immune response. Also, mice, when immunized with a human antigen, usually recognize highly immunogenic determinants. However, human tumor antigens may be weakly immunogenic and do not elicit a significant immune response in mice. Humans, on the other hand, may easily recognize these novel antigens and mount an immune response against them. Furthermore, human MAbs will tell us more about human polymorphic antigens, such as HLA, than MAbs from other species. This technology provides

investigators an opportunity to study the spectrum of the human B-lymphocyte repertoire, particularly those to tumor antigens, and may open up new
areas of investigation facilitating the diagnosis and treatment of human
cancers.

Acknowledgment

M. C G. is the recipient of an NIH Investigator Research Award.

References

Abrams, P. G., Knost, J. A., Clarke, G., Wilburn, S., Oldham, R. K., and Foon, K. A., 1983,
    Determination of the optimal human cell lines for development of human hybridomas, *J.
    Immunol.* **131:**1201.
Boss, B. D., Langman, R., Trowbridge, I., and Dulbecco, R. (eds.), 1983, *Monoclonal Antibodies and
    Cancer,* Academic Press, New York.
Carey, T. E., Takahashi, T., Resnick, L. A., Oettgen, H. F., and Old, L. J., 1976, Cell surface
    antigens of human malignant melanoma. I. Mixed hemadsorption assay for humoral immu-
    nity to cultured autologous melanoma cells, *Proc. Natl. Acad. Sci. USA* **73:**3278.
Chiorazzi, N., Wasserman, R. L., and Kunkel, H. G., 1982, Use of Epstein–Barr virus-trans-
    formed B cell lines for the generation of immunoglobulin-producing human B cell
    hybridomas, *J. Exp. Med.* **156:**930.
Cleveland, P. H., Richman, D., Oxman, M. N., Wickham, M. G., Binder, P. S., and Worthen, D.
    M., 1979, Immobilization of viral antigens on filter paper for a (^{125}I) staphylococcal protein
    A immunoassay, *J. Immunol. Meth.* **29:**369.
Cote, R. J., Morrissey, D. M., Houghton, A. N., Beattie, Jr., E. J., Oettgen, H. F., and Old, L. J.,
    1983, Generation of human monoclonal antibodies reactive with cellular antigens, *Proc. Natl.
    Acad. Sci. USA* **80:**2026.
Croce, C., Linnenbach, A., Hall, W., Steplewski, Z., and Koprowski, H., 1980, Production of
    human hybridomas secreting antibody to measles virus, *Nature* **288:**488.
Dillman, R. O., 1984, Monoclonal antibodies in the treatment of cancer, *CRC Crit. Rev. On-
    col./Hematol.* **1:**357.
Edwards, P. A. W., Smith, C. M., Neville, A. M., and O'Hare, M. J., 1982, A human–human
    hybridoma system based on a fast-growing mutant of the ARH-77 plasma cell leukemia-
    derived line, *Eur. J. Immunol.* **12:**641.
Glassy, M. C, and Ferrone, S., 1982, Differential segregation patterns of human chromosomes in
    somatic cell hybrids constructed with human B lymphocytes and human melanoma cells,
    Cancer Res. **42:**3971.
Glassy, M. C, and Handley, H. H., 1985, Monoclonal antibodies and enzyme immunofiltration,
    in: *Biotechnology Handbook* (P. N. Cheremisinoff and R. P. Ouelette, eds.), Technomic Publish-
    ing, Lancaster, Pennsylvania, p. 420.
Glassy, M. C, Handley, H., Seegmiller, J. E., and Royston, I., 1981, A lymphoblastoid B cell line
    useful for generating immunoglobulin secreting human–human hybridomas, *Fed. Proc.*
    40:996.
Glassy, M. C, Handley, H. H., Hagiwara, H., and Royston, I., 1983a, UC 729-6, a human
    lymphoblastoid B cell line useful for generating antibody-secreting human–human
    hybridomas, *Proc. Natl. Acad. Sci. USA* **80:**6327.

Glassy, M. C, Handley, H. H., Cleveland, P. H., and Royston, I., 1983b, An enzyme immunofiltration assay useful for detecting human monoclonal antibody, *J. Immunol. Meth.* **58**:119.

Glassy, M. C, Handley, H. H., Royston, I., and Lowe, D. H., 1983c, Human monoclonal antibodies to human cancers, in: *Monoclonal Antibodies and Cancer* (B. D. Boss, R. E. Langman, I. S. Trombridge, and R. Dulbecco, eds.), Academic Press, New York, p. 163.

Handley, H. H., and Royston, I., 1982, A human lymphoblastoid B cell line useful for generating immunoglobulin-secreting human hybridomas, in: *Hybridomas in Cancer Diagnosis and Treatment* (M. S. Mitchell and H. F. Oettgen, eds.) Raven Press, New York, p. 125.

Handley, H. H., Royston, I., and Glassy, M. C., 1983. The production of human monoclonal antibodies to human tumor associated antigens, in: *Intercellular Communication in Leukocyte Function*, Wiley-Interscience, New York, p. 617.

Hellstrom, K. E., and Brown, J. P. 1979, Tumor antigens, in: *The Antigens*, Volume 5 (M. Sela, ed.), Academic Press, New York, p. 1.

Houghton, A. N., Brooks, H., Cote, R. J., Taormina, M. C., Oettgen, H. F., and Old, L. J., 1983, Detection of cell surface and intracellular antigens by human monoclonal antibodies. Hybrid cell lines derived from lymphocytes of patients with malignant melanoma, *J. Exp. Med.* **158**:53.

Köhler, G., and Milstein, C., 1975, Continuous cultures of fused cells secreting antibody of predefined specificity, *Nature* **256**:495.

Lever, J. E., Nuki, G., and Seegmiller, J. E., 1974, Expression of purine overproduction in a series of 8-azaguanine-resistant diploid human lymphoblast lines, *Proc. Natl. Acad. Sci. USA* **71**:2679.

Levy, J. A., Virolainen, M., and Defendi, V., 1968, Human lymphoblastoid lines from lymph node and spleen, *Cancer* **22**:517.

Levy, J. A., Buell, D. N., Creech, C., Hirshaut, Y., and Silverberg, H., 1971, Further characteristics of the WIL-1 and WIL-2 lymphoblastoid lines, *J. Natl. Cancer Inst.* **46**:647.

Lowe, D. H., Handley, H. H., Schmidt, J., Royston, I., and Glassy, M. C, 1984, A human monoclonal antibody reactive with human prostate, *J. Urol.* **132**:780.

Olssen, L., and Kaplan, H. S., 1980, Human–human hybridomas producing monoclonal antibodies of predefined antigenic specificity, *Proc. Natl. Acad. Sci. USA* **77**:5429.

Ruddle, F. H., 1973, Linkage analysis in man by somatic cell genetics, *Nature* **242**:165.

Schlom, J., Wunderlich, D., and Teramoto, Y. A., 1980, Generation of human monoclonal antibodies reactive with human mammary carcinoma cells. *Proc. Natl. Acad. Sci. USA* **77**:6841.

Sikora, K., and Phillips, J., 1981, Human monoclonal antibodies to glioma cells, *Br. J. Cancer* **43**:105.

Sikora, K., and Wright, R., 1981, Human monoclonal antibodies to lung-cancer antigens, *Br. J. Cancer* **43**:696.

Taylor, I. W., 1980, A rapid single step staining technique for DNA analysis by flow microfluorimetry, *J. Histochem. Cytochem.* **28**:1021.

Ueda, R., Shiku, H., Pfreundschuh, M., Takahashi, T., Li, L. T. C., Whitmore, Jr., W., Oettgen, H. F., and Old, L. J., 1979, Cell surface antigens of human renal cancer defined by autologous typing, *J. Exp. Med.* **150**:564.

Webb, K. S., Ware, J. L., Parks, S. F., and Paulson, D. F., 1981, A serologic approach to the definition of human prostatic carcinoma antigens, *Prostate* **2**:369.

13

Human–Human Hybridoma Technology
Five Years of Technical Improvements, and Its Application in Cancer Biology

LENNART OLSSON AND PETER BRAMS

I. Introduction

Cloning and immortalization of antibody-producing human B lymphocytes are required to establish monoclonal cell lines that secrete human immunoglobulin of predefined specificity. Such cultures may be obtained either (1) by transformation of normal B lymphocytes, e.g., by virus, or (2) by somatic cell hybridization of normal B lymphocytes with malignant cells, resulting in cell hybrids that have preserved the secretion of specific antibody of the B lymphocyte and the growth properties of the malignant cells. The former method has been used almost exclusively with Epstein–Barr virus (EBV) as the transforming agent, and some human monoclonal antibodies with interesting specificity have been obtained by this method (Steinitz *et al.*, 1979; Zurawski *et al.*, 1978; Irie *et al.*, 1982; Watson *et al.*, 1983; Rosen *et al.*, 1983).

However, since the introduction of murine hybridoma technology almost 10 years ago, somatic cell hybridization of antibody-producing B lymphocytes with established cell lines of myeloma cells seems to be the method by which monoclonal antibodies of human origin can be produced conveniently. However, a number of technical obstacles have delayed the establishment of human–human (H–H) hybridoma technology as a routine procedure comparable to rodent hybridoma production. The majority of these technical

LENNART OLSSON AND PETER BRAMS • Cancer Biology Laboratory, State University Hospital (Rigshospitalet), DK-2100 Copenhagen, Denmark.

227

difficulties and their impact on the efficiency of procedures for establishment of antibody-secreting H–H hybridomas were reviewed recently (Olsson and Kaplan, 1983; Olsson, 1984).

About 5 years ago, two independent groups reported on successful generation of the first H–H hybridomas with predefined specificity (Olsson and Kaplan, 1980; Croce et al., 1980), but many laboratories had difficulties in using the reported malignant fusion partners for H–H hybridoma production. In fact, these negative results were a significant impetus for us to investigate the reasons for these negative results and also to initiate attempts to improve the H–H hybridoma technology. Now, more than 4 years later, the contributions of numerous laboratories have led to substantial technological improvements, so that human MAbs now are produced routinely in many laboratories. The various stages of this development have clearly underlined that successful production of MAbs by hybridoma technology relies on multiple technical steps, of which the failure of just one is sufficient to impair the whole procedure. The human malignant fusion partners were clearly inferior to the comparable mouse plasmacytomas. Only very few true human myeloma lines have been established. In our first report on H–H hybridomas (Olsson and Kaplan, 1980) we used a hypoxanthine phosphoribosyltransferase-negative (HPRT$^-$) variant of the U-266 myeloma cell line (Nilsson et al., 1970). This line has a relatively high population doubling time (PDT; ~40–50 hr) and a low cloning efficiency (CE; <0.1%) both in semisolid agar medium and by limiting dilution in liquid medium. Both growth parameters were found to be crucial for H–H hybridoma production (Olsson et al., 1983). Moreover, the original HPRT$^-$ variant of the U-266 myeloma line (SKO-007) was found to be mycoplasma-contaminated, which probably is the major reason almost 2 years elapsed before other investigators could confirm that the SKO-007 line could be used for H–H hybridoma production (Abrams et al., 1983; Cote et al., 1983; Houghton et al., 1983), although with very low fusion frequency. The cell line used by Croce et al. (1980), designated GM1500, was found not to be a true myeloma cell line, but an EBV-transformed B-lymphoblastoid line. This line also had low fusability, and the hybrids had low Ig secretion. Better malignant fusion partners were therefore clearly needed. Below we describe how we have approached this problem.

Another important factor in H–H hybridoma production is access to optimally antigen-primed human B lymphocytes, which for obvious reasons in most cases has to be done outside the human body. Moreover, such in vitro antigen priming systems are also important for conventional rodent hybridoma production. Several in vitro antigen priming systems have been described [for review, see Reading (1982)]. We describe below a system developed by van Ness et al. (1984) that has the advantages of (1) only requiring small amounts of antigen (~1 μg per ~5 × 10^7 lymphocytes) and (2) resulting in an immune response against phylogenetically highly conserved amino acid sequences.

Screening for antibody specificity of human MAbs follows the same principles as for murine MAbs. In our laboratory these screening methods have shifted from radioimmunoassays (RIA) and enzyme-linked immunosorbent assays (ELISA) to be based mainly on dot-blot analysis with immobilized antigen on nitrocellulose paper (Hawkes *et al.*, 1982; Pettijohn *et al.*, 1984).

Human–human hybridoma technology is a powerful tool in cancer biology to investigate whether humans can raise an immune response against autochthonous tumors. Such studies have already been reported for melanoma (Houghton *et al.*, 1983), breast cancer (Schlom *et al.*, 1980), and acute leukemia (Olsson *et al.*, 1984). Furthermore, experiments with murine MAbs have demonstrated that antigenic modulation is an important phenomenon. Here we show that human MAbs against tumor-associated antigens also may result in substantial antigenic modulation.

II. Improvement of Malignant Fusion Partners

More than ten different human cell lines have been reported useful malignant fusion partners for H–H hybridoma production. These cell lines fall into two categories: (1) true myeloma/B-lymphoma lines and (2) EBV-transformed B-lymphoblastoid lines. Most of these lines have been reviewed elsewhere (Kozbor and Roder, 1983; Olsson, 1984). Compared to the murine plasmacytoma lines, all these lines are hampered by low fusability, high degree of instability with respect to chromosome content and Ig secretion, and low cloning efficiency. Furthermore, most H–H hybrids produced by fusions of B lymphocytes with EBV-transformed lymphoblastoid lines also seem to have very low Ig secretion.

For the last 3 years we have used an HPRT$^-$ human B-lymphoma line (RH-L4) as malignant fusion partner (Olsson *et al.*, 1983). This line produces, but does not secrete, IgG(κ), and has resulted in stable, Ig-producing hybrids upon fusion to human lymphocytes (Olsson *et al.*, 1983, 1984). However, the growth rate and cloning efficiency of this line are low compared to similar murine B-lymphoma/plasmacytoma lines (PDT $\approx$ 40–50 hr and CE $\approx$ 0.04% vs. PDT $\approx$ 15–20 hr and CE $\approx$ 10% for murine lines). The possibility of establishing new myeloma/B-lymphoma cell lines with short PDT and high CE seemed poor, and therefore we decided to attempt to alter the growth properties of the RH-L4 line.

Phenotypic characteristics of malignant cells, including growth properties, can be assumed to be genetically determined. Human cell lines normally have higher PDT and lower CE than comparable mouse cell lines, and it has been unclear whether the human gene repertoire upon appropriate activation could result in growth properties comparable to rodent cell systems. A number of mechanisms are involved in gene regulation and activation [for reviews see Razin and Riggs (1980) and Doerfler (1983)]. In recent years it has become evident from studies of gene regulation in both prokaryotic and eukaryotic cells that 5-methylcytosine (m^5Cyt) is an important gene silencing factor, and that demethylation may lead to gene expression (Holliday and Pough, 1975; Razin and Riggs, 1980; Riggs and Jones, 1983; Doerfler, 1983). Profound alterations of cellular phenotypes have been observed after treatment of cells with 5-azacytidine (5-azaC), which results in demethylation of the genome when it is incorporated in place of cytosine, because 5-azaC cannot be methylated. Thus, malignant cells have been shown to change their immunogenicity (Frost *et al.*, 1984) and tumorigeneic, nonmetastatic cells have been shown to express the metastatic phenotype upon treatment with 5-azaC (Olsson and Forchhammer, 1984).

The RH-L4 B-lymphoma line was treated with 5-azaC in order to generate RH-L4 sublines with short PDT and high CE. Other human cell lines were also treated with 5-azaC to induce changes in proliferative activity; the details of the experimental procedures are described elsewhere (Olsson *et al.*, 1985). Briefly, RH-L4 cells were cultivated for 3 days in 3 μM 5-azaC, which was found to be nonmutagenic and nontoxic to RH-L4 cells. After the 3 days, the RH-L4 cells were transferred to ordinary culture medium, and samples were harvested each day and assayed for their clonability in semisolid agar medium. Forty-two individual clones were harvested at the day of maximal cloning efficiency, expanded in liquid medium, and the PDT and CE determined for each clone. Some of the clones had short PDT and/or high CE, and although a number of subclones with altered growth gradually reverted to values of the original clones, a few subclones remained changed in their growth properties even >1 yr after 5-azaC treatment and could therefore be tested repeatedly for their usefulness as malignant fusion partners.

Table I shows that subclone 14 was particularly suitable for H–H hybridoma production with respect to fusion frequency and cloning efficiency of hybrids both in semisolid agar medium and liquid medium, as well as with respect to Ig production. This line is now used routinely in our production of H–H hybridomas. Despite several attempts, we have not yet succeeded in

TABLE I

Qualities of Three Different Cell Lines as Malignant Fusion Partner for Human Hybridoma Production

Cell line	Fusion frequency[a] ($\times 10^{-7}$)	Ig secretion (μg/ml)
RH-L4	~10	0.1–10
RH-L4 subclone 14	~80	5.0–30
SKO-007	~40	1.0–20

[a]Fusion was done with pokeweed mitogen-stimulated lymphocytes as described previously (Olsson *et al.*, 1983).

isolating a variant of subclone 14 that does not produce Ig. A proportion of the Ig molecules secreted by the hybrids of B lymphocytes and subclone 14 cells are therefore permutated Ig products. However, the fraction of permutated Ig molecules is insignificant for most practical purposes, since the RH-L4 subclone 14 cells produce <100 ng Ig/10^6 cells per 24 hr and the hybrids normally >10 μg/10^6 cells per 24 hr. In conclusion, it seems that the 5-azaC treatment has resulted in a very significant improvement of the RH-L4 line for H–H hybridoma production. It is conceivable that the described procedure can be applied to other human myeloma or B-lymphoma cell lines and thereby result in even more suitable malignant fusion partners for H–H hybridoma production.

III. In Vitro Antigen Priming

Several *in vitro* antigen priming systems have been described both for murine and human lymphocytes [for review see Reading (1982)]. These attempts have mainly focused on the culture conditions for supporting B-lymphocyte proliferation, such as types of serum proteins, addition of hormones, or cell density. Normally, the specific antigen has simply been added in its purified form to the culture, and the antigen–cell interaction supposed to take place spontaneously. These procedures have resulted in a B-lymphocyte response to both soluble and particulate antigens and both with mouse and human B cells. However, most of these *in vitro* priming systems require rather significant amounts of antigen (normally >0.1 mg/10^7 lymphocytes), and in addition it is unclear whether these systems can be used to elicit a B-lymphocyte response against a broad antigenic spectrum.

Considerable efforts have been invested in producing MAbs against phylogenetically highly conserved insoluble cellular proteins, but these have met with very limited success. It therefore seems to be a substantial technical advance that van Ness *et al.* (1984) recently reported on an *in vitro* priming system that reproducibly allows generation of a B-lymphocyte immune response against phylogenetically conserved antigenic determinants on cellular proteins. We have recently used this system for *in vitro* antigen priming to produce murine MAbs against histone epitopes that are phylogenetically conserved and present on histones in tunicates, fish, rodents, and humans (Brams *et al.*, in preparation). A considerable advantage of the system is that it requires only low amounts of antigen (<1 μg/10^7 immune cells). Such amounts of antigen can often be obtained by simple elution from SDS–gels and therefore obtained in rather purified form as compared to a total cell extract. However, the use of denatured proteins as antigenic material excludes an immune response against most of the epitopes on the native proteins, since most epitopes in many systems seem determined by the *three-dimensional* structure of the *native* molecule (Lane and Koprowski, 1982).

The *in vitro* antigen priming system of van Ness *et al.* (1984) was found to work reproducibly in our laboratory for murine hybridoma work, and we have therefore attempted to adapt the system for H–H hybridoma work. However, the system could not readily be transferred to H–H hybridoma production, because human lymphocytes died within 24 hr after suspension in the culture medium used for *in vitro* priming. Two types of thymocyte-conditioned medium were prepared by incubating $(1-2) \times 10^8$ thymocytes/ml in RPMI 1640 + 50% FCS and in serum-free RPMI 1640 medium for 24 and 16 hr, respectively. Both media were supplemented with 1.0×10^{-4} M cimetidine, 1.0×10^{-6} M hydrocortisone, 10 μg/ml 1,1-dimethylhydrazine, 2×10^{-5} M β-mercaptoethanol, 2.0×10^{-5} M glutathione, 2.0×10^{-5} M each of adenosine, guanosine, uridine, and cytidine, 3.0×10^{-6} M thymidine, 3.0×10^{-5} M hypoxanthine, 2.0 mM sodium pyruvate, 1.0 mM sodium glutamine, and nonessential amino acids. The chosen pure antigen was conjugated to silica beads. Murine spleen cells and peritoneal macrophages taken from the same mice were mixed with silica beads in serum-free thymocyte-conditioned medium, and after 6–9 hr incubation, the serum containing thymocyte-conditioned medium was added to give a FCS percentage of approximately 16. The cells were subsequently cultivated for 5–7 days in 95% humidity and 5% CO_2, and then fused with the $HPRT^-$ myeloma cells. It was found that the supplements in the serum-free medium were toxic to human peripheral blood lymphocytes, and consequently they had to be adapted to human cells, which required reduction in the concentration of most supplements to 1/5–1/10 of the dose used for murine cells. Our current procedure for *in vitro* antigen priming of human cells is outlined in Fig. 1.

Most *in vitro* antigen priming systems result only in IgM-producing B lymphocytes, and the above procedure is no exception. It is a major obstacle to the generation of specific IgG-producing B lymphocytes by *in vitro* antigen priming procedures that the currently used culture conditions only permit B-lymphocyte propagation in culture for ~10 days, which is too short a period to result in specific IgG-producing B lymphocytes. However, it is conceivable that improved culture conditions may result in propagation of B lymphocytes for longer periods (weeks). We are currently attempting to obtain such B lymphocytes by (1) 5-azaC treatment of the cells 1–3 days after initiation of the priming in an attempt to obtain demethylation in some of the specific B lymphocytes, and thereby further propagation of some of these cells, (2) addition of conditioned medium from RH-L4 subclone 14, which seems to produce a growth factor for B-lymphocyte proliferation, and (3) addition of specific antigen plus/minus pokeweed mitogen 5–7 days after initiation of the priming to maintain the ongoing lymphoblast response against the specific antigen. It is hoped that these experiments within the next 4–6 months will result in the establishment of an *in vitro* priming system that can result in specific IgG-producing clones.

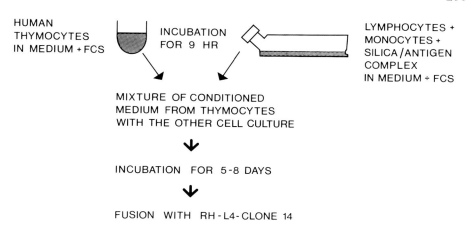

CULTURE MEDIUM : RPMI - 1640 , 2 mM SODIUM PYRUVATE , 1mM GLUTAMINE
1.1 - DIMETHYLHYDRAZINE , CIMETIDINE , HYDROCORTISONE .

FIGURE 1. Principles for the procedure of *in vitro* antigen priming of human lymphocytes [see also text and van Ness *et al.* (1984)]. Conditioned medium is prepared from thymocyte cultures and mixed with a culture that contains (1) the lymphocytes to be primed, (2) monocytes, and (3) the specific antigen conjugated to silica beads. The mixture is incubated for 5–8 days and the viable mononuclear cells fused with the malignant fusion partner (RH-L4 subclone 14).

IV. Fusion Procedures, Cultivation of Human–Human Hybrids, and Screening for Immunoglobulin Production

Table II shows the fusion frequency and number of Ig-producing hybrids when human peripheral blood lymphocytes (PBLs) were fused with RH-L4 subclone 14 cells after various types of pretreatment of the PBLs. Fusion frequencies were the same with lymphocytes pretreated by *in vitro* antigen priming or by pokeweed mitogen (PWM) stimulation, but the *in vitro* antigen priming was clearly superior with respect to the number of specific hybrids.

Manipulation of specific IgM-producing hybrids is another procedure for obtaining IgG-secreting hybrids. It was recently reported that UV-irradiation may result in chain switch from μ to γ in EBV-transformed lymphoblastoid cells (Rosen and Klein, 1983), but it remains to be seen whether this procedure is applicable to a variety of IgM-producing B lymphocytes.

A number of reports have shown that on the average, H–H hybridomas produce lower amounts of Ig than mouse hybridomas, both when they are

TABLE II

Yield of Human Hybridomas upon Fusion of Human Peripheral Blood Lymphocytes[a] (PBLs) with the RH-L4 Subclone 14 Line

Treatment of PBLs prior to fusion	Fusion frequency ($\times 10^{-7}$)	Percent hybrids secreting specific antibody[b]	Ig secreting (μg/ml)
None	~10	0	1.0–20.0
PWM stimulation for 5 days	~80	0.1	5.0–30
In vitro antigen priming for 7 days	~70	2.0	5.0–20
In vitro antigen priming for 7 days followed by PWM stimulation for 5 days	~70	2.3	5.0–25

[a]The PBLs were taken 5 days after an antigenic boost of a volunteer with tetanus toxoid.
[b]Determined as the percentage of wells with Ig-secreting hybrids that contained Ig with signficant binding to tetanus toxoid antigen as determined by dot-blot analysis.

created with myeloma cells or with EBV-transformed lymphoblastoid cells as malignant fusion partners. We have attempted to increase the Ig secretion of H–H hybrids by demethylation with 5-azaC treatment. About 40% of the antibody-producing H–H hybridomas had significantly increased Ig secretion after 5-azaC treatment, ~50% had unchanged Ig secretion, and ~10% had decreased Ig secretion (Table III). Induction of Ig secretion by 5-azaC has only been attempted in some nonsecretory variants of murine hybridomas, in which about 20% of the non Ig-secreting hybrids could be induced to produce Ig. Loss of Ig secretion in hybridomas is normally ascribed to loss of chromosomes encoding for Ig (heavy or light chains) or chromosomes encoding for factors that determine the Ig-secretory apparatus. Our results demonstrate that another important factor for loss of Ig secretion may be changes in DNA methylation. It seems therefore that the 5-azaC treatment should be attempted in those cases where a crucial hybridoma clone has lost its Ig secretion. We are currently investigating whether similar effects of 5-azaC can be obtained by treatment of H–H hybrids that have lost Ig secretion.

Polyethylene glycol (PEG) with different molecular weights and in different concentrations (w/v) have been used as fusogen (Table IV). A 37% (w/w) PEG with a molecular weight of 1000 resulted in the highest fusion frequency, although the fusion frequencies with PEG 1500 and 4000 were not substantially different. In contrast, a PEG with a molecular weight of ~6000 reduced significantly the yield of viable hybrids, probably due to a toxic effect of the PEG.

It has previously been reported that pokeweed mitogen (PWM) stimulation of human PBLs prior to fusion increased the amount of hybrids as compared to unstimulated PBLs (Olsson *et al.*, 1983). However, the amount of hybrids is not increased by mitogen stimulation of lymphocytes after *in vitro*

TABLE III

Effects of 5-Azacytidine on Ig-Secretion of Murine and Human Hybridomas

Number of murine (M) and human (H) hybrids	Ig secretion after 5-azaC treatment[a]					
	Decreased		Unchanged		Increased	
	M	H	M	H	M	H
M: 12, H: 11	1	2	6	5	5	4

[a]The hybridomas were incubated for 3 days in RPMI 1640 with 15% FCS, supplemented with 3 μM 5-azaC. Ten subclones were subsequently isolated per hybrid culture and the Ig secretion determined. If >3 subclones secreted more or less than 5 μg/ml Ig as compared to original clone, it was considered significant.

antigen priming and PWM stimulation was therefore omitted when *in vitro* antigen-primed cells were used.

In our hands propagation of H–H hybrids has required monocyte feeder cells, both when B-lymphoma and myeloma cells have been used as malignant fusion partners. However, the H–H hybrids produced with the RH-L4 subclone 14 as malignant fusion partner have been found to be independent of monocyte feeder cells both in the initial propagation of the hybrid cells after fusion as well as during cloning procedures by limiting dilution. It is unclear why the H–H hybrids produced with RH-L4 subclone 14 cells as malignant fusion partner are independent of monocyte feeder cells, but we are currently

TABLE IV

Number of Ig-Secreting Hybrids after Fusion of PWM-Stimulated Human PBLs with RH-L4 Subclone 14 with Different Types of Polyethylene Glycol (PEG)

Molecular weight of PEG	W/V	Fusion frequency[a] ($\times 10^{-7}$)
1000	37%	~70
	50%	~80
1500	37%	~60
	50%	~60
4000	37%	~50
	50%	~40
6000	37%	~10
	50%	~10

[a]As estimated from the number of viable hybrid clones 30–40 days after fusion.

testing for secretion of B-lymphocyte growth factors by the RH-L4 subclone 14. Thus, it seems that a careful study of the factors produced by the RH-L4 subclone 14 and supporting B-lymphocyte/B-lymphoma/H–H hybridoma growth has the potential to contribute to our understanding of the biological factors that control growth of B lymphocytes and their malignant counterparts.

Murine hybridomas normally can be identified in the cultures 10–14 days after fusion, whereas it has been characteristic of the H–H hybridomas generated in our laboratory that they first appear 20–35 days after fusion, and that screening for Ig 14–20 days after fusion normally is negative, in contrast to the mouse system. The screening system obviously has to be adapted to the antigen against which MAbs are generated. Many laboratories usually first screen for Ig secretion and subsequently for antigenic specificity. However, we have experienced in our work with both murine and human MAbs to cell surface constituents that such an approach for antibody screening may exclude interesting hybridomas. Screening for Ig secretion is normally done by solid-phase radioimmunoassay (RIA) or by enzyme-linked immunosorbent assay (ELISA). Both assays depend on the attachment of the MAbs to a plastic surface, and normally in competition with the proteins in the fetal calf serum that in conventional hybridoma systems are added to the culture medium in a final concentration of 10–15%. Most MAbs have a relatively high affinity to plastic as compared to serum proteins, but some do not bind firmly despite a relatively high affinity ($>10^7/M$) to the specific epitope. We therefore screen both for Ig secretion and specific reaction to antigen with the same supernatant. We have previously used RIA and/or ELISA for this purpose, but we have lately found that dot-blot analysis with immobilized antigen material on nitrocellulose paper provides a better sensitivity with respect to both Ig testing and reactivity with specific antigens. In particular, the background "noise" of this test system is minimal, whereas ELISA in particular often is impaired by a high nonspecific background reaction. We therefore now routinely screen hybridoma supernatants by dot-blot analysis. For cell surface constituents, we also use FACS analysis, because a number of MAbs are directed against epitopes that are created by the three-dimensional (3D) structure of the molecule and therefore often are eliminated upon denaturation. Table V shows the binding of 35 MAbs raised against cell surface constituents when analyzed by FACS on viable cells, by cell-binding ELISA, and by dot-blot. About two-thirds of the MAbs could only bind to non-denatured cell constituents. This indicates that analysis of MAbs reactive to cell surface constituents preferably should be done by FACS. Moreover, it is highly conceivable that denaturation also results in loss of epitopes on intracellular components, and that the initial screening for MAbs reactive with such structures also should include methods that do not imply denaturation.

It is also of importance that a number of cellular epitopes are created by carbohydrate or lipid structures, and that conventional screening procedures may not detect MAbs against structures simply because these substances do not attach to the plastic surface or nitrocellulose paper that normally is the

TABLE V
Effect of Denaturation on the Binding of 35 Monoclonal Antibodies to Cellular Constituents

Method of analysis	Number of MAbs binding/total MAbs
Fluorescence-activated cell sorter	35/35
Cell-binding ELISA	31/35
Dot-blot	16/35

basis for ELISA/RIA and dot-blot assays. Furthermore, since a number of MAbs against cell surface constituents have been found to react with carbohydrate/lipid structures (see below), it is obvious that screening systems including detection of carbohydrate/lipid structures should be included in the initial assay systems for antibody reactivity.

Cloning procedures for H–H hybridomas have been described elsewhere (Brodin *et al.*, 1983). However, H–H hybrids generated with RH-L4 subclone 14 do not require monocyte feeder cells, and this has largely facilitated cloning procedures. Two procedures can be applied for further expansion and large-scale production of a given H–H hybridoma antibody: (1) large-scale production of H–H cultures, and (2) propagation of H–H hybrids as ascites tumors in nude mice. Large-scale culture of H–H hybrids is our preferred method, partly because the subsequent antibody purification is simpler, provided the H–H hybrids first are adapted to serum-free culture conditions, and partly because it assures that the H–H hybrids remain free of endogenous murine infectious agents, such as viruses that may limit the use of human MAbs derived from such hybrids.

We have previously reported that growth of H–H hybridomas as tumors in nude mice can be facilitated by concomitant grafting of the hybridoma cells mixed with human foreskin fibroblasts. Table VI shows the efficiency of this procedure for seven different H–H hybridomas as compared to mere grafting of H–H hybrids without fibroblasts. Upon adaptation to ascites tumors in nude mice, not all tumors secreted large amounts of MAbs into the ascites fluid. The reason(s) for the lack of antibody titer in serum from several of the mice are unknown, but it is obviously another impetus for attempts to perform large-scale production entirely by *in vitro* procedures.

V. Human Monoclonal Antibodies against Tumor-Associated Antigens

A number of murine MAbs have already been generated against tumor-associated antigens (TAA) on tumors of both animal and human origin [for review, see the monograph edited by Mitchell and Oettgen (1983)]. Most of

Table VI

Heterotransplantation of Seven Human–Human Hybrids into Nude Mice and the Ig Production of Such Tumors upon Conversion from Subcutaneous Growing Tumors to Ascitic Tumors

Number of human–human hybridomas	Number of cells grafted	Route of injection[a]	Tumor cell inoculum mixed with 2×10^6 foreskin fibroblasts[b]	Take	Ig content in ascites fluid (μg/ml)
1	5×10^6	sc	−	−	—
			+	+	~10
		ip	−	−	—
			+	−	—
2	5×10^6	sc	−	−	—
			+	+	~60
		ip	−	−	—
			+	−	—
3	5×10^6	sc	−	+	50
			+	+	40
		ip	−	−	—
			+	−	—
4	5×10^6	sc	−	−	—
			+	+	~5
		ip	−	−	—
			+	−	—
5	5×10^6	sc	−	−	—
			+	+	200
		ip	−	−	—
			+	−	—
6	5×10^6	sc	−	−	—
			+	+	20
		ip	−	−	—
			+	−	—
7	5×10^6	sc	−	+	90
			+	+	130
		ip	−	−	—
			+	−	—

[a]sc, Subcutaneous; ip, intraperitoneal.
[b]The tumor cells and fibroblasts were mixed prior to injection.

these antibodies have been directed against antigens that typically fall into one of the following groups: (1) normal differentiation antigens, (2) embryonic antigens, (3) antigens with high tumor specificity. Monoclonal antibodies against all these types of antigens are useful in relation to experimental work, where it may contribute to a better understanding of malignant transformation. The various areas of cancer biology and oncology that can be expected to benefit from the development of MAbs against TAAs have been described elsewhere in more detail, including the perspectives for application of human MAbs (Kaplan *et al.*, 1982). However, the technical obstacles described above in relation to H–H hybridoma production have hampered significantly the generation of relevant human MAbs, and it is only within the last 2 or so years that substantial progress has been made in the development of human MAbs against TAAs. Reports on human MAbs reactive with melanoma cells (Houghton *et al.*, 1983), glioma cells (Sikora *et al.*, 1982), and leukemia cells (Olsson *et al.*, 1984) have shown that human MAbs can be generated against all three types of antigens. Houghton *et al.* (1983) thus described a set of human MAbs that reacted with both cell surface antigen and intracellular structures. Fusion of lymphocytes from patients with leukemia with the RH-L4 lymphoma line resulted in a H–H hybridoma clone that secreted a MAb with high specificity for human leukemia cells (Olsson *et al.*, 1984). This antigen could be demonstrated on leukemia cells from about one-third of patients with acute leukemia. The antigen was not specific for myeloid leukemia cells, since some samples from patients with acute lymphoblastic leukemia also reacted with the MAb. It is of particular interest that the epitope has not yet been found on nonmalignant human cells. Thus, our investigations on embryonic tissues have failed to demonstrate the presence of the antigen in fetal tissues, but further analysis is required to assess this firmly. Furthermore, despite many attempts, we have been unsuccessful in producing murine MAbs against this epitope. It is thus possible that the epitope cannot be recognized by the murine immune system, but only across an allogeneic barrier.

This emphasizes one of the most important potential roles of the H–H hybridoma system, namely to provide a tool to investigate whether humans can raise an immune reaction against autochthonous tumors. From the investigations of patients with melanomas or leukemias, it is indicated that patients can mount an immune reaction against their own cancer, and this suggests that some human cancer cells may express neoantigens on their surface.

The areas of application of human MAbs with high specificity for malignant tumors have been described elsewhere (Kaplan *et al.*, 1982; Olsson and Kaplan, 1983). Moreover, among the major obstacles of applying MAbs in tumor diagnosis and therapy is the pronounced intratumoral phenotypic diversity (IPD) that now has been described in a number of different experimental and human tumor systems (Olsson, 1983; Heppner, 1984). The biological implications of IPD have also been described recently, and it has been argued that IPD may be an important feature of malignancy (Olsson, 1983; Frost and Kerbel, 1983).

The biochemical nature of TAAs has only been well established for a minority of those antigens that have been identified as tumor-associated. Among those that have been somewhat characterized, a substantial proportion are directed against carbohydrates or glycolipids that often are associated with normal cellular proteins to form large (molecular weight typically >200,000), complex molecules. Some of these complexes have been found to be rare blood group antigens (Hansson *et al.*, 1983), whereas others seem to have high specificity for certain malignant tumors (Hakomori and Kannagi,

1983; Feizi, 1984; Bumol and Reisfeld, 1982; Hellström *et al.*, 1984; Ginsburg *et al.*, 1984). It is of considerable interest that a large number of abnormal epitopes are related to carbohydrate/carbohydrate–lipid structures, because it indicates that abnormal activity of glycosyltransferase(s) is taking place in these malignant cells.

Antigen modulation has been shown in the last few years to be an important and frequent phenomenon when antibodies interact with antigens on eukaryotic cell surfaces. Antigenic modulation was primarily demonstrated with respect to TL antigens on murine leukemia cells (Old *et al.*, 1968), and later in relation to the several antigens on human cells when incubated with specific MAbs (Ritz *et al.*, 1980; Antel *et al.*, 1982). Furthermore, *in vitro* therapy of leukemia with MAbs has demonstrated that such therapy also may result in antigenic modulation. Figure 2 illustrates our current method for analyzing for antigenic modulation. These procedures were applied for a leukemia-associated antigen detected by a human MAb (aml-18). It is seen from Fig. 3A that the antigenic modulation takes place very rapidly in this

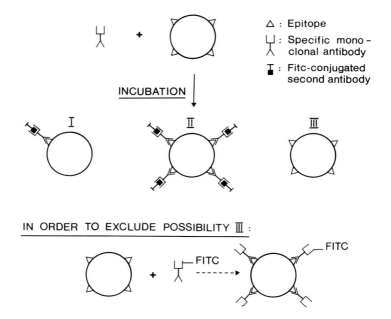

FIGURE 2. Procedures for analysis of antigenic modulation. The target cells are incubated with the specific antibody. After incubation a proportion of the cells are stained with (1) FITC-conjugated rabbit anti-mouse Ig to detect specific antibody on the cell surface, (2) FITC-conjugated specific antibody to analyze for expression of the specific epitope.

D. Applications to Autoimmunity

14

The Production of Monoclonal Antibodies by Human–Human Hybridomas
Their Application to Studies of Autoimmune Diseases

YEHUDA SHOENFELD AND ROBERT S. SCHWARTZ

I. Introduction

In this chapter we review our experience with the human–human hybridoma technology and compare our results with those of others. We also provide a brief review of our results in the analysis of human monoclonal lupus autoantibodies. A more comprehensive review of applications of hybridoma technology to studies of human autoimmune disease has been published elsewhere (Shoenfeld and Schwartz, 1984). Anyone just beginning to use the hybridoma method with human lymphocytes should appreciate that the technology is in a state of flux. Many of the methodological details are bound to change as new fusion partners and other improvements become introduced. Nothing written here should be considered as the final word on the topic.

The hybridoma method introduced by Köhler and Milstein (1975) has had an enormous impact on the biological sciences because it enables the production of monoclonal antibodies against almost any existing immunogen. The original technique has been improved by several modifications, such as

YEHUDA SHOENFELD • Department of Medicine "D" (Research Laboratory of Autoimmune Diseases), Beilinson Medical Center, Petach Tiqva, Israel. ROBERT S. SCHWARTZ • Hematology-Oncology Division, New England Medical Center, Boston, Massachusetts 02111.

the use of polyethylene glycol (PEG) instead of Sendai virus as the fusing agent and the development of nonsecreting myeloma cell lines (Shulman *et al.*, 1978; Ritts *et al.*, 1983). In addition, procedures to increase the yield of monoclonal antibodies by hybridomas have been developed (Milstein, 1980).

Until 1980, the hybridoma technique was applied almost exclusively to mouse cells. However, human monoclonal antibodies are highly desirable for the diagnosis and treatment of human disease. They will minimize the *in vivo* problems caused by foreign animal proteins, such as anaphylaxis and refractoriness to mouse monoclonal antibodies. Almost half the patients treated with murine monoclonal antibodies have developed an antibody response to mouse immunoglobulins (Kozbor and Roder, 1983; Miller and Levy, 1981; Ritz *et al.*, 1981; Miller and Levy, 1981; Cosimi *et al.*, 1981; Takahashi *et al.*, 1983). By contrast, sensitization to human immunoglobulins is unusual. From the biological standpoint, human monoclonal antibodies should reveal more information about certain human diseases than murine monoclonal antibodies. For example, monoclonal antibodies generated by the human–human hybridoma method may be more specific than those obtained by murine fusions in the case of tumor-associated antigens. Human monoclonal autoantibodies could also be used to select and develop anti-idiotypic antibodies, which may be useful for suppressing the response to autoantigens or allografts.

The short history of human hybridomas has been marked by technical difficulties, but several new human fusion partners may render the method more generally applicable than it has been (Table I). There have also been attempts to produce human monoclonal antibodies with mouse or rat fusion partners. However, the mixed-species hybridomas preferentially lose their human chromosomes and frequently eliminate the genes that code for immunoglobulin production. Since the chromosomal constitution of intraspecies hybrids is comparatively stable, human–human hybridomas are more likely than human–mouse fusions to be a consistently reliable source of human monoclonal antibodies.

TABLE I

Human Fusion Partners

Cell line	Ig secreted	Reference
GM 4672	IgG	Croce *et al.* (1980)
U-266	IgE	Nilsson *et al.* (1970)
UC729-6	IgM	Glassy *et al.* (1983)
UC729-HF2	None	Abrams *et al.* (1983)
RPMI-8226	—	Matsuoka *et al.* (1977)
8226AR/NIP4-1	None	Pickering and Gelder (1982)
RH-L4	None	Brodin *et al.* (1983)
SKO-007	IgE	Olsson and Kaplan (1980)
LICR-LON-HMy2	IgG	Edwards *et al.* (1982)
WIL2/729HF	—	Denis *et al.* (1983)

lymphoblastoid cells, such as those of the GM 4672 line. Similar results were demonstrated by others (H. S. Kaplan *et al.*, 1982; Chiorazzi *et al.*, 1982), but lipopolysaccharide was without effect (H. S. Kaplan *et al.*, 1982). The beneficial effect of PWM stimulation in the production of hybridomas depends on functioning T lymphocytes. Therefore, isolation of the B lymphocytes from other peripheral blood mononuclear cells prior to stimulation is not recommended. The time of incubation of the cells with PWM seems to affect the isotype of the immunoglobulin secreted by the hybridomas. The shorter the period of stimulation, the greater the percentage of cells secreting IgM, whereas longer incubations tend to favor IgG-secreting hybridomas (Y. Shoenfeld, unpublished data). The number of cells retrieved after 6 days of incubation with PWM, however, ranges between 25% to 85% of the original number.

C. In Vitro Stimulation with Antigen Prior to Fusion

This technique may improve the frequency of positive hybrids. In the murine system (Stahli *et al.*, 1980), the increase in blasts after immunization was shown to predict the successful generation of specific hybrids.

D. Cell Plating Density

The well size and cell plating concentration also affect the growth of hybridoma clones. The maximum yield of hybridomas was obtained in 2-ml wells that were plated with 4×10^5 cells (22.8% of wells demonstrated clones). Smaller wells (0.3 ml) plated with 2×10^5 and 1×10^5 cells/well produced clones in 12.2 and 7.2% of wells, respectively. The importance of cell density at the stage of seeding was also found by others (Olsson and Kaplan, 1980). Optimal concentrations of cells may have to be determined for each new human fusion partner.

E. Well Size

In contrast to the findings in mouse hybridomas, we (Shoenfeld *et al.*, 1982) as well as others (Croce *et al.*, 1980; Eisenbarth *et al.*, 1982; Massicote *et al.*, 1984; Sikora *et al.*, 1982) have found that the yield of hybridomas was higher when the fused cells were seeded into large wells (2 ml) instead of into conventional 96-well plates (0.15 ml). We found a yield of 32% of hybrids in 2-ml wells, whereas in only 1.8% of the 0.3-ml wells were hybrids formed, even though cell densities were similar in both cases. The large wells may be advantageous by providing a larger surface area for hybridoma growth than the small wells.

F. PEG Concentration

Most investigators have used PEG concentrations ranging between 38% and 50%. Of three different concentrations (38%, 44%, 50%), we found 44% to be optimal. Croce *et al.* (1980) used 50% PEG with GM 1500 cells, and Edwards *et al.* (1982) obtained 79% successful fusions with 50% PEG with the LICR-LON-HMy2 cell line. However, they exposed the cells to PEG for a shorter period of time than we did. The optimal PEG concentration may vary with the fusion partner used and on the length of time of exposure during the procedure.

G. HAT Medium

We grow the cells in HAT medium until visible clones are established. The practice of growing the cells thereafter in medium containing only HT medium was replaced by immediate transfer of the clones to complete RPMI 1640 medium with 20% FCS, and no effect on cell growth was found.

H. Tests to Authenticate the Hybridomas

We performed several tests to determine whether the cell lines we developed were actually hybridomas, rather than immortalized B cells that might result from infection with EBV (Steinitz *et al.*, 1977).

1. Chromosomal analysis showed that 6–42% of cells from 11 different lines were hyperdiploid. The number of chromosomes ranged from 52 to 92, and along with hyperdiploid cells, diploid and hypodiploid cells were also present. This heterogeneity was caused by loss of chromosomes during repeated passage of the hybridomas in tissue culture. The closer to the fusion date the hybridoma was examined, the more hyperdiploid cells were found (Y. Shoenfeld, unpublished data).

2. Analysis of biosynthetically labeled immunoglobulins secreted by our hybridomas demonstrated that all of them produced both IgM (5–25 μg/ml) and IgG (2–16 ng/ml). The presence of both parental immunoglobulins indicated that the cloned growths were the product of a cell fusion.

3. HLA analysis also substantiated the hybridoma nature of our fusion products. Twelve cell lines reacted in immunofluorescence tests with monoclonal antibodies directed against HLA-A2, which is expressed by the GM 4672 cells, and with HLA-B5, which occurs in about 60% of Caucasians, but not in the GM 4672 line.

Edwards *et al.* (1982) also confirmed the hybridoma nature of their cell lines, but in contrast to our cells, the hyperdiploid modal number of their karyotypes remained stable over 30 passages. An additional method to ensure the hybridoma characteristic of the cells was reported by Sikora *et al.* (1982), who measured the DNA content of lymphocytes, myeloma cells, and hybrid cells. The DNA content of the hybrid cells was approximately the sum of that of the two parent cells.

I. Immunoglobulin Secretion

Our cell lines produce 5–25 μg of Ig/ml (in a cell concentration of 2×10^6/ml). Similar results were reported in other human hybridomas. Attempts to transfer the hybridomas to nude mice or to immunosuppressed (irradiated and treated with corticosteroids) BALB/c mice have failed. However, the use of large culture flasks (1 liter) with continuous magnetic stirring was found to be a useful means of harvesting large amounts of hybridoma tissue culture fluid (Feder and Tolber, 1983).

J. Isotype of Hybridoma Antibodies

All of our antibodies have the IgM isotype. We believe that this restriction is due to either the duration of the PWM stimulation or the greater tendency of human cells with surface IgM to fuse. Most human hybridomas thus far reported produce IgM. However, there are exceptions. Handley et al. (1982) obtained hybrids from draining lymph node cells of cancer patients that secreted IgG. Similar results were obtained by us recently (Y. Shoenfeld, unpublished data). Cote et al. (1983) found a high proportion of IgA-secreting clones from a fusion with axillary lymph nodes, whereas fusions with peripheral blood lymphocytes yielded IgM-secreting clones. Success in producing IgA, IgG, and IgM monoclonal antibodies against sheep red blood cells was reported by fusing WIL2/729HF cells with tonsilar lymphocytes that had been immunized in vitro (Strike et al., 1982).

The secretion of immunoglobulin by the parental myeloma cell line dilutes the specific antibody of interest and adds an additional difficulty to the procedure for isolation of the antibody. In the murine system this difficulty was overcome by the development of nonsecreting myeloma cell lines (Shulman et al., 1978). A new nonsecreting human fusion partner has been reported (Table I).

K. Source of Lymphocytes

We have used peripheral blood lymphocytes as well as splenic lymphocytes obtained from splenectomized patients. Several investigators (Sikora et al., 1982; Cote et al., 1983) have also reported on the successful use of lymphocytes from lymph nodes or tumors.

L. Feeder Layer

Our hybrids do not require a feeder layer, either in the stage of the primary growth or in the limiting dilution procedure. However, other investigators have found an absolute necessity for a feeder layer for their cells (Cote *et al.*, 1983). Brodin *et al.* (1983) described the use of human monocytes as a feeder layer. Our method of using all the mononuclear cells from the peripheral blood at the time of the fusion may explain why we do not need a feeder layer. Eisenbarth *et al.* (1982) also succeeded in growing hybrids without a feeder layer with the GM 4672 cell line.

M. Epstein–Barr Virus

Fusion partners established from malignant lymphocytes are often infected with this virus. Nevertheless, repeated tests of our GM 4672 cell lines for the presence of EBNA, a diagnostic antigen of the Epstein–Barr virus, were negative. A novel method, which is reported to yield high numbers of human hybrids, entails the fusion of EBV-transformed B cells with a human fusion partner (Kozbor and Reder, 1983). The transformed cells were found to be 36-fold more susceptible to hybridization than resting lymphocytes. An additional advantage of EBV-infected lymphocytes lies in their continuous growth in tissue culture. This property allows the flexibility of repeating the fusion experiments at any time.

N. Mycoplasma

Infection of cell cultures with mycoplasma has serious consequences and can destroy irreplaceable cell lines. The unfortunate experience with the SKO- human fusion partner is an example of the problem. The infection is insidious and affects both the growth and the functional activity of cultured cells, including hybridomas. Failure to obtain fusions may be due to mycoplasma and not any lack of skill. The organism is difficult to detect. Many tests have been proposed, but all of them have drawbacks. We have discovered mycoplasma in some of our cultures only by electron microscopy when bacteriologic cultures and fluorescent dye tests were repeatedly negative. A new method that involves thymidine incorporation by culture supernatants (where the organisms thrive) seems superior to electron microscopy and fluorescent dye staining (D. R. Kaplan *et al.*, 1984).

Mycoplasma deprives cells of thymidine and arginine. If infection is suspected, cells can be "rescued" by growing them in medium that is supplemented with these two constituents. We have found that antibiotics are useless. An elaborate and expensive cloning technique may have to be employed to rid a cell line of the organism. No degree of vigilance can be too extreme to guard against this destructive organism.

Chiorazzi, N., Wasserman, R. J., and Kunkel, H. G., 1982, Use of EB virus transformed B cell lines for the generation of immunoglobulin-producing B cell hybridomas, *J. Exp. Med.* **156:**930–935.

Cleveland, W. L., Wood, I., and Erlanger, R., 1983, Routine large-scale production of monoclonal antibodies in a protein-free culture medium, *J. Immunol. Meth.* **56:**221–234.

Cosimsi, A. B., Colvin, R., Burton, R. C., Rubin, R., Goldstei, G., Kunk, P., Hansen, W. P., Delmonico, F., and Russel, F., 1981, Use of monoclonal antibody to T-cell subsets for immunologic monitoring and treatment of recipient of renal allografts, *N. Engl. J. Med.* **305:**318–314.

Cote, B. J., Morrissey, D. M., Houghton, A. N., Beattie, E. J., Oettgen, H. F., and Old, L. J., 1983, Generation of human monoclonal antibodies reactive with cellular antigens, *Proc. Natl. Acad. Sci. USA* **80:**2026–2030.

Croce, C. M., Linnenback, A., Hall, W., Steplewski, Z., and Koprowski, H., 1980, Production of human hybridomas secreting antibodies to measles virus, *Nature* **288:**488–489.

Denis, K. A., Wall, R., and Saxon, A., 1983, Human–human B cell hybridomas from *in vitro* stimulated lymphocytes of patients with common variable immunodeficiency, *J. Immunol.* **131:**2273–2276.

Edwards, P. A., Smith, C. M., Neville, A. M., and O'Hare, M. J., 1982, A human–human hybridoma system based on a fast growing mutant of the ARH-77 plasma cell leukemia derived line, *Eur. J. Immunol.* **12:**641–648.

Eisenbarth, G. S., Linnenbach, A., Jackson, R., Scearce, R., and Croce, C. M., 1982, Human hybridomas secreting anti-islet autoantibodies, *Nature* **300:**264–267.

Feder, J., and Tolbert, R. W., 1983, The larger scale cultivation of mammalian cells, *Sci. Am.* **248:**36–43.

Glassy, M. C., Handley, H. H., Hagiwara, H., and Royston, I., 1983, UC 729-6, a human lymphoblastoid B cell line useful for generating antibody-secreting human–human hybridomas, *Proc. Natl. Acad. Sci. USA* **80:**6327–6331.

Handley, H. H., and Royston, I., 1982, A human lymphoblastoid B-cell line useful for generating immunoglobulin-secreting human hybridomas, in: *Hybridomas in Cancer Diagnosis and Treatment* (M. S. Mitchell and H. F. Oettgen, eds.), Raven Press, New York, pp. 125–132.

Harris, E. N., Boey, M. L., Mackworth-Young, C. G., Gharavi, A. E., Patel, B. M., and Loizou, S., 1983, Anticardiolipin antibodies; detection by radioimmunoassay and association with thrombosis in SLE, *Lancet* **2:**1211–1214.

Hsu-Lin, S. H., Shoenfeld, Y., Furie, B., Schwartz, R. S., and Furie, B. C., 1982, Human hybridoma produced monoclonal autoantibodies that bind to platelets, *Blood* **60:**187A (abstract).

Isenberg, D. A., Shoenfeld, Y., Madaio, M. P., Rauch, J., Reichlin, M., Stollar, B. D., and Schwartz, R. S., 1984a, Measurement of anti DNA antibody idiotypes in systemic lupuserythematosus, *Lancet* **2:**417–421.

Isenberg, D. A., Shoenfeld, Y., and Schwartz, R. S., 1984b, Multiple serologic reactions and their relationship to clinical activity in SLE; A study of 56 patients, *Arthritis Rheum.* **17:**132–138.

Kaplan, D. R., Henkel, T. J., Braciale, V., and Braciale, T. J., 1984, Mycoplasma infection of cell cultures; Thymidine incorporation of culture supernatants as a screening test, *J. Immunol.* **132:**9–11.

Kaplan, H. S., Olsson, L., and Raubitschek, A., 1982, Monoclonal human antibodies. A recent development with wide ranging clinical potential, in: *Monoclonal Antibodies in Clinical Medicine* (A. J. McMichael and J. W. Fabre, eds.), Academic Press, London, pp. 17–35.

Köhler, G., and Milstein, C., 1975, Continuous cultures of fused cells secreting antibody of predefined specificity, *Nature* **256:**495–497.

Kozbor, D., and Roder, J. C., 1983, The production of monoclonal antibodies from human lymphocytes, *Immunol. Today* **4:**772–779.

Lafer, E. M., Rauch, J., Andrzejewski, C. J., Mudd, D., Furie, B., Furie, B. D., Schwartz, R. S., and Stollar, B. D., 1981, Polyspecific monoclonal lupus autoantibodies reactive with both polynucleotides and phospholipids, *J. Exp. Med.* **153:**897–909.

Massicote, H., Rauch, J., Shoenfeld, Y., and Tannenbaum, H., 1984, Delineation of optimal conditions for the production of human–human hybridomas secreting anti-DNA autoantibodies from patients with systemic lupus erythematosus, *Hybridoma* **3**:215–222.

Matsuoka, Y., Moore, G. E., Yagi, Y., and Prenman, D., 1977, Production of free light chains of immunoglobulin by a hematopoetic cell line derived from a patient with multiple myeloma, *Proc. Soc. Exp. Biol. Med.* **125**:1246–1252.

Miller, R. A., and Levy, R., 1981, Response of cutaneous T cell lymphoma to therapy with hybridoma monoclonal antibody, *Lancet* **2**:226–230.

Milstein, C., 1980, Monoclonal antibodies, *Sci. Am.* **243**:66–74.

Nilsson, K., Bennick, H., Johansson, S. G. P., and Pontén, J., 1970, Established immunoglobulin producing myeloma (IgE) and lymphoblastoid (IgG) myeloma patient, *Clin. Exp. Immunol.* **7**:447–452.

Olsson, L., and Kaplan, H. S., 1980, Human–human hybridomas producing monoclonal antibodies of predefined antigenic specificity, *Proc. Natl. Acad. Sci. USA* **77**:5429–5431.

Osband, M., Cavagnaw, J., and Kupchik, H. Z., 1982, Successful production of human–human hybridoma IgG antibodies against RH (D) antigen, *Blood* **60**(5, Suppl. 1):81a.

Pickering, J. W., and Gelder, F. B., 1982, A human cell line that does not express immunoglobulins but yields a high frequency of antibody secreting hybridomas, *J. Immunol.* **129**:406–412.

Ritts, R. E., Ruiz-Arguelles, A., Weyl, K. G., Bradley, A. L., Weihmeir, B., Jacobson, D. J., and Strehlo, B., 1983, Establishment and characterization of human non-secretory plasmacytoid cell line and its hybridization with human B cells, *Int. J. Cancer* **31**:133–141.

Ritz, J. M., Sallman, S., Clavell, L., Notis, M., McConaty, J., Rosenthal, P., and Schlossman, S., 1981, Serotherapy of acute lymphoblastic leukemia with monoclonal antibody, *Blood* **58**:78–86.

Schwartz, R. S., 1983, Monoclonal lupus autoantibodies, *Immunol. Today* **4**:68–69.

Seidman, J. G., Leder, A., Nau, M., Norman, B., and Leder, P., 1978, Antibody diversity, *Science* **202**:11–17.

Shoenfeld, Y., and Schwartz, R. S., 1984, Immunologic and genetic aspects of autoimmune diseases, *N. Engl. J. Med.* **311**:1019–1029.

Shoenfeld, Y., Hsu Lin, S. C., Gabriels, J. E., Silberstein, L. E., Furie, B. C., Furie, B., Stollar, B. D., and Schwartz, R. S., 1982, Production of autoantibodies by human–human hybridomas, *J. Clin. Invest.* **70**:205–208.

Shoenfeld, Y., Rauch, J., Massicote, H., Datta, S. K., André-Schwartz, J., Stollar, B. D., and Schwartz, R., 1983, Polyspecificity of monoclonal autoantibodies produced by human–human hybridomas, *N. Engl. J. Med.* **308**:414–420.

Shulman, M., Wilde, C. D., and Köhler, G., 1978, A better cell line for making hybridoma secreting specific antibodies, *Nature* **276**:269–271.

Sikora, K., Alderson, T., Phillips, J., and Watson, J. V., 1982, Human hybridomas from malignant gliomas, *Lancet* **1**:11–14.

Silberstein, L. E., Shoenfeld, Y., Schwartz, R. S., and Berkman, E. M., 1985, A combination of IgG and IgM autoantibodies in chronic cold agglutinin disease: Immunologic studies and response to splenectomy, *Vox Sang.* **48**:105–109.

Stahli, C., Staehelin, T., Miggiano, V., Schmidt, J., and Haring, P., 1980, High frequency of antigen specific hybridomas; Dependence on immunization parameters and prediction by spleen cell analysis, *J. Immunol. Meth.* **32**:297–304.

Steinitz, M., Klein, G., Koskimies, S., and Makela, O., 1977, EB virus-induced B lymphocyte cell lines producing specific antibody, *Nature* **269**:420–422.

Strike, L., Dvens, B. H., Lundak, R. L., 1982, in: *Proceedings 15th International Leucocyte Culture Conference*, p. 272.

Takahashi, H., Okazaki, H., Terasaki, P. I., Iwaki, Y., Kinukawa, T., Taguchi, Y., Chia, D., Hardiwidjaja, S., Miura, K., Ishizaka, M., and Billing, R., 1983, Reversal of transplant rejection of monoclonal antiblast antibody, *Lancet* **2**:1155–1158.

15

Human Monoclonal Autoantibodies Reactive with Multiple Organs

FLOYD TAUB, JO SATOH, CARLO GARZELLI, KARIM ESSANI, AND ABNER LOUIS NOTKINS

I. Introduction

Human monoclonal antibodies that react with normal tissues (autoantibodies) have recently been prepared from peripheral blood lymphocytes (PBLs) of patients with insulin-dependent diabetes mellitus (IDDM) and thyroiditis. This chapter describes the methods by which these monoclonal autoantibodies have been obtained and evaluates their reactivity with normal tissue antigens. In addition, the capacity of these monoclonal autoantibodies to react with antigens in multiple organs is described.

II. Establishment of Continuous Cell Lines Producing Autoantibodies

A. Human–Mouse Hybridomas

Human–mouse hybridomas were prepared by fusion of unfractionated PBLs with non-immunoglobulin-secreting, BALB/c, 8-azaguanine-resistant

FLOYD TAUB, JO SATOH, CARLO GARZELLI, KARIM ESSANI, AND ABNER LOUIS NOTKINS • Laboratory of Oral Medicine, National Institute of Dental Research, National Institutes of Health, Bethesda, Maryland 20205.

myeloma cell line Sp-2 (Lane *et al.*, 1982; Satoh *et al.*, 1983). PBLs were isolated from heparinized blood by a Ficoll–Hypaque gradient. After washing, Sp-2 cells and PBLs were mixed at the ratio of 1:1 or 1:2, and centrifuged in a conical tube. The ratio of 1:2 yielded the highest frequency of hybridomas. Between 0.6 and 1.0 ml of 50% (w/v) polyethylene glycol 1000 (pH 7.2) at 37°C was added to the cell pellet and then gradually diluted with RPMI 1640 medium. Fused cells were resuspended in complete medium consisting of RPMI 1640, 20% fetal bovine serum, glutamine, sodium pyruvate, and antibiotics. One-tenth milliliter of this suspension was added to each well of a 96-well microculture plate. In our hands, 1×10^5 or 2×10^5 cells/well produced the highest frequency of hybridomas (approximately five hybridomas per 10^6 lymphocytes). Higher concentrations of cells were much less efficient. Therefore, 2×10^5 cells were generally seeded in each well. Twenty-four hours after fusion, 0.1 ml of HAT medium (complete medium supplemented with 1×10^{-4} M hypoxanthine, 4×10^{-7} M aminopterin, and 3×10^{-10} M thymidine) was added to each well. Half (0.1 ml) the culture supernatant was replaced with fresh HAT medium every 3 or 4 days for 4 weeks. The addition of feeder cells was found to be unnecessary for growth of the fused cells.

When hybridomas had grown to confluence, generally 2–4 weeks after fusion, culture supernatants were screened for human immunoglobulin (Ig) production by an enzyme-linked immunosorbent assay (ELISA). The supernatant fluids that contained more than 1.0 μg/ml of human Ig were tested for reactivity with normal human tissues (see below).

Hybridomas producing autoantibodies were cloned by a limiting dilution method (McKearn, 1980). One hybridoma cell/well was cultured with 5×10^3 peritoneal macrophages from BALB/c mice. In the presence of macrophages as feeder cells, cloning efficiency varied from 5 to 50%. The cloning efficiency and rate of growth varied among hybridomas. Cloning efficiency without feeder cells was extremely low.

B. Human/Human Hybridomas

Human myeloma cell line GK-5 (kindly provided by Dr. J. F. Kearney, Tumor Institute and Comprehensive Cancer Center, University of Alabama) was used as the fusion partner (Kearney, 1984). GK-5 is 6-thioguanine-resistant. It does not produce heavy chain, but a small amount (approximately 10 ng/ml) of κ chain is secreted. GK-5 was fused with PBLs, and fused cells were cultured by the same procedure as for human–mouse hybridomas. Approximately 6–8 weeks after fusion, human–human hybridomas became confluent in the wells. When the wells were confluent, the culture supernatants were screened by ELISA for human Ig using heavy-chain-specific antisera. For cloning, one hybridoma cell/well was cultured with 5×10^3 human embryo fibroblasts irradiated with 2000 R as feeder cells.

C. Epstein–Barr Virus (EBV) Transformation

Continuous human cell lines producing monoclonal autoantibodies have been generated *in vitro* by transformation with EBV (Garzelli *et al.*, 1984). Since EBV-induced antigens can generate cytotoxic T lymphocytes and NK cells capable of inhibiting the growth of EBV-transformed B cells (Bird *et al.*, 1981; Takasugi *et al.*, 1982), T cells were separated prior to viral infection by passage through a nylon wool column (Trizio and Cudkowicz, 1974). Five million nylon-adherent (i.e., B-lymphocyte-enriched) cells, suspended in 1 ml of culture medium, were infected by incubation for 2 hr at 37°C with 0.5 ml of supernatant of the EBV-producer B95-8 marmoset cell line (Miller and Lipman, 1973). After one wash, 5×10^4 EBV-infected cells were seeded in each well of a 96-well plate and incubated in a humidified atmosphere in the presence of 7.5% CO_2. Usually, the EBV-infected B lymphocytes were cultured in the presence of 1×10^5 feeder cells/well consisting of autologous T lymphocytes treated with mitomycin C (25 μg/ml, 30 min, 37°C). The cells were fed twice a week by replacing half of the culture medium. Evidence that the cells were transformed included formation of cell colonies, acid production, increase in cell number, and the ability of cells to be successfully subcultured (Miller and Lipman, 1973).

Three to four weeks after EBV infection, the cell cultures were screened for Ig concentration and tissue-reacting autoantibodies. Lymphoblastoid cell cultures producing autoantibodies were cloned using a limiting dilution method (McKearn, 1980). Human allogeneic peripheral blood mononuclear cells (10^5 cells/well of a microtiter plate) treated with mitomycin C were used as feeder cells.

III. Comparison of Methods for Generating Monoclonal Autoantibodies

A comparison of the three different methods is given in Table I. In our experience, EBV transformation was the most efficient method of obtaining continuous cell lines. EBV-transformed B-cell lines were generated in 100% of the wells seeded with as low as 1×10^4 nylon-adherent, B-lymphocyte-enriched cells. This corresponds to a transformation efficiency greater than 1×10^{-4}. However, the cloning of these cells by seeding at a density of one cell/well led to the growth of cells in only 2–6% of the wells.

Hybridomas were produced at much lower efficiency than EBV-transformed lines. Approximately three out of 10^6 or three out of 10^7 human lymphocytes formed growing hybridomas when fused with mouse or human myeloma cells, respectively. The cloning of hybridoma cells by limiting dilution was generally more successful than cloning EBV-transformed B cells, although the cloning efficiency was quite variable.

TABLE I

Comparison of Methods of Generating Monoclonal Autoantibodies

	Human–mouse hybridoma	Human–human hybridoma	EBV transformation
Frequency of establishing cell lines[a,b]	3.3×10^{-6}	3.4×10^{-7}	$>1 \times 10^{-4}$
Immunoglobulin production[c] (%)	18	75	73
Autoantibody production[d] (%)	23	13	69
Cloning efficiency[e]	28	18	3
(Range) (%)	(5–49)	(0–50)	(2–6)

[a]Number of wells containing hybridomas was divided by total PBLs used for fusion. A total of 26 human–mouse and 53 human–human fusion experiments were performed.
[b]EBV transformation has been consistently obtained in 100% of wells seeded with as few as 1×10^4 nylon-adherent, B-lymphocyte-enriched cells.
[c]Percentage of wells with hybridomas or EBV-transformed cells that contained more than 1 µg/ml of Ig when confluent.
[d]Percentage of wells with >1 µg/ml Ig that contained tissue-reactive antibody, detected by avidin–biotin complex immunoperoxidase staining.
[e]Percentage of wells with growth when one hybridoma or EBV-transformed cell was seeded in each well.

High proportions of human–human hybridomas and EBV-transformed B-cell cultures (75 and 73%, respectively) produced more than 1 µg/ml of Ig, whereas only 18% of human–mouse heterohybridomas produced that amount of Ig.

Autoantibodies reacting with normal tissues were frequently found in EBV-transformed cell cultures. In fact, when wells with ≥1 µg/ml of Ig were assayed, 69% of the EBV-transformed cell cultures produced autoantibodies, whereas only 23% of human–mouse hybrids and 13% of human–human hybrids produced autoantibodies.

IV. Methods of Screening for Autoantibodies

Ideally, screening for autoantibodies would allow the identification of reactions with specific antigens in the form in which they normally exist, even if present in small amounts. Unfortunately, such an ideal method does not exist. Microscopic examination of tissue sections, however, can identify very specific reactions, including reactions with rare components of the tissue. Since many tissue sections can be rapidly viewed, an extremely large number of antigens can be easily screened.

Tissue sections, however, have their limitations. Frozen sections allow many antigens to diffuse out. Thus, reactions with soluble molecules, such as hormones, should be sought by other methods. This is true even though frozen sections are generally fixed on the slides using a combination of drying and chemicals (e.g., acetone or alcohol). More vigorous fixation (e.g., aldehyde cross-linkers such as formaldehyde or gluteraldehyde and coagulative fixatives such as Bouin's or Zamboni's) biochemically alters tissue antigens so that they cannot diffuse out. Although these fixatives are frequently used, especially prior to embedding specimens in hard media for sectioning, it should be remembered that antigens in tissue sections may not be in the same form as they were in the living cell and that the antigenicity may vary significantly depending on the method of fixation. In our studies the monoclonal antibodies were tested on sections of monkey and/or human tissues. Monkey tissues were often used because they were a convenient source of fresh, well-preserved specimens. In general, no difference in the reactivity of the antibodies was found on monkey as compared to well-preserved human tissues.

The binding of an unlabeled monoclonal antibody to tissue sections can be identified by reaction of that antibody with a labeled second antibody. The simplest second antibody is anti-human Ig conjugated to fluoresceinisothiocyanate. The binding of this antibody may be directly visualized by fluorescent microscopy. An alternative approach is to use anti-human Ig conjugated to an enzyme, usually peroxidase. The enzyme can then be detected by simple light microscopy following formation of a colored precipitate at sites of enzyme localization in the presence of a suitable substrate. The sensitivity of this latter method may be increased by the avidin–biotin complex (ABC) technique (Hsu *et al.*, 1980). This technique uses secondary antibodies conjugated to biotin. The tissue-bound biotinylated antibody is then reacted with a complex of avidin, biotin, and peroxidase. Enhanced sensitivity occurs because many peroxidase molecules are bound to each complex and several complexes may bind to each biotin-labeled antibody. In our experience ABC methodology can detect monoclonal autoantibody at concentrations 5–10 times lower than detected by indirect immunofluorescence.

V. Evaluation of Tissue Reactivity of Monoclonal Autoantibodies

The procedures described above have been applied for producing and studying human monoclonal autoantibodies. A number of clones producing tissue-reacting IgM monoclonal autoantibodies have been isolated and found to react with specific cell types in many organs, including pancreas, thyroid, parathyroid, lung, gall bladder, stomach, spleen, thymus, urinary bladder, and brain (Figs. 1–3).

By testing these autoantibodies against a panel of normal tissues, we found that many of them react with antigens in more than one organ. We refer to these multiple-organ-reactive antibodies as MOR antibodies. However, each antibody showed a peculiar and individual pattern of tissue reactivity. The partial reactivity pattern of three of these monoclonal autoantibodies is shown in Table II and Figs. 1–3. Monoclonal MOR JW H10, produced by EBV transformation, reacted with a variety of tissues, including thyroid acinar cells, pancreatic acinar cells and ducts, smooth muscle (Fig. 1D), basement membrane of stratified squamous epithelium, axons of peripheral nerve, bladder mucosa (Fig. 1B), and parathyroid cells (Fig. 1F). Monoclonal antibody MOR-h12, produced by human–human fusion, also reacted with a variety of tissues, but not with thyroid or stratified squamous epithelium. It did, however, react with islets and ductules in the pancreas (Fig. 2B), smooth muscle, bronchial mucosa (Fig. 2D), chondrocytes (Fig. 2D), gall bladder mucosa (Fig. 2F), stellate or dendritic-shaped cells in the white pulp of the spleen (Fig. 2I), and sinusoids in red pulp (Fig. 2J) of the spleen. Monoclonal antibody MOR-h1, produced by human–mouse fusion, also showed its own unique tissue pattern, reacting with pituitary (Fig. 3A), thyroid acinar cells (Fig. 3B), some cells in the gastric mucosa (Fig. 3C), and pancreatic islet cells and ductules (Fig. 3D).

The ability to produce monoclonal MOR antibodies by the three different methods indicates that MOR reactivity is not due to a particular method of preparation. Moreover, detecting MOR reactivity is not dependent upon the method of screening; reactivity with multiple organs is detected when either frozen (Fig. 1) or paraffin-embedded (Figs. 2 and 3) tissues are used as antigens. MOR activity is also detected when antibodies are selected for reaction with fixed cultured cells rather than tissue sections (C. Garzelli and F. Taub, unpublished observations). The peculiar reactivity of one such antibody (MOR LA G9) with the surface and nuclei of cells in the stratified squamous epithelium of the esophagous is illustrated in Fig. 1H.

Initially, we thought that MOR antibodies were unusual and rare. As a result of more extensive screening procedures, we are now finding many MOR antibodies. In fact, MOR antibodies are turning out to be the rule rather than the exception.

VI. Purification of Human Autoantigens by Immunoaffinity Chromatography

The availability of large quantities of monoclonal autoantibodies has made it possible to isolate autoantigens from normal tissues by immunoaffinity chromatography. This is illustrated with MOR-h1, which reacts with the thyroid, stomach, pituitary, and pancreas. An immunoaffinity column was prepared by conjugating affinity-purified MOR-h1 with CNBr-activated Sepharose 4B. Tissue extracts were passed through the affinity column and bound antigens were eluted and analyzed by SDS–PAGE (Satoh et al., 1984). As seen in Fig. 4A,B, thyroid and stomach extracts yielded one major polypeptide with an apparent molecular weight of 35,000 (35K). This polypeptide (35K) was also detected in the pituitary (Fig. 4C). These three antigens reacted strongly with MOR-h1 by ELISA (data not shown). A second

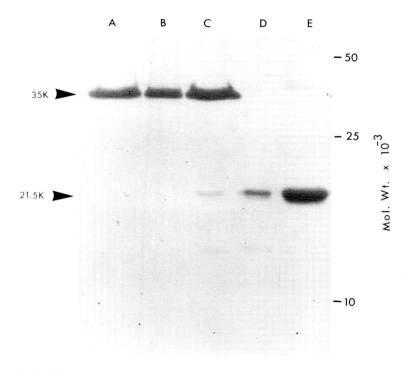

FIGURE 4. Isolation of human autoantigens. Tissue extracts were passed through an MOR-h1 affinity column, and the bound antigens were eluted, concentrated, and electrophoresed on 15% SDS–polyacrylamide. A 35K polypeptide was isolated from (A) thyroid, (B) stomach, and (C) pituitary. The pituitary extract also contained an additional polypeptide of 21.5K (lane C). This polypeptide has an electrophoretic mobility identical to that of (D) natural growth hormone and (E) cloned synthetic growth hormone. [From Satoh et al. (1984).]

ence, EBV transformation is the most effective method for establishing continuous B-cell lines. EBV-transformed B-cell lines were produced at 100-fold higher efficiency than human–mouse and 1000-fold higher efficiency than human–human hybridomas. EBV-transformed cultures were 3–5 times more likely to produce autoantibodies than hybridomas. However, cloning of hybridoma cells was more efficient than cloning of EBV-transformed cells.

Both hybridoma technology and EBV transformation led to isolation of clones producing monoclonal IgM autoantibodies. EBV-transformed B-lymphocyte cultures also produced tissue-reactive IgG (Garzelli et al., 1984). Cloning yielded IgG-producing cell lines; however, the antibodies produced by these clones did not react with tissues. Similarly, human hybridomas producing IgG have been obtained, but they also failed to react with normal tissues.

Most studies on monoclonal antibodies have been concerned with identifying antibodies that react with the specific antigen(s) used for immunization. In contrast, we searched for autoantibodies that reacted with any one of the perhaps thousands of epitopes present in tissue sections of various organs.

This broad type of screening has allowed us to detect reactivities that would have been missed by more limited assay procedures. In fact, this analysis has shown that multiple organ reactivity is very common. Similar types of observations are being made in other laboratories. For example, human monoclonal lupus autoantibodies, selected for the ability to react with DNA, can react with different polynucleotides and cardiolipin (Shoenfeld *et al.*, 1983). More recently, IgM monoclonal rheumatoid factors have been isolated that react not only with IgG molecules, but also with DNA and cytoskeletal elements (Rubin *et al.*, 1984).

Some of the monoclonal autoantibodies we isolated from patients with autoimmune diseases show some reactivities characteristic of the disease. For example, monoclonal autoantibodies reacting with thyroid acinar cells and colloid have been isolated by EBV transformation from a patient with Hashimoto's thyroiditis (Garzelli *et al.*, 1984), and monoclonal autoantibodies reacting with pancreatic islet cells have been isolated by preparing hybridoma or by EBV transformation of lymphocytes from patients with IDDM (Satoh *et al.*, 1983; Garzelli *et al.*, 1984). However, it is not yet clear whether the cloned autoantibodies are identical or related to any of the autoantibodies found in patients' sera.

Recently, we have produced autoantibodies from lymphocytes of normal individuals by EBV transformation (Garzelli *et al.*, 1984). We have also generated monoclonal MOR autoantibodies from normal mice (Prabhakar *et al.*, 1984). These findings are consistent with the hypothesis that the normal B-lymphocyte repertoire has the capability of making a variety of autoantibodies, but *in vivo* this is under the strict control of the immunoregulatory system. Cell fusion or EBV transformation allows B lymphocytes to divide and secrete autoantibodies. Regardless of how they are obtained, these human monoclonal autoantibodies should prove to be useful reagents for diagnostic purposes, for studying development or differentiation, and for isolating human autoantigens.

References

Bird, G., Britton, S., Ernberg, I., and Nilsson, K., 1981, Characteristics of Epstein–Barr virus activation of human B lymphocytes, *J. Exp. Med.* **154:**832–839.

Garzelli, C., Taub, F. E., Scharff, J. E., Prabhakar, B. S., Ginsberg-Fellner, F., and Notkins, A. L., 1984, Epstein–Barr virus transformed lymphocytes produce monoclonal autoantibodies that react with antigens in multiple organs, *J. Virol.* **52:**722–725.

Haspel, M. V., Onodera, T., Prabhakar, B. S., McClintock, P. R., Essani, K., Ray, U. R., Yagihashi, S., and Notkins, A. L., 1983, Multiple organ-reactive monoclonal autoantibodies, *Nature* **304:**73–76.

Hsu, S. M., Raine, L., and Fanger, H., 1981, The use of avidin–biotin–peroxidase complex (ABC) in immunoperoxidase techniques: A comparison between ABC and unlabeled antibody (PAP) procedures, *J. Histochem. Cytochem.* **29:**577–580.

Kearney, J. F., 1984, Hybridomas and monoclonal antibodies, in: *Fundamental Immunology* (W. E. Paul, ed.), Raven Press, New York, pp. 751–766.

Lane, H. C., Shelhamer, J. H., Mostowski, H. S., and Fauci, A. S., 1982, Human monoclonal anti-keyhole limpet hemocyanin antibody-secreting hybridoma produced from peripheral blood B lymphocytes of a keyhole limpet hemocyanin-immune individual, *J. Exp. Med.* **155**:333–338.

McKearn, T. J., 1980, Cloning of hybridoma cells by limiting dilution in fluid phase, in: *Monoclonal Antibodies* (R. H. Kennett, T. J. McKearn, and K. B. Bechtol, eds.), Plenum Press, New York, p. 374.

Miller, G., and Lipman, M., 1973, Release of infectious Epstein–Barr virus by transformed marmoset leukocytes, *Proc. Natl. Acad. Sci. USA* **70**:90–194.

Prabhakar, B. S., Saegusa, J., Onodera, T., and Notkins, A. L., 1984, Lymphocytes capable of making monoclonal autoantibodies that react with multiple organs are a common feature of the normal B cell repertoire, *J. Immunol.* **133**:2815–2817.

Rubin, R. L., Balderas, R. S., Tan, E. M., Dixon, F. J., and Theofilopoulos, A. N., 1984, Multiple autoantigen binding capabilities of mouse monoclonal antibodies selected for rheumatoid factor activity, *J. Exp. Med.* **159**:1429–1440.

Satoh, J., Prabhakar, B. S., Haspel, M. V., Ginsberg-Fellner, F., and Notkins, A. L., 1983, Human monoclonal autoantibodies that react with multiple endocrine organs, *N. Engl. J. Med.* **309**:217–220.

Satoh, J., Essani, K., McClintock, P. R., and Notkins, A. L., 1984, Human multiple organ-reactive monoclonal autoantibody recognizes growth hormone and a 35K protein, *J. Clin. Invest.* **74**:1526–1531.

Shoenfeld, Y., Rauch, J., Massicotte, H., Datta, S. K., André-Schwartz, J., Stollar, B. D., and Schwartz, R. S., 1983, Polyspecificity of monoclonal lupus autoantibodies produced by human–human hybridomas, *N. Engl. J. Med.* **308**:414–420.

Takasugi, M., Mickey, M. R., and Levine, P. H., 1982, Natural and antibody-dependent cell-mediated cytotoxicity to cultured target cells superinfected with Epstein–Barr virus, *Cancer Res.* **42**:1208–1214.

Trizio, D., and Cudkowicz, G., 1974, Separation of T and B lymphocytes by nylon wool columns: Evaluation of efficacy by functional assay *in vivo, J. Immunol.* **113**:1093–1097.

Monocyte-conditioned medium used as a source of IL-1 (Finelt and Hoffmann, 1979) is a beneficial but not essential component of our culture system. It enhances antibody production 2–10 times but its primary effect may be seen in the stabilization of culture conditions. Upon repeated testing of PBMs from the same donor, consistent results were obtained only if monocyte-conditioned medium was added to the cultures.

With these modifications of the Mishell–Dutton system, human PBM cultures can be induced to produce antibody against red blood cell-bound antigenic determinants. The response is antigen-specific as defined by cross-sensitization to unrelated antigens (Table I) and by inhibition with antibody directed against the immunogen (Fig. 1). The response of antigen-reactive B cells depends on the function of helper T cells (Table II) and is negatively influenced by suppressor cells.

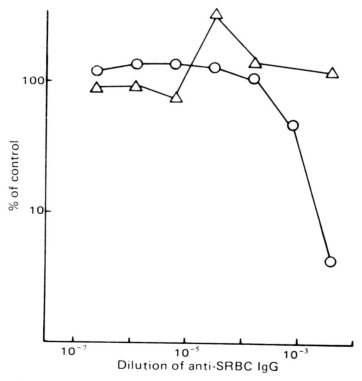

FIGURE 1. Inhibition of rabbit anti-SRBC serum of immunization with SRBC IgG. PBMs were cultured in the presence or absence of anti-SRBC IgG and immunized with SRBC and burro red blood cells conjugated with TNP (BRBC-TNP). The data are expressed as percent of the plaque-forming cell response obtained in the absence of antibody to SRBC. Each value was determined from a pool of eight cultures harvested on day 6.

TABLE II
Dependence of Antibody Production by Human Peripheral Blood B Cells on T-Cell Function

| Number of cells in culture ($\times 10^{-5}$) | | PFC/10^6 cultured cells | |
Nonrosetting (B cells)	Rosetting (T cells)	Anti-SRBC	Anti-TNP
1.2	0	0	0
0	3	110	0
0	1	185	0
0	0.3	0	0
1.2	3	660	670
1.2	1	490	1160
1.2	0.3	80	210

[a]PBMs separated into SRBC-rosetting and SRBC-nonrosetting fractions (Weiner *et al.*, 1973) were cultured in the combinations indicated and immunized with SRBC and BRBC-TNP. Antibody-forming cells were determined on day 6; each value was determined from a pool of eight cultures. The response of the T-cell fraction to SRBC may be attributed to the rosetting of SRBC-specific B cells (Hoffman, 1980).

V. The Role of Suppressor Cells in the Generation of Antibody-Forming Cells in Vitro

The activity of suppressor cells was a primary concern in developing the culture system for human PBMs. Extraordinarily strong suppressor cell activity was consistently found in PBMs from cancer patients (Hoffmann *et al.*, 1982). We investigated this phenomenon and found that suppressor cells can be conveniently removed from PBMs by passage over Sephadex G-10 columns (Fig. 2) (Hoffmann *et al.*, 1982). Sephadex G-10 column filtration was introduced by Ly and Mishell (1974) as a way to remove macrophages from lymphoid cell suspensions. The column, however, also retains antibody-secreting B lymphocytes (Ly and Mishell, 1974) and activated suppressor T lymphocytes from mouse spleen cells (Pickel and Hoffmann, 1977a). The suppressor cell trapped on the column following passage of PBMs from patients with advanced cancer was shown to express the T8 cell-surface marker (Hoffmann *et al.*, 1982) and is thus considered to be a suppressor T cell (Fig. 3) (Rheinherz *et al.*, 1980). Phenotypic analysis of column-separated PBMs revealed that column filtration did not significantly alter the proportion of T8-positive cells (Table III), suggesting that the active suppressor cells represent a small fraction of the T8-positive PBM population and that the active cells are retained on the column due to size or other changes (Hoffmann *et al.*, 1982).

With this information we investigated whether Sephadex G-10 filtration

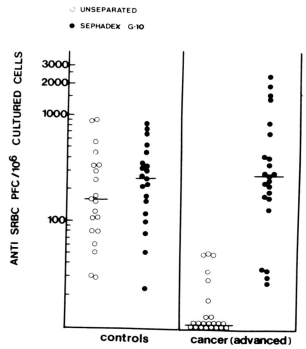

FIGURE 2. Effect of Sephadex G-10 column filtration on the generation of plaque-forming cells (PFC) in cultures of PBMs from healthy donors and from melanoma patients. PBM cells were cultured (○) unseparated or (●) following passage over Sephadex G-10 columns, and PFC counted 6 days later. All cultures were immunized with SRBCs.

alleviated suppressor cell influences in cultures of PBMs from healthy donors. Table IV shows that PBMs eluted from the column respond well when human serum is added without delay to the culture. This finding suggests that the inhibitory effect of early human serum addition requires cells that are retained on the column. SAC, the polyclonal B-cell stimulus (Schurman *et al.*, 1980) initially introduced with the intention to help B cells overcome suppressor cell effects, was no longer an essential component; it merely enhanced the response (Table V). These observations demonstrate that passage of human PBMs over Sephadex G-10 columns is an effective means to reduce the influence of peripheral blood suppressor cells (Hoffmann *et al.*, 1982).

Other procedures for the removal of suppressor cells have been suggested in the literature. The cytolytic removal of T cells that express the T8 marker (Rheinharz *et al.*, 1980) did not, in our experiments, increase the antibody formation by PBMs. This could be explained if T8-positive lymphocytes consist of more than one subpopulation, one of which is acting as an amplifier cell. Cavagnaro and Osband (1983) suggested that suppressor cells

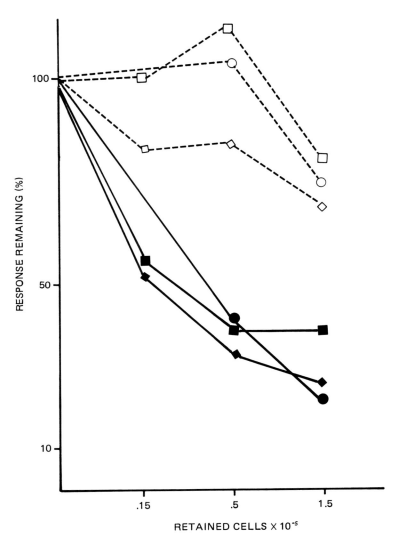

FIGURE 3. Sensitivity of column-retained suppressor cells to treatment with OKT8 antibody and complement. PBMs retained on Sephadex G-10 columns were added in graded numbers (as indicated) to 2.5×10^5 PBM cells eluted from the column. Number of plaque-forming cells was determined 6 days later from pools of eight cultures. Column-retained cells were treated with (closed symbols) NMS and complement or (open symbols) OKT8 antibody and complement. Data shown were obtained with PBMs from three cancer patients.

Ly, I. A., and Mishell, R. I., 1974, Separation of mouse spleen cells by passage through columns of Sephadex G-10, *J. Immunol. Meth.* **5**:239–247.

Marrack, P., Graham, S. D., Jr., Kushnir, E., Leibson, H. J., Roehm, N., and Kappler, J. W., 1982, Nonspecific factors in B cell responses, *Immunol. Rev.* **63**:33–49.

Mishell, R. I., and Dutton, R. W., 1967, Immunization of dissociated spleen cell cultures from normal mice, *J. Exp. Med.* **126**:423–442.

Muchmore, A. U., Kosi, I., Dooley, N., and Blaese, R. M., 1976, Artifactual plaque formation *in vitro* and *in vivo* due to passive transfer of specific antibody, *J. Immunol.* **116**:1016–1019.

Pickel, K., and Hoffmann, M. K., 1977a, Suppressor T cells arising in mice undergoing a graft-vs-host response, *J. Immunol.* **118**:653–656.

Pickel, K., and Hoffmann, M. K., 1977b, The Iy phenotype of suppressor T cells arising in mice subjected to a graft versus host reaction, *J. Exp. Med.* **145**:1169–1175.

Ralph, P., Welte, K., Levi, E., Nakoinz, I., Litcofsky, P. B., Mertelsmann, R. H., and Moore, M. A. S., 1984, Human B cell-inducing factor(s) for production of IgM, IgG and IgA: independence from Il 2, *J. Immunol.* **132**:1858–1862.

Rheinherz, E. L., Kung, P. C., Goldstein, G., and Schlossman, S. F., 1979, Further characterization of the human inducer T cell subset by monoclonal antibody, *J. Immunol.* **123**:2894–2896.

Rheinherz, E. L., Kung, P. C., Goldstein, G., and Schlossman, S. F., 1980, A monoclonal antibody reactive with the human cytotoxic/suppressor T cell subset defined by a heteroantiserum termed TH$_2$, *J. Immunol.* **124**:1301–1307.

Roehm, N. W., Marrack, P., and Kappler, J. W., 1983, Helper signals in the plaque-forming cell response to protein-bound haptens, *J. Exp. Med.* **158**:317–333.

Schimpl, A. J., and Wecker, E., 1975, A third signal in B cell activation given by TRF, *Transplant Rev.* **23**:176–188.

Schimpl, A., Hübner, A., Wong, L., and Wecker, E., 1980, Characteristics of late acting T cell replacing factor, *Behring Inst. Mitt.* **67**:221–229.

Schurman, R. K. B., Gelfand, E. B., and Dosh, H. M., 1980, Polyclonal activation of human lymphocytes *in vitro*. I. Characterization of the lymphocyte response to a T cell-independent B cell mitogen, *J. Immunol.* **125**:820–826.

Weiner, M. S., Bianco, C., and Nussenzweig, U., 1973, Enhanced binding of neuraminidase-treated sheep erythrocytes to human T lymphocytes, *Blood* **42**:939–946.

E. Special Topics

17

Human–Human Hybridomas in the Study of Immunodeficiencies

KATHLEEN A. DENIS, RANDOLPH WALL, AND ANDREW SAXON

I. Introduction

The majority of B-lymphocyte hybridomas, whether rodent–rodent, rodent–human, or human–human, are produced to use the resulting antibodies as tools. These monoclonal antibody products of hybridomas have been used successfully to purify proteins, define antigenic structures on normal and malignant cells, characterize viruses and microorganisms, and numerous other related tasks (Kennett *et al.*, 1980; Yelton and Scharff, 1981). Certainly one of the major goals of human–human hybridoma technology is to use human monoclonal antibodies in the diagnosis and therapy of a wide range of human disease states.

Hybridomas can also be useful in the immortalization of lymphoid cells for the purpose of studying these cell types in detail. This is particularly valuable if the subset of lymphoid cells is present in low numbers, is highly contaminated with other cell types, or is difficult to obtain. Hybridomas derived from fetal and neonatal B lymphocytes have been used in murine systems to better characterize early cell lineages and their immunoglobulin gene expression (Burrows *et al.*, 1979; Perry *et al.*, 1981; Denis and Klinman, 1983).

KATHLEEN A. DENIS AND RANDOLPH WALL • Departments of Microbiology and Immunology, UCLA School of Medicine, Los Angeles, California 90024. ANDREW SAXON • Department of Medicine, UCLA School of Medicine, Los Angeles, California 90024.

Mouse–human hybridomas have been used to study the structure of human immunoglobulin genes (Dolby *et al.*, 1980), to characterize the immunoglobulins expressed by human B-cell tumors (Levy *et al.*, 1980) and to examine the cellular defects present in agammaglobulinemia (Schwaber and Rosen, 1978).

It has been our interest to establish human–human hybridomas to better study the B-cell defects present in several human immunodeficiency states (Denis *et al.*, 1983). B lymphocytes from these patients are difficult to obtain in large enough quantity for biochemical and molecular studies. Even after numerous separation steps, the population of B cells obtained will still be contaminated with other cell types. Furthermore, such enriched B cells still represent a very heterogeneous mixture of cells at different stages of development as well as committed to different isotype production. The B lymphocytes from immunodeficiency patients are often unresponsive to mitogens and therefore cannot be selectively expanded by mitogenic stimulation (de la Concha *et al.*, 1976; Ashman *et al.*, 1980). Viral transformation of certain B-lymphocyte populations is possible; however, these cell lines are difficult to clone (Schwaber *et al.*, 1978) and B cells from certain immunodeficiency patients lack receptors for Epstein–Barr virus (Schwaber *et al.*, 1980). In addition, chromosomal translocations and DNA rearrangements are often observed in transformed lymphoid cells, many of these involving the immunoglobulin heavy chain locus (Klein, 1983). For these reasons, human–human hybridomas provided an improved approach to the study of B-cell function in humoral immunodeficiencies. The large number of clonally derived cells that could be obtained by this technique enables studies at the cellular, protein, and nucleic acid levels, which will aid in our understanding of the B-lymphocyte defects present in immunodeficiencies.

II. Immunodeficiency Patients Used in Hybridoma Formation

Two types of immunodeficiency patients were chosen for our initial studies of immunodeficiencies using human–human hybridomas. Adult patients with either common variable immunodeficiency (CVI) or selective IgA deficiency were used as lymphocyte donors for hybridoma formation. Common variable immunodeficiency typically has its onset in adolescent or adult life. CVI patients usually have normal numbers of circulating surface immunoglobulins (sIg)-positive B lymphocytes (Geha *et al.*, 1974; Gupta and Good, 1980). In general, these patients' B lymphocytes fail to mature into immunoglobulin-secreting cells *in vivo* and the serum Ig levels in these patients are very low, although not absent. Stimulation of the B lymphocytes from these patients with mitogens or antigens usually does not induce the cell proliferation and Ig secretion seen in normal individuals (de la Concha *et al.*, 1976; Stevens *et al.*, 1980). Cell separation and reconstitution *in vitro* have implicated inherent B-cell defects in the majority of patients with CVI (Geha *et al.*, 1974; Ashman *et al.*, 1980; De Gast *et al.*, 1980; Mitsuya *et al.*, 1981), but the molecular defects in these cells have been difficult to study.

Selective IgA deficiency is the most common of primary B-cell immunodeficiencies and, like CVI, probably represents a heterogeneous group of disorders in both its probable causes and its clinical manifestations. While many patients with selective IgA deficiency are asymptomatic, as a group they are subject to increased respiratory infections and gastrointestinal disorders (Ammann and Hong, 1971). This immunodeficiency syndrome is characterized by very low to absent serum IgA levels with normal levels of other immunoglobulins. However, B cells with surface IgA are present in these patients, although whether the number of such sIgA$^+$ cells is normal or decreased is controversial (Lawton *et al.*, 1972). Thus, as in the CVI patients, there does not appear to be an absence of the structural genes encoding the immunoglobulin heavy chains in these patients. Certain selective IgA deficiencies have been attributed to the lack of T-cell help or excess T-cell suppression (Waldmann, 1976), but many of these patients have intrinsic B-cell defects in the full maturation to IgA-secreting cells.

The patients that were used in the studies described here had normal percentages of sIg$^+$ B cells and E-rosetting T cells (Table I). Their serum immunoglobulin levels were consistent with their diagnosis of either CVI or selective IgA deficiency. In addition, cell separation and reconstitution experiments involving these patients had shown their defects to be related to B-cell function and not due to lack of helper T cells or an excess of T-cell suppression (Ashman *et al.*, 1980, and A. Saxon, unpublished observations). Clonally derived human–human hybridoma B-cell lines from these patients have allowed the study of potential cellular and molecular defects in these immunodeficiency states.

TABLE I

Clinical Characteristics of Immunodeficiency Patients[a]

Patient code	Diagnosis	Percent sIg$^+$ lymphocytes	Percent E-rosetting lymphocytes	Serum Ig (mg/dl)		
				IgM	IgG	IgA
A	CVI	4	77	2	93	2
C	CVI	4	73	2	145	5
D	CVI	6	65	27	143	2
F	CVI	17	65	3	106	0
G	CVI	ND	75	5	99	0
H	CVI	5	70	25	52	0
I	CVI	ND	60	21	6	24
J	IgA deficiency	8	67	124	940	0
K	IgA deficiency	ND	ND	234	1320	0
—	Normals	2–8	66–72	50–271	566–1313	79–366

[a]ND, Not determined.

III. Lymphocyte Activation and Hybridization

The B-lymphoblastoid line WIL2/729 HF (obtained from Dr. R. Lundak, University of California at Riverside) was used as the malignant parent in the creation of these hybridomas. This cell line is deficient in the enzyme HGPRT and can be selected against using HAT medium. Peripheral blood lymphocytes (PBLs) from these immunodeficiency patients separated by Ficoll–Hypaque gradients (Boyum, 1968) were used as the other partner in the fusions. Several attempts to hybridize the unstimulated peripheral blood lymphocytes resulted in failure to obtain any viable fusion products (Denis *et al.*, 1983). In addition, a 5-day exposure to various mitogens such as PWM and EBV also failed to generate cells capable of successful hybridization. However, mitogens often fail to stimulate PBLs from immunodeficiency patients to proliferate and secrete immunoglobulin (Mitsuya *et al.*, 1981). Their failure of cells to form hybrids was likely a reflection of the absence of activated B cells needed for successful fusion (Köhler and Milstein, 1976). Proper stimulation of these cells was obtained with a combination of PWM and Cowan I (Lipsky, 1980; Saiki and Ralph, 1981) as outlined in Fig. 1. Ficoll–Hypaque-purified PBLs from the immunodeficiency patients were cultured *in vitro* in the presence of 0.25 μl/ml PWM and 0.001% Cowan I in RPMI 1640 medium supplemented with 15% fetal calf serum. The cells were at a density of 10^6/ml. After 5 days, the mononuclear cells were counted and mixed with an equal number of WIL2/729 HF cells. These cells were then fused by an 8-min exposure to 30% PEG 1000 (Kennett *et al.*, 1978). The cells were plated in microtiter wells (3×10^5/well) and hybrids selected with HAT medium (13.6 μg/ml hypoxanthine, 0.18 μg/ml aminopterin, and 7.6 μg/ml thymidine) (Littlefield, 1964). After 2–3 weeks, growing hybrids were visible and the supernatants from these were assayed for human immunoglobulin production by radioimmunoassay. Hybridization results after PWM plus Cowan I treatment are shown in Table II. The success of the mitogen treatment is seen in the excellent cell recoveries obtained on day 5. It is of interest to note that these cells did not mature to immunoglobulin secretion with this stimulation (Denis *et al.*, 1983). These cells had a rather low fusion frequency, less than $1/10^6$, but an average of 33% of the hybridomas produced human immunoglobulin. From these Ig-producing hybridomas, 18 lines were obtained by limiting dilution cloning for further characterization.

IV. Characterization of the Hybridomas Obtained from the Peripheral Blood B Cells of Immunodeficiency Patients

The hybridomas from immunodeficient B lymphocytes produced only IgM, whether derived from CVI patients or IgA-deficiency patients. Karyotype analysis of three of the hybridomas showed them to be approximately

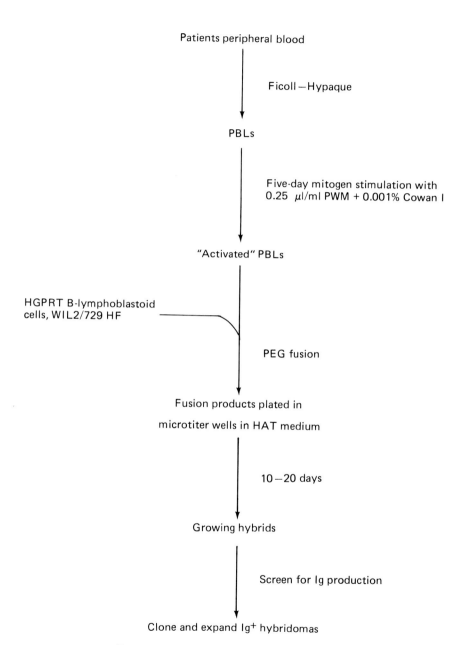

FIGURE 1. Scheme for hybridoma formation.

TABLE II
Hybridization Results

Patient	Number of PBLs ($\times$ 10^6)	Percent recovered on day 5	Hybridization frequency (per 10^6 PBLs)	Percent immunoglobulin secretors (number)
A	25	64	0.56	22 (2)
C	50	120	0.95	49 (28)
D	42	52	0.54	33 (4)
F	50	96	0.83	67 (27)
G	72	83	0.31	21 (4)
H	55	76	0.57	25 (6)
I	50	86	0.67	31 (9)
J	42	118	0.51	24 (6)
K	36	63	0.46	21 (2)

tetraploid, with modal chromosome numbers of 91, 92, and 92 (Denis *et al.*, 1983). All hybridomas were mycoplasma-free as determined by fluorescent DNA staining (Russell *et al.*, 1975).

It has been noted that hybridomas derived from lymphoblastoid fusion partners secrete much less immunoglobulin than those derived from myeloma fusion partners, due to the intrinsic character of these cell types (Kozbor and Roder, 1983). However, we observed a distinct difference in the levels of immunoglobulin secretion between hybridomas derived from these two types of immunodeficiency patients. Hybridomas derived from IgA-deficiency patients secreted IgM in the range of 120 to >400 ng/ml culture fluid (Table III). These secretion levels are comparable to those seen with hybri-

TABLE III
IgM Secretion by Cloned Hybridomas from Immunodeficiency Patients

Patient	Diagnosis	Clone number	IgM secreted[a] (ng/ml culture fluid)
C	CVI	18.F2	6
F	CVI	28.5	10
		32.15	20
G	CVI	6.4	20
		8.6	50
H	CVI	3.1	5
I	CVI	6.4	5
		10.1	60
J	IgA deficiency	8.6	400
		15.1	400
		25.1	120

[a]WIL2/729 HF secretes <1 ng/ml of IgM in culture.

domas derived from normal peripheral blood lymphocytes (data not shown). In contrast, the Ig-secreting hybridomas derived from CVI patients have IgM secretion levels of only 5–60 ng/ml of culture fluid (Table III). The hybridomas obtained from the lymphocytes of CVI patients have consistently lower levels of immunoglobulin secretion when compared to other hybridomas derived in the same manner and grown under the same conditions. Thus, the CVI hybridomas appear to have retained an intrinsic defect in immunoglobulin secretion despite the contribution of the lymphoblastoid cell parent.

V. Immunoglobulin Gene Analysis of the Hybridomas Derived from Immunodeficiency Patients

The process by which a B lymphocyte rearranges a variety of segments of DNA to create an intact gene for an immunoglobulin heavy or light chain has been well characterized [reviewed by Leder (1982); Honjo (1983); Tonegawa (1983)]. The DNA segments encoding the V, D, and J regions of the heavy chain are separated from the C-region DNA by stretches of intervening DNA in the germ-line state. Early in B-cell development the V_H and D segments rearrange adjacent to the J_H region to form a functional μ heavy chain gene. Light chain rearrangement takes place in a similar manner subsequent to this. Following these events at the DNA level, a B cell is capable of producing an intact IgM molecule.

To confirm that the production of IgM in the hybridoma cells was derived from the Ig genes of the immunodeficiency patients' B cells, DNA rearrangements at the heavy chain locus were examined. High-molecular weight DNA was extracted from human sperm, WIL2/729 HF, and the hybridoma lines by the method outlined in Fig. 2. Southern blots (Southern, 1975) of the restriction-enzyme-digested DNA were probed with a radiolabeled segment of DNA corresponding to the μ constant region (Fig. 3). The results of this analysis are published elsewhere (Denis et al., 1983). In summary, it was demonstrated that each hybridoma had a unique rearranged μ gene contributed by the immunodeficiency patients' cells in addition to the two rearranged μ genes of the non-IgM-secreting lymphoblastoid cell parent. Thus, IgM produced by these hybridomas is encoded by the patients' DNA, and this provides additional confirmation that the structural genes for IgM molecules are intact in these patients.

In addition, similar restriction analysis was performed using probes for the α and ϵ constant regions (Fig. 3) on the DNA from the IgA-deficiency patients. Again, no gross abnormalities were seen in these structural genes (Fig. 4).

A possible explanation for the failure of these immunodeficiency cells to express immunoglobulin properly would be alteration of the heavy chain switch region. This facilitates isotype switching to heavy chain classes other

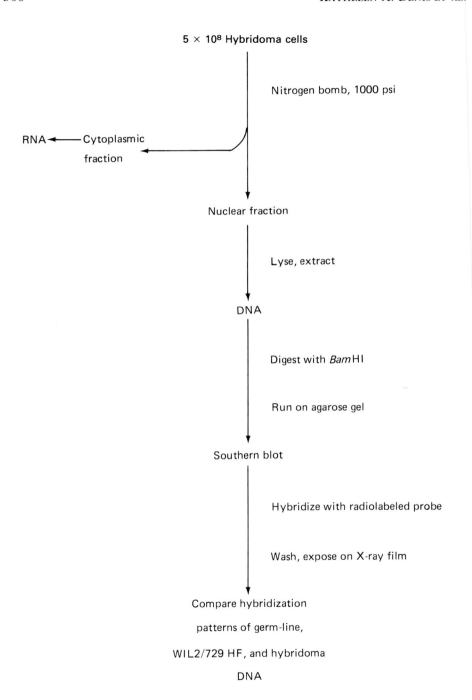

FIGURE 2. Nucleic acid extraction and analysis procedure.

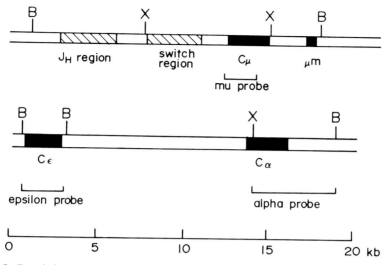

FIGURE 3. Restriction enzyme digests and DNA probes used in analysis of human immunoglobulin heavy chain genes. The germ-line DNA configuration of the μ, ε, and α immunoglobulin heavy chain genes and the corresponding DNA probes are shown. *Bam*HI digests of high-molecular weight DNA from the hybridomas were used to analyze rearrangements at the J_H locus as well as the presence of the ε and α genes. An *Xba*I digest was used to assess the integrity of the switch and μ constant region loci. B = *Bam*HI, X = *Xba*I.

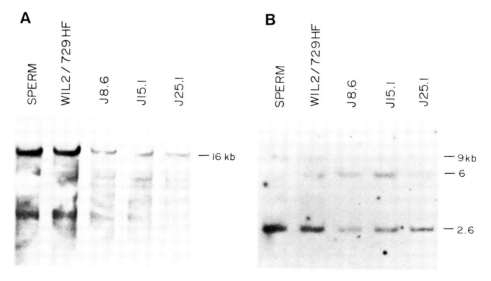

FIGURE 4. Southern blot analysis of α and ε immunoglobulin heavy chain genes in IgA-deficiency hybridomas. *Bam*HI-digested high-molecular weight DNA from these cells was electrophoresed in agarose and blotted onto nitrocellulose. The blots were hybridized to either radiolabeled (A) α or (B) ε probes (see Fig. 3). All hybridomas show only the normal 16-kb band of α hybridization (panel A) (Flanagan and Rabbitts, 1982) and the normal 9-, 6- and 2.6-kb bands of ε hybridization (panel B) (Max *et al.*, 1982). These bands were identical to those seen in the germ-line control (human sperm DNA).

than IgM and IgD. Deletions in the switch region were probed using an *Xba*I digest of the hybridoma DNA and the μ constant region probe (see Fig. 3). An intact switch region would give a 7.5-kb hybridizing band; all of the hybridomas displayed only this 7.5-kb band in their DNA (Fig. 5). This result indicates no major structural alterations in the switch region that could account for the B-cell immunodeficiencies.

Such restriction digests of DNA from the hybridomas derived from the immunodeficiency patients are limited in their ability to diagnose defects. Point mutations or very small deletions in the DNA regions analyzed would not be detected. However, it does appear that there are no gross alterations of the genes coding for the immunoglobulin μ constant regions or the switch region in these patients' DNA. In addition, the IgA-deficiency patients' DNA appears to contain intact immunoglobulin α and ε constant region genes, which are the deficient isotypes in these patients.

VI. RNA Processing of μ Heavy Chain Message in the Hybridomas Derived from Immunodeficiency Patients

The RNA processing events that generate immunoglobulin heavy chain proteins from messenger RNA transcribed from the rearranged heavy chain genes have been studied for several years [reviewed by Wall and Kuehl (1983)]. The membrane and the secreted heavy chains of each immunoglobulin isotype are encoded by a complex transcription unit, which can generate both proteins from a single heavy chain gene. The relative levels of production of the two proteins are governed by control mechanisms that are poorly understood. Approximately 20–50% of immunoglobulin μ heavy chain is of the secreted form in normal pre-B and immature B cells, although this protein is not secreted by these cells (Mains and Sibley, 1982). The ratio of secreted to membrane μ mRNA as well as μ protein then increases as the B cell matures.

The level of μ heavy chain mRNA and the ratio of membrane to secreted μ mRNA were analyzed in these immunodeficiency hybridomas using Northern blot analysis (Thomas, 1980). The lymphoblastoid parent WIL2/729 HF had barely detectable μ heavy chain mRNA (Fig. 6), which was of the 2.3-kb membrane form. This result was expected from the extremely low amount of IgM secreted by these cells in culture (less than 1 ng/ml; see Table III). Hybridomas derived from the peripheral blood lymphocytes of selective IgA-deficiency patients possessed equal amounts of membrane and secreted μ heavy chain mRNA (J8.6 and J25.1, Fig. 6). Hybridomas derived from the peripheral blood lymphocytes of normal individuals had a similar ratio of these two μ mRNA forms (not shown). In contrast, hybridomas derived from the peripheral blood lymphocytes of CVI patients showed a decreased level of

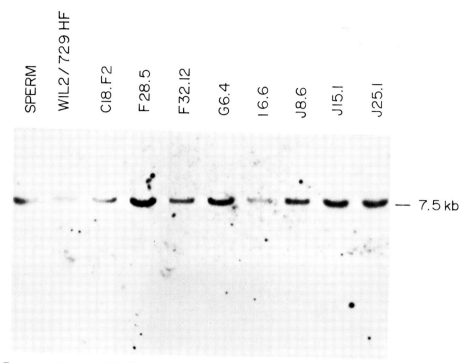

FIGURE 5. Immunoglobulin heavy chain switch region analysis. High-molecular weight DNA from the hybridomas was digested with XbaI and Southern blot analysis performed using a radiolabeled μ probe (see Fig. 3). A single band of hybridization was present at 7.5 kb in all hybridoma cells as well as the germ-line control (human sperm DNA).

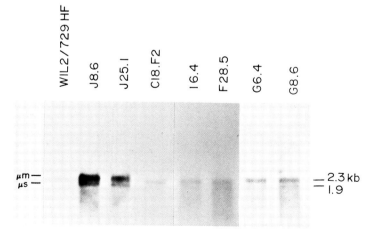

FIGURE 6. Northern blot analysis of μ heavy chain mRNA. Poly A-selected RNA (5 μg; 20 μg of WIL2/729 HF mRNA) was treated with glyoxyl, electrophoresed in agarose, and transferred to nitrocellulose (Thomas, 1980). The blot was hybridized to a radioactive μ probe (see Fig. 3) that detects both the membrane and secreted forms of μ mRNA.

μ mRNA, with a marked predominance of the membrane form of μ heavy chain mRNA (Fig. 6). It is important to note that these hybridomas were selected on the basis of optimal immunoglobulin secretion. Despite this selection at the protein level, all CVI patient-derived hybridomas had very low levels of secreted μ mRNA, low levels of total μ heavy chain mRNA, and an increased ratio of membrane to secreted μ mRNA when compared to other hybridomas (Fig. 6). This directly reinforces the observation of decreased levels of IgM secretion in the CVI hybridomas when compared to other hybridomas (see Table III). Taken together, these results indicate an inability of the CVI lymphocytes to secrete immunoglobulin efficiently, which appears to be related to a defect in RNA processing resulting in preferential production of membrane μ mRNA over secreted μ mRNA.

VII. Discussion

The elucidation of the molecular basis for many immunodeficiencies has been hindered by the lack of suitable tissue for study. Often, the only affected cell type is a small subpopulation of lymphocytes, which are difficult to isolate in sufficient numbers or purity for extensive study. Human–human hybridomas have provided an alternate approach to the study of these diseases. Normal lymphocytes isolated from these patients can be fused to a continuously cultured cell line and the resulting hybridomas cloned and characterized.

In this study we have examined hybridomas derived from patients with common variable immunodeficiency and selective IgA deficiency. A single lymphoblastoid cell line was used as the malignant parent for these hybridomas; thus, comparisons could be made among the hybridomas. The hybridomas made from the peripheral blood lymphocytes of selective IgA-deficiency patients were very similar to hybridomas made from the peripheral blood lymphocytes of normal individuals in the amount of IgM secreted and in the levels and proportions of μ heavy chain mRNA. Indeed, selective IgA-deficiency patients have normal numbers of surface immunoglobulin-positive cells as well as normal levels of serum IgM. This group of hybridomas was used as a basis for comparison of the CVI patient-derived hybridomas, since any influence of the lymphoblastoid parent would be equal.

The lack of genetic inheritance and the overall nature of these two immunodeficiencies made it unlikely that they were caused by an absence or gross change of the immunoglobulin structural genes. The limited DNA analysis presented in this study has already provided confirmation for this. However, the regulation of μ immunoglobulin heavy chain gene and its protein products appears to differ between the CVI-derived hybridomas and the IgA-deficiency-derived hybridomas in at least two ways. First, the overall transcription of μ heavy chain mRNA is much lower in the CVI-derived hybridomas when compared to other hybridomas. Second, the processing of the heavy chain mRNA precursors results in a much higher ratio of membrane to secreted μ mRNA in the CVI-derived hybridomas. The final result of these two changes is a much decreased level of IgM secretion by the hybridoma. It is possible that similar events lead to the very low levels of serum IgM (as well as other isotypes) in the CVI patients.

It is interesting to speculate whether these changes in the CVI hybridomas are due to a lack of positive signals for the switch to secretion or the presence of inappropriate negative signals that prevent these events. This could be addressed by the fusion of the CVI peripheral blood lymphocytes to a cell type with strong positive signals for immunoglobulin secretion, such as a myeloma cell. Examination of the resulting hybridomas would show whether the dominant secretory phenotype of the myeloma could overcome the CVI defect or if any negative regulatory events in the CVI lymphocyte would affect secretion of the myeloma protein. It would also be possible that these types of regulation could not act in a *trans* manner and the hybridoma would retain good secretion of the myeloma protein and poor secretion of the CVI immunoglobulin. Alternatively, the hybridomas described in this study could be subjected to lymphocyte growth and maturation factors (Howard and Paul, 1983) or nonspecific transcription-enhancing drugs (Boyd and Schrader, 1982) and monitored for increased immunoglobulin secretion.

The hybridomas derived from selective IgA-deficiency patients in this study were indistinguishable from those derived from normal individuals. However, all of the hybridomas secreted IgM, an isotype not affected in this disease. Perhaps other lymphocyte activation schemes could be used to provide IgA-expressing hybridomas, which could be used to better study this disease.

Human–human hybridomas have provided a new and promising approach to the study of immunodeficiencies. Future studies such as this and others (Schwaber *et al.*, 1983) should contribute enormously to our understanding and our ability to treat these diseases.

ACKNOWLEDGMENTS

Our thanks to Ann Fisher and Carla Carter for technical help and to Kay Vasley for manuscript preparation. K. A. D. was supported by USPHS CA 09120. This work was supported by USPHS grants AI 13410, AI 15251, and CA 12800 and NSF grant PCM 79-24876.

References

Ammann, A. J., and Hong, R., 1971, Selective IgA deficiency: Presentation of 30 cases and a review of the literature, *Medicine* **50**:223.

Ashman, R. F., Saxon, A., and Stevens, R. H., 1980, Profile of multiple lymphocyte functional defects in acquired hypogammaglobulinemia, derived from *in vitro* cell recombination analysis, *J. Allergy Clin. Immunol.* **65**:242–256.

Boyd, A. W., and Schrader, J. W., 1982, Derivation of macrophage-like lines from the pre-B lymphoma ABLS 8.1 using 5-azacytidine, *Nature* **297**:691–693.

Boyum, A., 1968, Isolation of mononuclear cells and granulocytes from human blood, *Scand. J. Clin. Lab. Invest. (Suppl).* **97**:77.

Burrows, P., LeJeune, M., and Kearney, J. F., 1979, Evidence that murine pre-B cells synthesize μ heavy chain but no light chains, *Nature* **280**:838–841.

De Gast, G. C., Wilkins, S. R., Webster, A. B. D., Rickinson, A. and Platts-Mills, T. A. E., 1980, Functional "immaturity" of isolated B cells from patients with hypogammaglobulinemia, *Clin. Exp. Immunol.* **42**:535–544.

de la Concha, E. G., Oldman, G., Webster, A. D. B., Asherson, G. I., and Platts-Mills, T. A. E., 1976, Quantitative measurements of T and B cell function in variable primary hypogammaglobulinemia: Evidence for a consistent B-cell defect, *Clin. Exp. Immunol.* **27**:208.

Denis, K. A., and Klinman, N. R., 1983, Genetic and temporal control of neonatal antibody expression, *J. Exp. Med.* **157**:1170–1183.

Denis, K. A., Wall, R., and Saxon, A., 1983, Human–human B cell hybridomas from *in vitro* stimulated lymphocytes of patients with common variable immunodeficiency, *J. Immunol.* **131**:2273–2278.

Dolby, T. W., Devuono, J., and Croce, C. M., 1980, Cloning and partial nucleotide sequence of human immunoglobulin μ chain cDNA from B cells and mouse–human hybridomas, *Proc. Natl. Acad. Sci. USA* **77**:6027–6031.

Flanagan, J. G., and Rabbitts, T. H., 1982, Arrangement of human immunoglobulin heavy chain constant region genes implies evolutionary duplication of a segment containing ε, γ, and α genes, *Nature* **300**:709–713.

Geha, R. S., Schneeberger, E., Merler, E., and Rosen, F. S., 1974, Heterogeneity of "acquired" or common variable agammablobulinemia, *N. Engl. J. Med.* **291**:1–6.

Gupta, S., and Good, R. A., 1980, Markers of human lymphocyte subpopulations in primary immunodeficiency and lymphoproliferative disorders, *Sem. Hematol.* **17**:1–29.

Honjo, T., 1983, Immunoglobulin genes, *Annu. Rev. Immunol.* **1**:499–528.

Howard, M., and Paul, W. E., 1983, Regulation of B-cell growth and differentiation by soluble factors, *Annu. Rev. Immunol.* **1**:307–33.

Kennett, R. H., Denis, K. A., Tung, A. S., and Klinman, N. R., 1978, Hybrid plasmacytoma production: Fusions with adult spleen cells, monoclonal spleen fragments, neonatal spleen cells and human spleen cells, *Curr. Top. Microbiol. Immunol.* **81**:77–91.

Kennett, R. H., McKearn, T. J., and Bechtol, K. B., 1980, *Monoclonal Antibodies*, Plenum Press, New York.

Klein, G., 1983, Specific chromosomal translocations and the genesis of B-cell derived tumors in mice and men, *Cell* **32**:311–312.

Köhler, G., and Milstein, C., 1976, Derivation of specific antibody-producing tissue culture and tumor lines by cell fusion, *Eur. J. Immunol.* **6**:511–519.

Kozbor, D., and Roder, J. C., 1983, The production of monoclonal antibodies from human lymphocytes, *Immunol. Today* **4**:72–79.

Lawton, A. R., Royal, S. A., Self, K. S., and Cooper, M. D., 1972, IgA determinants on B lymphocytes in patients with deficiency of circulating IgA, *J. Lab. Clin. Med.* **80**:26–33.

Leder, P., 1982, The genetics of antibody diversity, *Sci. Amer.* **246**:102–115.

Levy, R., Dilley, J., Brown, S., and Bergman, Y., 1980, Mouse × human hybridomas, in: *Monoclonal Antibodies* (R. H. Kennett, T. J. McKearn, and K. B. Bechtol, eds.), Plenum Press, New York, pp. 137–153.

Lipsky, P. E., 1980, Staphylococcal protein A, a T cell-regulated polyclonal activator of human B cells, *J. Immunol.* **125**:155–162.

Littlefield, J. W., 1964, Selection of hybrids from matings of fibroblasts *in vitro* and their presumed recombinants, *Science* **145**:709.

Mains, P. E., and Sibley, C. H., 1982, Control of IgM synthesis in the murine pre-B cell line, 70Z/3, *J. Immunol.* **128**:1664–1670.

Max, E. E., Battey, J., Ney, R., Kirsch, I. R., and Leder, P., 1982, Duplication and deletion in the human immunoglobulin genes, *Cell* **29**:691–699.

Mitsuya, H., Osaki, K., Tomino, S., Katsuki, T., and Kishimoto, S., 1981, Pathophysiologic analysis of peripheral blood lymphocytes from patients with primary immunodeficiency. I. Ig synthesis by peripheral blood lymphocytes stimulated with either PWM or EBV *in vitro, J. Immunol.* **127**:311–315.

Perry, R. P., Kelley, D. E., Coleclough, C., and Kearney, J. F., 1981, Organization and expression of immunoglobulin genes in fetal liver hybridomas, *Proc. Natl. Acad. Sci. USA* **78**:247–251.

Russell, W. C., Newman, C., and Williamson, D. H., 1975, A simple cytochemical technique for demonstration of DNA in cells infected with mycoplasmas and viruses, *Nature* **253**:461–462.

Saiki, O., and Ralph, P., 1981, Induction of human immunoglobulin secretion. I. Synergistic effect of B cell mitogen Cowan I plus T cell mitogens or factors, *J. Immunol.* **127**:1044–1047.

Schwaber, J. F., and Rosen, F. S., 1978, Induction of human immunoglobulin synthesis and secretion in somatic cell hybrids of mouse myeloma and human B lymphocytes from patients with agammaglobulinemia, *J. Exp. Med.* **148**:974–986.

Schwaber, J., Lazarus, H., and Rosen, F., 1978, Bone marrow-derived lymphoid cell lines from patients with agammaglobulinemia, *J. Clin. Invest.* **62**:302–310.

Schwaber, J. F., Klein, G., Ernberg, I., Rosen, A., Lazarus, H., and Rosen, F. S., 1980, Deficiency of Epstein–Barr virus (EBV) receptors on B lymphocytes from certain patients with common varied agammaglobulinemia, *J. Immunol.* **24**:2191–2196.

Schwaber, J., Molgaard, H., Orkin, S. H., Gould, H. J., and Rosen, F. S., 1983, Early pre-B cells from normal and X-linked agammaglobulinemia produce Cu without an attached V$_H$ region, *Nature* **304**:355–358.

Southern, E. M., 1975, Detection of specific sequences among DNA fragments separated by gel electrophoresis, *J. Mol. Bio.* **98**:503–517.

Stevens, R. H., Tamaroff, M., and Saxon, A., 1980, Inability of patients with common variable hypogammaglobulinemia to generate lymphoblastoid B cells following booster immunization, *Clin. Immunol. Immunopathol.* **16**:336–343.

Thomas, P. S., 1980, Hybridization of denatured DNA and small DNA fragments transferred to nitrocellulose, *Proc. Natl. Acad. Sci. USA* **77**:5201–5205.

Tonegawa, S., 1983, Somatic generation of antibody diversity, *Nature* **302**:575–581.

Waldmann, T. A., 1976, Defect in IgA secretion in IgA specific suppressor cells in patients with selective IgA deficiency, *Trans. Assoc. Am. Physicians* **89**:215.

Wall, R., and Kuehl, M., 1983, Biosynthesis and regulation of immunoglobulins, *Annu. Rev. Immunol.* **1**:393–422.

Yelton, D. E., and Scharff, M. D., 1981, Monoclonal antibodies: A powerful new look in biology and medicine, *Annu. Rev. Biochem.* **50**:657–680.

TABLE I

Human Mononuclear Leukocyte Lineages Identified by Murine Monoclonal Antibodies[a]

Lineage	Surface markers
T	Leu 1, 4, 5 (T1, 3, 11)
B	sIg, HLA DR, Leu 12
Monocytes	Leu M3, OKM1, HLA DR
Natural killer	Leu 11 (Fc γ receptor)

[a]The antibodies listed identify all or nearly all cells within a lineage. Although most of the markers listed are not absolutely lineage-specific, in many instances they can be used to identify or isolate a desired cell type. In all or nearly all instances, these markers mediate important immunologic functions.

antigen] and suppressor/cytotoxic cells [which express the Leu 2 (T8) antigen] (Reinherz *et al.*, 1979, 1980; Evans *et al.*, 1981; Kotzin *et al.*, 1981; Gatenby *et al.*, 1981). Like their Lyt-2$^+$ and Lyt-2$^-$ counterparts in mice (Cantor and Boyse, 1977), the two human subsets were initially thought to have non-overlapping functions. However, it is now known that both subsets contain cells capable of maturing into cytotoxic effector cells. In fact, recent studies suggest that the Leu 2$^+$ or Leu 3$^+$ surface phenotype may be primarily associated with the capacity of T cells to recognize particular products of genes within the major histocompatibility complex (MHC) (Engleman *et al.*, 1981a). Thus, the Leu 3 subset includes cells that can proliferate in response to MHC class II alloantigens (HLA DP, DQ, DR) or soluble antigens presented in association with class II determinants on antigen-presenting cells. Once

TABLE II

Functional Subsets of Human T Cells Identified with Murine Monoclonal Antibodies

Monoclonal antibody	Percent of circulating T cells	Functional cell type identified
Leu 2/T$_8$	25–40	Suppressor and cytotoxic T cells
Leu 3/T$_4$	50–65	Helper and inducer T cells
Leu 8	75–85	Distinguishes helper (Leu 3$^+$, 8$^-$) and suppressor/inducer (Leu 3$^+$, 8$^+$) T cells; stains other cell types as well
9.3	70–90	Distinguishes cytotoxic (Leu 2$^+$, 9.3$^+$) and suppressor (Leu 2$^+$, 9.3$^-$) T cells; stains all Leu 3$^+$ T cells

activated, Leu 3$^+$ cells can activate B cells and Leu 2$^+$ cytotoxic and suppressor cells (Reinherz *et al.*, 1979, 1980; Evans *et al.*, 1981; Kotzin *et al.*, 1981; Gatenby *et al.*, 1981), or become cytotoxic effector cells that are specific for determinants on class II molecules (Krensky *et al.*, 1982; Meuer *et al.*, 1982a). By contrast, in the absence of Leu 3$^+$ cells or their soluble products, Leu 2$^+$ cells cannot proliferate in response to soluble antigens or class II determinants (Engleman *et al.*, 1981a), but can differentiate under the influence of Leu-3$^+$ cells into either suppressor cells or cytotoxic effector cells, usually with restriction for class I (HLA-A, -B, -C) molecules (Meuer *et al.*, 1982a; Damle *et al.*, 1984). Recently, evidence has accumulated to suggest that the Leu 2 and Leu 3 molecules may serve as associative recognitive elements with specificity for class I and II MHC determinants, respectively (Engleman *et al.*, 1981b; Meuer *et al.*, 1982b; Engleman *et al.*, 1983). Such a role for these cell surface structures may account for the genetically restricted functions of each subset.

Although T cells within each major lineage may share a common receptor for MHC, as noted above, each subset includes cells that mediate a variety of functions. Conceivably, a given T cell may be able to perform the entire repertoire of immune functions, depending on factors external to the cells, such as the nature of the antigenic stimulus. Alternatively, a given T cell may be genetically programmed for a more restricted set of functional capabilities. The results of our studies indicate the existence of functionally distinct subsets within each of the two major T-cell lineages. Although the existence of multifunctional T cells cannot be excluded, it appears that most T cells perform narrowly defined functions, which correlate well with surface phenotype. Thus, for example, monoclonal antibody to the Leu 8 surface molecule can be used to distinguish Leu 3$^+$ cells capable of activating suppressor cells (Leu 3$^+$, 8$^+$) from Leu 3$^+$ cells capable of inducing B cells to secrete antibody (Leu 3$^+$, 8$^-$) (Gatenby *et al.*, 1982; Mohagheghpour *et al.*, 1983; Damle *et al.*, 1984a). Another monoclonal antibody, designated 9.3, can be used to separate precursors of Leu 2$^+$ cytolytic cells (Leu 2$^+$, 9.3$^+$) from suppressor cells (Leu 2$^+$, 9.3$^-$) (Meuer *et al.*, 1983).

The availability of the monoclonal antibodies anti-Leu 8 and 9.3 has enabled us to explore the basis of suppressor cell activation. The results of our studies indicate that at least one type of suppressor T cell recognizes and responds in a specific manner to antigen-activated inducer cells rather than directly to antigen. Following maturation and clonal expansion, such suppressor T cells (Ts) interact with antigen receptors on T helper/inducer cells to downregulate the helper/inducer response to antigen. The experimental data in support of this conclusion were obtained as follows. Leu 3$^+$ inducer T cells were activated with antigen for 1 week, washed extensively, and then used as irradiated stimulators in cultures with fresh autologous Leu 2$^+$ cells. Following this second culture, the activated Leu 2$^+$ cells were reisolated and tested for their ability to inhibit the response of fresh Leu 3$^+$ cells to antigen. In these studies antigen-primed Leu 3$^+$ cells were capable of activating Ts cells in the absence of antigen (Damle and Engleman, 1983; Damle *et al.*, 1984a). Suppression of the response of fresh autologous T cells was specific for the original antigenic stimulus, and the target of suppression was the helper/inducer population of T cells rather than antigen-presenting cells (Damle and Engleman, 1983; Damle *et al.*, 1984a). At no point during their activation were Ts cells exposed directly to antigen.

Apparently, Ts precursors interact with molecules either expressed on or secreted by activated inducer cells and this interaction initiates maturation and clonal expansion of Ts cells. To determine which molecules are involved in such interactions, activated inducer cells were incubated, in the absence of complement, with a panel of monoclonal antibodies directed at defined cell surface antigens, then washed extensively and tested for their ability to activate Ts cells. Antibodies directed against the T3 (Leu 4) complex (which includes the T-cell antigen receptor) (Meuer *et al.*, 1983) or HLA class I determinants on Leu 3^+ cells blocked the activation of suppressor cells, whereas antibodies to a variety of other cell surface antigens had no effect (Damle *et al.*, 1984b). Incubation of Leu 2^+ Ts precursors with the same antibodies revealed that anti-T3 blocked the generation of suppressor cells. Cell mixing experiments showed that whereas activation of suppressor/inducer cells is restricted by class II HLA determinants, both the interaction between Ts precursors and T inducer cells and that between Ts effectors and T helper/inducer cells are restricted by class I HLA antigens (Damle *et al.*, 1984b). Thus, it appears that T3-associated antigen receptors on precursors of Ts cells interact with antigen recognition structures on suppressor/inducer cells, and the apparent specificity of suppression for the priming antigen reflects specificity for "idiotypic" determinants on antigen-reactive helper/inducer cells.

Although suppressor circuits of the type described above have been shown to regulate the response to both soluble and cellular antigens *in vitro*, it is not yet known whether such circuits are active *in vivo*. Similarly, it remains to be shown which of the multiple steps in the circuit are mediated by soluble factors. The generation of T–T hybrids with the functional characteristics of each cell type involved in the circuit should be useful in the pursuit of answers to these questions.

III. The Role of Lymphokines in Immunoregulation

While it is beyond the scope of this chapter to attempt a detailed discussion of the numerous lymphokines described to date, it is important to consider briefly the role of some of the better defined lymphokines in immunoregulation. As mentioned earlier, many T-cell functions are mediated by soluble immunoregulatory factors. Therefore, an understanding of the mechanisms of action of these lymphokines is essential to our overall understanding of immunoregulation. Moreover, since they are active at extremely low concentrations and are relatively stable in the presence of serum, they represent exciting candidates for use as a new class of immunotherapeutic agents. On this basis, an intense effort has been ongoing in many laboratories to isolate and characterize lymphokines.

Clarification of the roles of lymphokines in regulation of the human immune response has resulted primarily from studies of *in vitro* systems. These model systems allow direct studies of defined immunologic processes, including B-cell differentiation and antibody formation, cytotoxic T-cell activation and function, suppressor cell induction and function, and natural killer cell activation and function. Maturation of B cells into immunoglobulin-secreting cells appears to require several distinct T-helper products, including B-cell growth factors, B-cell differentiation factors, and probably interleukin 1 and interferon γ (Moller, 1984; Okada *et al.*, 1983; Falkoff *et al.*, 1983). Maturation of cytolytic T cells requires interleukin 2, secreted principally by activated helper/inducer T cells, and possibly additional differentiation factors derived from non-T cells or cytolytic cells themselves (Moller, 1982; Finke *et al.*, 1981). The factors necessary for the activation of suppressor T cells are perhaps the least well understood. In addition to a presumed role for classical lymphokines such as interleukins 1 and 2, substances such as histamine clearly affect the formation of suppressor cells (Sansoni *et al.*, 1985). Additional T-cell factors are thought to transmit antigen-specific helper and suppressor signals (Webb *et al.*, 1983), although the failure to date to isolate such factors in quantities sufficient for detailed structural analysis has led to uncertainty regarding their physiological significance. Clearly, however, there continues to be great interest in such specific factors, since they offer the theoretical potential of manipulating the immune response in *vivo* in an antigen-specific manner. Other T-cell-derived factors include several that regulate hematopoiesis and others that appear to lyse tumor cells but not normal cells. It is likely that T cells elaborate many more factors than have been defined to date, and that such factors probably affect a wide variety of target cells and functions.

IV. Human T–T Hybridomas

The construction of T–T hybrids is a natural extension of the technology originally developed by Köhler and Milstein (1975) for the purpose of producing monoclonal antibodies of desired specificity from B–B hybridomas. The initial impetus for the production of T-cell hybrids was the inadequacy of available sources of lymphokines for detailed functional and biochemical characterization. Bulk cultures of mitogen-stimulated lymphocytes were the major source of lymphokines for investigative studies, but such cultures contain many different cell types and, consequently, also contain a great many lymphokines, often with opposing or synergistic effects on immunity. Tech-

Meuer, S. C., Hussey, R. E., Hodgdon, J. C., Hercend, T., and Schlossman, S. F., 1982b, Surface structures involved in target recognition by human cytotoxic T lymphocytes, *Science* **218**:471.

Meuer, S. C., Acuto, O., Hussey, R. E., Hodsdon, J. C., Fitzgerald, K. A., Schlossman, and Reinherz, E. L., 1983, Evidence for the T3-associated 90k heterodimer as the T cell antigen receptor, *Nature* **303**:808.

Mitsuya, H., Guo, H.-G., Cossman, J., Megson, M., Reitz, M. S., and Broder, S., 1984, Functional properties of antigen-specific T cells injected by human T-cell leukemia-lymphoma virus (HTL^v-1), *Science* **225**:1484.

Mohagheghpour, N., Benike, C. J., Kansas, G. S., Bieber, C., and Engleman, E. G., 1983, Activation of antigen specific suppressor T cells in the presence of cyclosporin requires interactions between T cells of inducer and suppressor lineage, *J. Clin. Invest.* **72**:2092.

Moller, G. (ed.), 1982, Interleukins and lymphocyte activation, *Immunol. Rev.* **63**.

Moller, G. (ed.), 1984, B cell growth and differentiation factors, *Immunol. Rev.* **78.**

Okada, M., Sakaguchi, N., Yoshimura, N., Hara, H., Shimuzu, K., Yoshida, N., Yoshizaki, K., Kishimoto, S., Yamamura, Y., and Kishimoto, T., 1983, B cell growth factors and B cell differentiation factor from human T hybridomas. Two distinct kinds of B cell growth factor and their synergism in B cell proliferation, *J. Exp. Med.* **157**:583.

Reinherz, E. L., Kung, P. C., Goldstein, G., and Schlossman, S. F., 1979, Separation of functional subsets of human T cells by a monoclonal antibody, *Proc. Natl. Acad. Sci. USA* **76**:4061.

Reinherz, E. L., Kung, P. C., Goldstein, G., and Schlossman, S. F., 1980, A monoclonal antibody reactive with the human cytotoxic/suppressor T cell subset previously defined by a heteroantiserum termed TH_2, *J. Immunol.* **124**:1301.

Sansoni, P., Silverman, E. D., Khan, M. M., Melmon, K. L., and Engleman, E. G., 1985, Immunoregulatory T cells in man. Histamine-induced suppressor T cells are derived from a Leu 2+ (T8+) subpopulation distinct from that which gives rise to cytotoxic T cells, *J. Clin. Invest.* **75**:650.

Webb, D. R., Kapp, J. A., and Pierce, C. W., 1983. The biochemistry of antigen-specific T cell factors, *Annu. Rev. Immunol.* **1**:423.

19

Production of Human T-Cell Hybridomas by Electrofusion

C. Gravekamp, S. J. L. Bol, A. Hagemeijer, and R. L. H. Bolhuis

I. Introduction

The somatic cell hybridization technique provides a means for the immortalization of specific cellular functions. Köhler and Milstein (1975) were the first to be successful in the immortalization of the production of specific immunoglobulins by cell fusion. They prepared a continuously immunoglobulin-secreting hybridoma cell line by fusion of mouse myeloma cells with spleen cells of an immunized mouse in the presence of inactivated Sendai virus. In addition to Sendai virus, polyethylene glycol (PEG) has also been widely used for cell fusion. During the past 10 years, an explosive development of hybridoma technology has taken place in many laboratories for the *in vitro* production of mouse monoclonal antibodies [for a review, see Reading (1982)]. It was later demonstrated that other cellular functions can also be immortalized by cell fusion. For example, mouse T-cell hybridomas that secrete immunoregulatory molecules such as interleukin 2 (IL-2) or T-cell replacing factor (TRF) have been produced. Other mouse T-cell hybrids expressing helper or suppressor functions have been established [for a review, see Malissen and Zeurthen (1982)]. More recently, several laboratories have directed their attention to xenogeneic and human–human hybrids exerting specific immunologic functions with a view to their potential clinical application. However, the preparation of human hybrids has generally appeared to

C. Gravekamp, S. J. L. Bol, and R. L. H. Bolhuis • Rotterdam Radiotherapeutic Institute, Rotterdam, The Netherlands. A. Hagemeijer • Department of Cell Biology and Genetics, Erasmus University, Rotterdam, The Netherlands.

be more difficult than that of murine hybrids. Initial growth of the fused cells (for human T–T and for some human B–B cell hybridomas) is difficult to achieve and often it takes more than a month before proliferation of fused cells can be observed (Greene *et al.*, 1982; Grillot-Courvalin and Brouet, 1981; Sikora *et al.*, 1982; Chiorazzi *et al.*, 1982). Moreover, human–human hybridomas frequently show chromosomal instability (Foung *et al.*, 1982; Kozbor and Roder, 1983). In this respect, the choice of fusion agent could be an important factor. PEG has a number of disadvantages that might be drawbacks in the production of a larger repertoire of hybrid cells.

1. The number of available human tumor cell lines suitable as fusion partners is limited. PEG-mediated fusion products require HAT (hypoxanthine–aminopterin–thymidine) medium to select the hybrid cells. Therefore, HAT-sensitive tumor cell lines are required and these are tedious to prepare. Many cell lines have to be tested for suitability because the chromosomal array of the tumor cell line is frequently incompatible with that of the lymphocytes (Kozbor and Roder, 1983; Foung *et al.*, 1982). Thus, the number of available tumor cell lines that have to be tested is limited by the requirement of HAT sensitivity.

2. Not every tumor cell line can be fused by use of PEG. It appears that aggregation of intermembrane particles (IMP), which could be necessary for cell fusion, does not occur in fusion-deficient cells (Roos *et al.*, 1983).

3. The fusion process cannot be monitored by microscopic observation.

To circumvent these problems, the electric field-induced cell fusion technique developed by Zimmermann (1982) may quite possibly be an efficient alternative to PEG-induced cell fusion. With this technique, close membrane contact is established between cells in an electrical field and fusion is induced by the application of a pulse of high field intensity. Electrofusion can be performed with relatively low cell numbers and the fusion process can be monitored microscopically. Although not performed in this study, visualization of the fusion procedure offers the possibility to isolate single fusion products and to culture them without HAT medium. In this chapter, we report on the efficiency of electrofusion in comparison with PEG fusion for the production of human T-cell hybridomas. In particular, we were interested in the possibilities of preparing human T-cell hybrids with cytolytic activity against tumor cells.

II. Fusion Partners in Polyethylene Glycol Fusion and Electrofusion

HSB-2, a human T-lymphoma cell line deficient for thymidine kinase and resistant to bromodeoxyuridine, was used for PEG fusion and electrofusion. The human cytotoxic T lymphocytes (CTLs) used for immortalization were derived from three sources:

1. Fresh peripheral blood lymphocytes (PBLs) isolated from the blood of a healthy donor by centrifugation in Ficoll–Paque (d = 1.077 g/cm^3).
2. Phytohemagglutinin (PHA)-stimulated lymphocytes obtained by stimulation of PBLs with 10 μg PHA/10^6 cells per ml during 48 hr.
3. Cloned cytotoxic T lymphocytes (clone 4) produced in our laboratory (Van de Griend and Bolhuis, 1984).

CTLs are able to recognize and subsequently lyse tumor cells [for a recent review, see Berke (1983)]. The PBLs and PHA-stimulated lymphocytes that we used for fusion exert nonspecific lytic activity against HSB-2, MOLT, K562, and K562 coated with PHA (lectin-dependent cytotoxicity) (data not shown). Clone 4 exerted strong allospecific cytotoxicity against an allogeneic EBV-transformed B-cell line (APD). This B-cell line was originally used as the stimulator cell of clone 4.

III. Polyethylene Glycol Fusion

Mechanisms for membrane fusion in mammalian cells involving either specific interactions between particle-rich membrane areas (Burwen and Satir, 1977) or nonspecific lipid–lipid interaction between particle-free areas in closely apposed cells have been proposed (Ahkong et al., 1975). One effect of PEG may be the alteration of the membrane structure in such a way that fusion is induced. Roose et al. (1983) observed aggregation of intermembrane particles (IMP) in cooled samples (4°C) of fused cells. No aggregation of IMPs was observed in samples of fusion-deficient cells, although aggregation of IMPs should not be absolutely required for PEG-mediated cell fusion. PEG could interact directly with membrane proteins or lipids, but could also act indirectly by induction of changes in pH or by effective hydration of the membrane.

During the past few years, human–human T-cell hybridomas secreting factors of immunologic interest also have been prepared by use of PEG (Malissen and Zeurthen, 1982). No human–human T-cell hybrids with cytolytic activity have been established up to now, although several attempts have been made. The failures were generally attributed to nonspecific lysis of the tumor cells by the CTLs during the fusion procedure (Kaufmann et al., 1981). At present, only a few murine hybridomas with cytolytic activity have been reported (Nabholz et al., 1980; Kaufmann et al., 1981; Berebbi et al., 1983) and one human T-cell–mouse B-cell cytotoxic hybridoma (Mukherji and Cieplinski, 1983). However, PEG fusion cannot be checked by microscope examination to see whether the tumor cells were actually lysed by the CTLs during the fusion procedure. Other explanations (chromosomal instability or fusion deficiency) for the failure to extablish human cytotoxic T-cell hybridomas cannot be ruled out. Nevertheless, due to the possibility of nonspecific lysis, we transiently reduced the cytotoxic activity of the PBLs and PHA-stimulated lymphocytes by heat shock according to Kaufmann *et al.* (1981) at 46°C during 10 min prior to fusion (reversible reduction was, respectively, 78 and 46%). Nontreated PBLs and PHA-stimulated lymphocytes have cytolytic activity (respectively, 49 and 48%) were used as controls in our attempts to produce hybridomas. Clone 4 does not lyse HSB-2; therefore, heat shock was not necessary.

Immediately after heat treatment, the CTLs were fused with HSB-2 at various ratios (5:1 to 2:1). The fusion procedure described by Oi and Herzenberg (1980) for B–B cell fusions was used, with minor modifications (see Section VI. A). After PEG fusion, the cells were resuspended in RPMI 1640 supplemented with 20% FCS, 4 mM glutamine, and 1% nonessential amino acids (Flow Lab) and cultured (6 × 10⁴ cells/100 μl per well) in microtiter wells. For the induction of initial growth of the hybrid cells, irradiated (40 Gy) murine bone marrow cells (4 × 10⁴ cells/100 μl per well) were added as feeder cells. Then, selection of hybrid cells was begun. Since the presence of thymidine in the HAT medium could have an inhibitory effect on the outgrowth of the fused cells, azaserine–hypoxanthine (AH) was used for selection of the hybrid cells according to Foung *et al.* (1982). One day later, the culture medium was supplemented with 100 μl AH (1 μl/ml azaserine, 10^{-5} M hypoxanthine) of double strength. After 14 days, the medium was altered by removing the azaserine. Proliferating cells were observed at 4–6 weeks after fusion (Table I). Heat-treated PBLs fused with HSB-2 yielded 11% of wells with proliferating cells, in contrast to nontreated PBLs, which showed no growth. However, neither treated nor nontreated PHA-stimulated lymphocytes yielded proliferating cells after fusion with HSB-2. The reason for the lack of growth is not clear. The best results were obtained with clone 4, which

Table I

Proliferating Cells after PEG Fusion[a]

Human CTL	Pretreatment of CTL	Human T-lymphoma line	Percent of wells with proliferating cells
PBL	None	HSB-2	0
PBL	Heat shock	HSB-2	11
PHA-ly	None	HSB-2	0
PHA-ly	Heat shock	HSB-2	0
Clone 4	None	HSB-2	29

[a]50 × 10⁶ PBL were fused with 10 × 10⁶ T-lymphoma cells, 50 × 10⁶ PHA-stimulated lymphocytes (PHA-ly) were fused with 10 × 10⁶ T-lymphoma cells, and 20 × 10⁶ clone 4 were fused with 10 × 10⁶ T-lymphoma cells. About 6 × 10⁴ fused cells were seeded per well and 4 × 10⁴ irradiated mouse bone marrow cells per well were used as feeder cells.

yielded 29% of wells with proliferating cells after fusion with HSB-2. As controls for the AH sensitivity of HSB-2, HSB-2 × HSB-2 fusions and HSB-2 plus CTL mixtures were cultured under the same conditions as were the lymphocyte × tumor fusions. In these control experiments (AH sensitivity of HSB-2), no proliferation was observed.

IV. Electrofusion

A. Technique

The experimental setup we used for electrofusion is shown in Fig. 2. It consists of a fusion chamber, a function generator (type 7707, P. Toellner Electronic), and a pulse generator (type 521, Devices).

A variety of cell fusion equipments, such as the Cell Fusion Apparatus (Krüss), Electrofusion Cell Generator (BTX), and Cell Fusion Apparatus (CGA) are commercially available.

The fusion chamber (Fig. 1) consists of two platinum wires (diameter 0.2 mm) mounted in parallel on a Perspex slide at a distance of 0.2 mm. This chamber is connected to the function generator, which is used as the voltage source for an alternating electrical field. A pulse generator is connected in parallel for the application of square pulses of high field intensities.

The electrofusion process can be divided into two stages:

1. *"Pearl chain" formation.* Cells are brought into close contact with each other in a nonuniform alternating electrical field of low intensity (field strength 100–250 V/cm; frequency 1–5 MHz). In the alternating electrical field, a dipole moment is induced in the cells because of charge separation or because of orientation of dipoles in the membrane. Cells then migrate in the nonuniform electrical field because the field intensity is not equal on both sides of the cells. This phenomenon is known

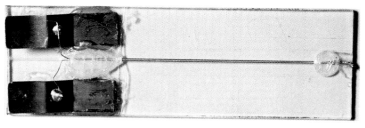

FIGURE 1. A fusion chamber. Two platinum wires (diameter 0.2 mm) are mounted in parallel on a Perspex slide at a distance of 0.2 mm.

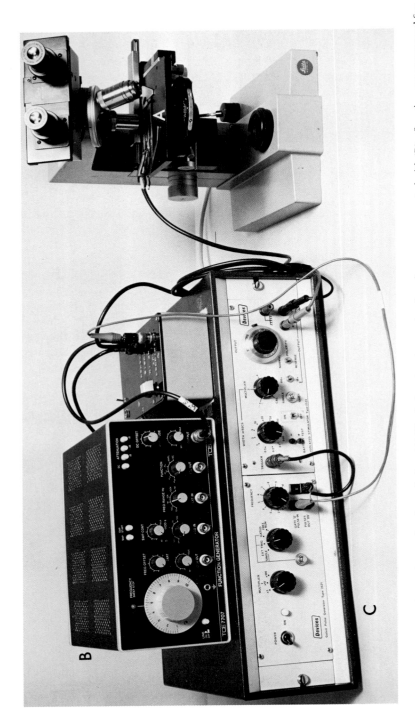

Figure 2. The experimental setup for electrofusion. (A) The fusion chamber, under the microscope, connected with (B) a function generator used for pearl chain formation. (C) Pulse generator, connected in parallel with the function generator, for induction of the electrical breakdown.

as dielectrophoresis. Migration of the dipole-induced cells occurs in the direction of the highest field intensity (Fig. 3).

2. *Fusion.* Fusion is induced by the application of a pulse of high field intensity (3000–5000 V/cm) and of short duration (10–50 μsec). An electrical breakdown takes place on that part of the membrane (lipid domains) where the cells have come into contact with each other (Fig. 4). Fusion takes place within seconds to minutes, depending on the cell type and species. The fusion process is shown in detail in Fig. 5.

B. Fusion Procedure

To reduce the conductivity of the cell suspension without substantially affecting the proper osmolarity, tumor cells and lymphocytes were washed

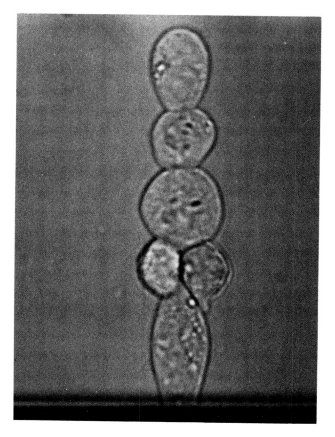

FIGURE 3. "Pearl chain" formation of human tumor cells and human lymphocytes in an alternating nonuniform electrical field. Large tumor cell comes into contact with small lymphocytes.

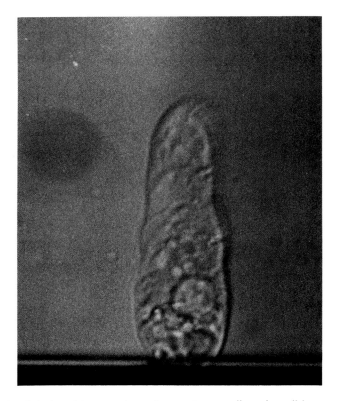

FIGURE 4. Fusion is induced between large human tumor cells and small human lymphocytes after application of the electrical breakdown pulse.

three times in a 0.3 M mannitol solution before fusion. However, cell aggregates were formed as a result of cell death. After 1 hr, the viability of the cells in the mannitol solution was 50%. Therefore, the washing procedure was reduced in time and carried out at 4°C to lower the cell metabolism. Furthermore, other sugars, such as glucose (essential for survival of many cells) and sorbitol in the washing procedures, were also tested. A 0.3 M mannitol–glucose solution [8:1.25 (v/v)] appeared to be suitable.

Formation of lipid domains (particle-free areas) is required for "pearl chain" formation and fusion. It is in these membrane areas that cell–cell contact and electrical breakdown take place. To create lipid domains in the membrane, cells were pretreated with pronase (1 mg/ml). The proteolytic activity of pronase causes partial degradation of membrane proteins, so that

FIGURE 5. A large human tumor cell comes into contact with a small lymphocyte in an alternating nonuniform electrical field. Fusion is induced by the application of the electrical breakdown pulse.

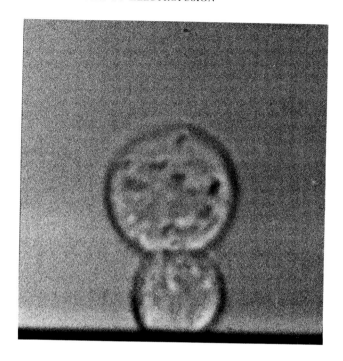

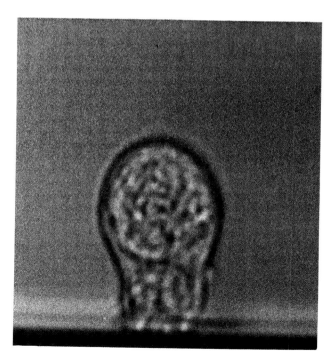

mobility of the remaining proteins increases (Vienken et al., 1983). This increase in the mobility may facilitate the emergence of lipid domains in the membrane during the exposure to the electrical field. Other enzymes, such as dispase and neuraminidase, had no effect. After the washing procedure and pretreatment, the cells were transferred to the fusion chamber.

Pearl chain formation was induced by a field strength of 250 V/cm and a frequency of 5 MHz. The intensity of the field pulse applied to induce fusion appears to be critical for subsequent proliferation of the cells. Although successful cell fusions were obtained by using pulses of 5000 V/cm during 10 μsec, no proliferation of cells could be induced. Lower pulses of prolonged duration were tested. Pulses of 4000 V/cm during 25 μsec were found to be suitable. Taking the factors mentioned above into account, an electrofusion protocol was designed (see Section VI.B) and successful fusions were achieved between human CTLs and HSB-2. PBLs, PHA-stimulated lymphocytes, and clone 4 (2×10^6) were fused with HSB-2 (1×10^6) by electrofusion. Immediately after fusion, the cells were transferred to RPMI 1640 containing 20% FCS, 4 mM glutamine, and 1% nonessential amino acids. The fused cells ($6 \times 10^4/100$ μl per well) were then distributed over the microtiter plates. Irradiated (40 Gy) murine bone marrow cells ($4 \times 10^4/100$ μl per well) were added as feeder cells. One day later, the culture medium was supplemented with 100 μl AH medium of double strength. As controls for AH sensitivity, HSB-2 × HSB-2 fusions and lymphocyte plus tumor mixtures were cultured under the same conditions as were the lymphocyte × tumor fusions. As observed by microscope examination, high fusion frequencies were obtained between PBLs and HSB-2. Lower frequencies were seen between clone 4 and HSB-2. The fusion frequency of PHA-stimulated lymphocytes and HSB-2 was considerably lower than that of PBLs or clone 4 with HSB-2. The fusion frequencies are reflected in the number of proliferating cells (Table II). High percentages of wells with proliferating cells of PBL × HSB-2 fusions and clone 4 × HSB-2 fusions (respectively, 99 and 69%) were obtained at 4–6 weeks after fusion. However, fusion of PHA-stimulated lymphocytes with HSB-2 yielded only 1%

TABLE II
Proliferating Cells after Electrofusion[a]

Human CTL	Pretreatment of CTL	Human T-lymphoma line	Percent of wells with proliferating cells
PBL	None	HSB-2	99
PHA-ly	None	HSB-2	1
Clone 4	None	HSB-2	69

[a]2×10^6 lymphocytes were fused with 1×10^6 T-lymphoma cells. About 6×10^4 fused cells were seeded per well and 4×10^4 irradiated mouse bone marrow cells per well were added as feeder cells.

of wells with proliferating cells. This is in accord with the fusion frequency observed between PHA-stimulated lymphocytes and HSB-2. No proliferation was observed in the control experiments (AH sensitivity of HSB-2).

V. Characterization of Fusion Products Obtained by Polyethylene Glycol and Electrofusion

A. Cytotoxic Activity

All fusion products obtained either by electrofusion or by PEG fusion were tested for cytolytic activity in the ^{51}Cr-release assay against K562, K562 coated with PHA, MOLT, and APD at an effector/target ratio of 150/1 and with 1000 target cells per well. Electrofusion of clone 4 with HSB-2 resulted in at least three of 200 cultures with cytotoxic activity of $10\% \pm 0.8$ (mean $\pm$ SD) only against APD, the original stimulator cell of clone 4. No cytolytic activity was found in CTL × tumor fusion products prepared with PEG. It is unlikely that the fusion procedure itself reduced the cytolytic activity, since no effect on cytolytic activity was shown in control experiments, i.e., treatment of the CTLs with PEG before or after electrofusion. The low level of cytolytic activity (10% lysis of target cells) may be explained by the fact that no limiting dilution procedure was done before the ^{51}Cr-release assay, and consequently the number of nonlytic hybridomas may have been higher or showed a higher proliferative capacity, thereby diluting the cytotoxic hybrid cells.

B. Chromosome Analysis of Parental Cell Lines and Hybrid Cells

Chromosome preparations were made from the parental cell lines and the fusion products by standard methods. Chromosomes were identified using R-bands obtained by heat denaturation and acridine orange staining. The karyotype of the HSB-2 cell line used in these experiments showed a sharp peak at 45–46 chromosomes, with a subpopulation (10%) of 90–92 chromosomes. It was characterized by two reciprocal translocations, t(1;7) (p35;q35), as described by Hayata et al. (1975), and a t(12;15) (q12;q21), as observed by us. Chromosome 15 as well as chromosome 21 showed strong fluorescent satellites. The cells with 45 chromosomes showed the loss of a Y chromosome or, randomly, an autosome. The karyotypes of the T-cell donor were normal diploid 46 XX or 46 XY. Centromeric and satellite polymorphisms were observed. Fusion products were karyotyped at some months after removal from the selection medium. The translocations derived from the HSB-2 parental cell line were always found in the fusion products. The number of chromosomes varied between 44 and 105, with two peaks around the diploid (45–46) and the tetraploid (90–94; more than 10% of the population) number of chromosomes. Specific polymorphic marker chromosomes from the T-cell donor were not identified at that time. Nevertheless, in some fusion products, newly found consistent markers (absent from the HSB-2 and the diploid donor) were observed.

C. Antigen Expression on the Membrane of Parental Cell Lines and Hybrid Cells

Parental cell lines and hybrid cells were phenotyped by use of monoclonal antibodies (MAbs) against OKT3 antigen expressed by mature T cells, OKT4 antigen expressed by helper/inducer T cells, and OKT8 antigen expressed by cytotoxic/suppressor T cells. In addition, an anti-TAC MAb (Uchiyama *et al.*, 1981) was used for detection of IL-2 receptors. HNK-1 (Abo *et al.*, 1981) is a MAb prepared against HSB-2. This membrane phenotyping was carried out by indirect immunofluorescence. As a second label, we used FITC-labeled goat anti-mouse IgG or IgM (Nordic, Tilburg, The Netherlands). After washing, the cell samples were analyzed with a fluorescence-activated cell sorter (FACS II, Becton-Dickinson, Sunnyvale, California) or by fluorescence microscope. HSB-2 expressed HNK-1 antigens on their membrane, but no OKT3, 4, or 8 antigens and no IL-2 receptors (before and after PHA or allogeneic stimulation). PBLs (fresh) expressed OKT3, 4, or 8 antigens and HNK-1 antigens, but no IL-2 receptors. Clone 4 expressed IL-2 receptors and OKT3 and 4 antigens, but no OKT8 and HNK-1 antigens. All hybrids obtained by PEG or electrofusion expressed HNK-1 antigens, but none of the lymphocyte markers. The expression of these markers (OKT3, 4, and 8 and IL-2) is probably genetically repressed by HSB-2. A negative influence of the fusion procedure could be excluded, because products of CTL × CTL fusions (PEG or electrofusion) did not have altered antigen expression of OKT 3, 4, or 8 or IL-2 receptors in comparison with unfused CTLs.

VI. Fusion Protocols

A. PEG Fusion

1. Materials

1. Polyethylene glycol 4000 (Merck) 40% (v/v) dissolved in distilled water containing 5% dimethylsulfoxide (DMSO)
2. Azaserine (A) (Sigma) 100× stock
   10 mg/100 ml; filter to sterilize and store at −20°C

3. Hypoxanthine (H) (Sigma) 100× stock
   136 mg/100 ml. To dissolve H, add 1 N NaOH until H is dissolved
   and neutralize pH with HCl.
   Filter to sterilize and store at −20°C.
4. DMEM:
   Dulbecco's Minimal Essential Medium
   4 mM glutamine
5. Hybridoma culture medium:
   RPMI 1640
   20% fetal calf serum (FCS)
   4 mM glutamine
   1% nonessential amino acids (Flow Lab)
6. RPMI 1640:
   RPMI 1640
   10% FCS
   4 mM glutamine

2. Lymphocytes

The human cytotoxic T lymphocytes (CTLs) used for PEG fusion and electrofusion are derived from three sources:

1. Fresh peripheral blood lymphocytes (PBLs), isolated from blood of a healthy donor by centrifugation in Ficoll–Paque ($d = 1.077$ g/cm^3).
2. Phytohemagglutinin (PHA)-stimulated lymphocytes, obtained by stimulation of PBLs with 10 μg PHA/10^6 cells per ml during 48 hr.
3. Cloned cytotoxic T lymphocytes (clone 4), generated at our laboratory (van de Griend and Bolhuis, 1984).

3. Murine Bone Marrow Cells

Bone marrow cells are collected on the day of fusion by injecting RPMI 1640 with force through the femurs. The number of cells recovered from one femur is usually 15×10^6. Wash the cells one time in RPMI 1640.

4. Tumor Cells

HSB-2, a human T-lymphoma cell line deficient for thymidine kinase and resistant to bromodeoxyuridine, is used for PEG and electrofusion.

5. Fusion Method

1. Wash tumor cells and lymphocytes 3 times in DMEM by centrifugation at $400 \times g$.
2. Mix tumor cells (10×10^6) with the lymphocytes ($20–50 \times 10^6$) and spin the cells down at $400 \times g$.
3.a. Add 1 ml PEG (40%) of 37°C to the cell mixture during 1 min.
   b. Stir the cells carefully during 1 min.
   c. Dilute the cell mixture with 1 ml DMEM of 37°C during 1 min.

    d. Then, add 8 ml DMEM of 37°C to the cell mixture during 1 min.
4. The fused cells are pelleted at 400 × g and resuspended in the hybridoma culture medium containing feeder cells. Then, the hybridoma culture medium with the fused cells (6 × 10^4/100 μl per well) and feeder cells (4 × 10^4/100 μl/per well) is distributed over the microtiter plates.
5. On the next day, 100 μl AH of double strength is added.
6. At one week after fusion, the hybridoma culture medium supplemented with AH is refreshed.
7. At two weeks after fusion, the hybridoma culture medium containing AH is altered by removing the azaserine.
8. At three weeks after fusion, the cells are cultured in hybridoma medium.
9. Proliferating cells are observed at 4–6 weeks after AH selection.

B. *Electrofusion Protocol*

1. *Materials*

1. Mannitol solution 0.3 M (Sigma)
   Glucose solution 0.3 M (Merck)
   Mix 8 volumes mannitol solution with 1.25 volumes glucose solution (man/glu solution).
2. Pronase 1 mg/ml (Merck)
3. Hybridoma culture medium and AH selection; see materials for PEG fusion

2. *Apparatus*

1. Fusion chamber
2. Function generator (type 7707, P. Toellner Electronic)
   AC peak voltage range: 0–10, steps 0.5
   AC frequency range: 0–10, steps 1
3. Pulse generator (type 521; Devices)
   DC voltage range: 0–100, steps 1
   DC pulse duration: 0–50, steps 5

The fusion chamber consists of two platinum wires (diameter 0.2 mm) mounted in parallel on a Perspex slide at a distance of 0.2 mm. This chamber is connected to the function generator, which is used as the voltage source for an alternating electrical field. A pulse generator is connected in parallel for the application of square pulses of high field intensity.

3. Fusion Method

1. Wash the tumor cells and the lymphocytes two times in man/glu solution at 4°C. The same tumor cells and lymphocytes were used as for PEG fusion.
2. Tumor cells and lymphocytes are pretreated with pronase (5–20 min).
   a. Add 100 μl pronase (1 mg/ml) to 100 μl man/glu solution containing the tumor cells or lymphocytes.
   b. Mix 100 μl pronase-treated tumor cells (1×10^6) with 100 μl pronase-treated lymphocytes (2×10^6).
3. Place 50 μl of the cell mixture in the fusion chamber.
4. Pearl chain formation of the cells is induced at 250 V/cm and 5 MHz by using the function generator. To induce fusion, one square pulse of 4000 V/cm during 10 μsec is applied by using the pulse generator.
5. Immediately after fusion, the voltage is decreased to zero. The cells are then collected and transferred to the hybridoma culture medium.
6. Repeat steps 3–5 three times.
7. Distribute the fused cells ($6 \times 10^4/100$ μl per well) in the hybridoma culture medium with the feeder cells ($4 \times 10^4/100$ μl per well) over the microtiter plates.
8. Fused cells are cultured in the same way as after PEG fusion.

VII. Discussion

Our first experiments with PEG and electrofusion of human CTLs with HSB-2 resulted in proliferating cells after AH selection. Electrofusion has a number of advantages in comparison with PEG fusions. The efficiency of electrofusion is considerably higher than that of PEG fusion, since more proliferating cells were obtained after electrofusion. This could be a result of higher fusion frequencies or better survival of the fusion products after electrofusion. In contrast to PEG fusion, electrofusion can be visualized by microscope. Visualization of the fusion process offers a number of possibilities:

1. The success rate of the fusion procedure can be determined. Lack of cell fusion as observed with PHA-stimulated lymphocyte × HSB-2 fusions was correlated with the lack of growth. However, failure in the establishment of hybridomas can also be due to unsuitable fusion partners (loss of chromosomes or genetic repression of genes involving growth).
2. Each cell line has its own membrane composition. Manipulation of the cell membrane (e.g., by enzymes) and adaptation of the fusion procedure can be performed in such a way that theoretically every cell

type is fusable in an electrical field. Optimal fusion conditions can be analyzed by microscope examination.
3. Single fusion products can be isolated by micromanipulation and cultured without the need of AH selection. Therefore, AH-sensitive cell lines are no longer required when applying electrofusion. In principle, every available tumor cell line can now be tested for its suitability as fusion partner.

With respect to the immortalization of human CTLs, one of the main problems appeared to be unsuitability of the fusion partners. In our experiments, the number of cytotoxic hybridomas was low (three of 200 cultures). Problems arose in the characterization of the fusion products. No lymphocyte membrane antigen expression of OKT3, 4, or 8 or IL-2 receptors was observed in the fusion products and no specific marker chromosomes of the lymphocytes could be identified. Nevertheless, the fusion products showed a more variable number of chromosomes (44–105) than did the HSB-2 (45–46 or 90–92), and newly formed markers that are absent in the parental cell lines and HSB-2 × HSB-2 fusion products were found. With the possibility of isolating and culturing single fusion products without the need of AH selection, many more T and non-T tumor cell lines can now be tested for their suitability as fusion partners. For this purpose, experiments are now in progress. Furthermore, electrofusion offers the possibility of accumulating lymphocyte properties in tumor cells by repeated fusions of lymphocyte × tumor fusion products with the same lymphocytes. It appears that lymphocyte × tumor fusion products are highly efficient as fusion partners (B. Härfast, personal communication, Biocell, Sweden). When PEG fusion is applied, the fusion products would have to be mutated for AH sensitivity, which is difficult to achieve.

In conclusion, we anticipate that the application and further development of electric field-induced cell fusion will greatly increase the versatility of hybridoma technology in the near future.

Acknowledgments

We would like to thank R. Vreugdenhil for excellent technical assistance, D. Monnikendam and C. Ronteltap for phenotyping of the fusion partners of the membrane antigens, and Dr. R. J. van de Griend for supplying the cloned cytotoxic T cells. We also thank J. S. Groen for supplying the electronics and R. Lipovitch for designing the fusion chamber. We are grateful to Dr. J. J. Haaijman and Dr. R. J. van de Griend for a critical reading of the manuscript, Dr. A. C. Ford for editing the English text, and M. van der Sman for typing the manuscript.

References

Abo, T., and Balch, T., 1981, A differentiation antigen of human NK and K cells identified by a monoclonal antibody (HNK-1), *J. Immunol.* **127**:1024–1029.

Ahkong, Q. F., Fisher, D., Tampion, W., and Lucy, A. J., 1975, Mechanisms of cell fusion, *Nature* **253**:194–196.

Berebbi, M., Foa, C., Imbert, E., Fabre, I., and Lidcey, C., 1983, Cytolytically active murine T lymphocyte/polyoma virus transformed fibroblast hybrids, *Exp. Cell Res.* **145**:357–368.

Berke, G., 1983, Cytotoxic T lymphocytes, how do they function? *Immunol. Rev.* **72**:5–42.

Burwen, S. J., and Satir, B. H., 1977, A freeze-fracture study of early membrane events during mast cell secretion, *J. Cell. Biol.* **73**:660–671.

Chiorazzi, N., Wasserman, R. J., and Kunkel, H. G., 1982, Use of Epstein–Barr-virus transformed B cell lines for the generation of immunoglobulin-producing human B cell hybridoma, *J. Exp. Med.* **156**:930–935.

Foung, S. H. K., Sasaki, D. T., Grumet, F. C., and Engleman, E. G., 1982, Production of functional human T–T cell hybridomas in selection medium lacking aminopterin and thymidine, *Proc. Natl. Acad. Sci. USA* **79**:7484–7488.

Greene, W. C., Fleisher, A., Nelson, D. L., and Waldmann, T. A., 1982, Production of human T suppressor hybridomas, *J. Immunol.* **129**(5):1986–1992.

Grillot-Courvalin, C., and Brouet, J. C., 1981, Establishment of a human T cell hybrid line with suppressive activity, *Nature* **292**(27):844–845.

Hayata, M., Oshimura, J., Minowada, J., and Sandberg, A. A., 1975, Chromosomal banding of cultured T and B lymphocytes, *In Vitro* **11**(6):361–368.

Kaufmann, Y., Berke, G., and Eshhar, Z., 1981, Functional cytotoxic T lymphocyte hybridomas, *Transplant. Proc.* **XIII**(1):1170–1174.

Köhler, G., and Milstein, C., 1975, Continuous cultures of fused cells secreting antibodies of predefined specificity, *Nature* **256**:495.

Kozbor, D., and Roder, J. C., 1983, The production of monoclonal antibodies from human lymphocytes, *Immunol. Today* **4**(3):72–79.

Malissen, B., and Zeurthen, J., 1982, Immortalizing T-cell function, *Immunol. Today* **3**(4):94–95.

Mukherji, B., and Cieplinski, W., 1983, Functional hybrids between human cytotoxic T and mouse myeloma cells, *Hybridoma* **2**(4):383–392.

Nabholz, M., Cianfriglia, M., Acuto, O., Conzelmann, A., Haas, W., Boehmer, H. V., McDonald, H. R., Pohlit, H., and Johnson, J. P., 1980, Cytolytically active murine T cell hybrids, *Nature* **287**:437–439.

Oi, V. T., and Herzenberg, L. A., 1980, Immunoglobulin-producing hybrid cell lines, in: *Selected Methods in Cellular Immunology* (B. B. Mishell and S. M., Shigii, eds.), Freeman, San Francisco, pp. 351–372.

Reading, C. L., 1982, Theory and methods for immunization in culture and monoclonal antibody production, *J. Immunol. Meth.* **53**:261–291.

Roos, S. D., Robinson, J. M., and Davidson, R. L., 1983, Cell fusion and intramembrane particle distribution in polyethelene glycol resistant cells, *J. Cell Biol.* **97**:909–917.

Sikora, K., Alderson, T., Phillips, J., and Watson, J. V., 1982, Human hybridomas from malignant gliomas, *Lancet* **i**:11–14.

Uchiyama, T., Broder, S., and Waldman, T. A., 1981, A monoclonal antibody (anti-TAC) reactive with activated and functionally mature human T cells, *J. Immunol.* **126**:1393.

Van de Griend, R. J., and Bolhuis, R. L. H., 1984, Rapid expansion of allospecific cytotoxic T cell clones using nonspecific feeder cell lines without further addition of exogenous IL-2, *Transplantation*, **38**(4):401–406.

Vienken, J., Zimmermann, U., Fouchard, M., and Zagury, D., 1983, Electrofusion of myeloma cells on the single level, *FEBS Lett.* **163**(1):54–56.

Zimmermann, U., 1982, Electric field mediated fusion and related electrical phenomena, *Biochim. Biophys. Acta* **694**:227–277.

TABLE II

Characteristics of BCGF Secreted by a Human T-Cell Hybridoma (2B$_{11}$)

Molecular weight	18,000–20,000
Isoelectric point	6.3, 6.6
Thermal stability	37°C for 12 hr; 70°C for 15 min
pH Stability	4.0–10.0
Enzymatic senstivity	Trypsin and chymotrypsin; resistant to DNase, RNase, and neuraminidase
Sensitivity to 2-mercaptoethanol	Resistant to 0.76 M 2-mercaptoethanol
Sensitivity to urea	Destroyed by 10 M urea

hybridoma 2B$_{11}$ was subjected to various thermal, chemical, and enzymatic conditions (Table II). BCGF activity was stable at 37°C for 12 hr and at 70°C for 15 min and was not destroyed by incubation with solutions over a pH range of 4–10. The effects of chemical reduction and denaturation on BCGF activity were studied by incubating 2B$_{11}$ supernatant with 2-mercaptoethanol and urea, respectively. There was no loss of BCGF activity following exposure to 2-mercapthoethanol in concentrations as high as 0.75 M. In addition, BCGF activity was stable after treatment with 5 M urea but was sensitive to incubation with 10 M solutions. All BCGF activity was destroyed by incubation with trypsin or chymotrypsin, confirming the protein nature of the BCGF molecule; however, activity was resistant to DNase, RNase, or neuraminidase. The isoelectric points of this BCGF, as determined by the technique of chromatofocusing, were 6.3 and 6.6 (Fig. 1).

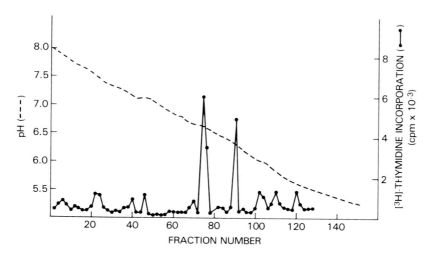

FIGURE 1. pI determination of 2B$_{11}$ B-cell growth factor (BCGF) by chromatofocusing. Sephadex G-100 column fractions containing BCGF activity were pooled and dialyzed against 0.025 M Tris–acetate buffer (pH 8.3) before being applied onto a Pharmacia PBE-94 column (1.0 × 38 cm). The column was eluted with 400 ml of buffer solution [7% (v/v) of polybuffer 74 and 3% (v/v) of polybuffer 96] adjusted to pH 5.0. Fractions were collected and dialyzed against phosphate-buffered saline before BCGF activity was determined.

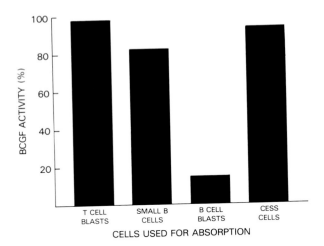

FIGURE 2. Absorption of B-cell growth factor (BCGF) activity by target cells. One-half-milliliter aliquots of $2B_{11}$ supernatant were absorbed for 4 hr at 4°C with 1×10^7 of the following target cells: phytohemagglutinin-stimulated T-cell blasts, small B cells, anti-μ-stimulated B cells, or CESS cells. Following absorption, the target cells were removed by centrifugation, and the supernatants were assayed for BCGF activity.

Absorption experiments were performed to identify the target cells capable of removing BCGF activity from the $2B_{11}$ hybridoma supernatant. As shown in Fig. 2, BCGF activity was absorbed following incubation with anit-μ-stumulated tonsillar B-cell blasts. In contrast, small, resting B cells separated from the B-cell-enriched population on the basis of size by counterflow centrifugation elutriation failed to remove significant amounts of BCGF activity. PHA-stimulated T-cell blasts also failed to remove BCGF activity, as did CESS cells. Thus, these data agree with a previous report (Okada et al., 1983) and suggest the presence of BCGF receptors on large, activated B cells but not on small, resting B cells or T-cell blasts.

V. Development of a Human T-Cell Hybridoma Secreting Both B-Cell Growth Factor and B-Cell Differentiation Factor

Four T-cell hybridization experiments were performed in an attempt to establish a BCDF-secreting hybridoma. Fifty-six wells from an initial number of 600 grew to confluence after 6 weeks, and one hybridoma supernatant (7D5) was found to contain both BCGF and BCDF activities (Butler et al., 1984b) (Fig. 3). In addition, this hybridoma supernatant was negative in assays for IL-2 and interferon. The 7D5 BCGF and BCDF activities were found to reside in protein fractions with molecular weights of 20,000 and 32,000, respectively (Fig. 4). Next, these active gel filtration column fractions were applied to a chromatofocusing column and samples collected and assayed for BCGF and BCDF activity (Fig. 5). BCGF activity was present in fractions with a pI of 6.6. In contrast, BCDF activity eluted in separate fractions with a pI of 5.9, similar to the findings of Yoshizaki et al. (1983).

To confirm the separateness of these two lymphokines, absorption studies were performed. As shown in Fig. 6, incubation of 7B5 supernatant with anti-μ-activated B cells removed BCGF activity but did not significantly decrease BCDF activity whereas incubation of the same supernatant with CESS cells removed BCDF activity without absorbing BCGF activity. No BCGF or BCDF activity was removed from hybridoma supernatant by incubation with PHA-stimulated T-cell blasts. Thus, the data presented above demonstrate

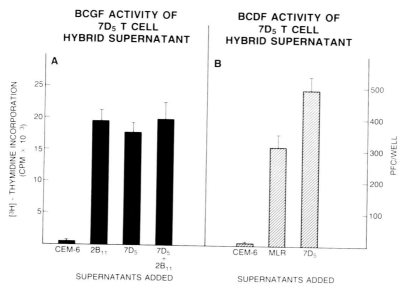

FIGURE 3. (A) B-cell growth factor (BCGF) activity in the supernatant from hybrid clone 7D5. Anti-μ-stimulated B cells (5 × 10⁴ cells/well) were cultured for 72 hr with supernatants (25% v/v) derived from the CEM-6 cell line, 2B₁₁ BCGF-producing human T-cell hybridoma, or 7D5 human T-cell hybridoma. Proliferation was measured by tritiated thymidine incorporation. Data represent the mean (±SEM) of triplicate experiments. (B) B-cell differentiation factor (BCDF) activity in the supernatant from hybrid clone 7D5. B cells were activated by SAC (10⁻³% v/v) for 72 hr, washed, and resuspended (3 × 10⁴ cells/well). The cells were cultured with supernatants (15% v/v) from the CEM-6 cell line, a BCDF-containing mixed lymphocyte culture supernatant, BCGF-containing 2B₁₁ supernatant, or 7D5 supernatant. The number of plaque-forming cells (PFC) per well was determined after an additional 3 days of culture. Data represent the mean (±SEM) of triplicate experiments.

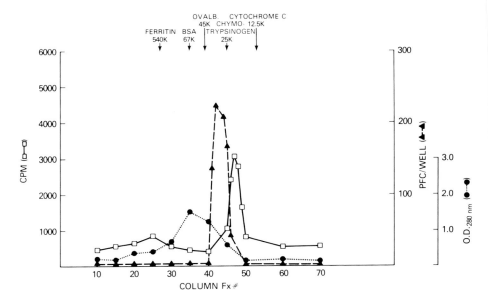

FIGURE 4. Molecular weight determination of 7D5 B-cell growth factor (BCGF) and B-cell differentiation factor (BCDF). Concentrated hybridoma supernatant was applied onto a Sephadex G-100 column (1.6 × 90 cm). The column was eluted with phosphate-buffered saline, and fractions were assayed for BCGF and BCDF activities as previously described. The results are expressed as (□) cpm of tritiated thymidine incorporation and (▲) number of plaque-forming cells (PFC) per culture well, respectively. (●) Protein concentration of the collected fractions measured by absorbance at 280 nm.

the selective absorption of either BCGF or BCDF by specific target cells and confirm that 7D5 supernatant contains two biochemically distinct molecules with different functional activities.

VI. Application of T-Cell Hybridoma-Derived B-Cell Growth Factor and B-Cell Differentiation Factor to the Study of Human B-Cell Immunoregulation

B cells are known to exist in a variety of activation and differentiation states, with the transition between these states dependent on different signals. The development of reliable assays for B-cell-specific lymphokines and the production of human T-cell hybridomas secreting large amounts of these lymphokines have provided the tools necessary to extend our knowledge of these B-cell regulatory events. Studies were performed in our laboratory to investigate the differential sensitivity of B-cell subpopulations to activation signals and to the signals provided by BCGF and BCDF.

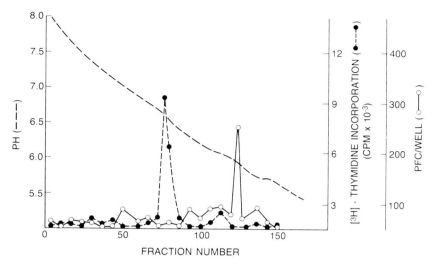

FIGURE 5. pI determination of 7D5 B-cell growth factor (BCGF) and B-cell differentiation factor (BCDF) by chromatofocusing. Fractions of 7D5 supernatant containing BCGF or BCDF activity were separately applied to a chromatofocusing column as described in the legend to Fig. 1. Fractions were collected and assayed for (●) BCGF and (○) BCDF activities.

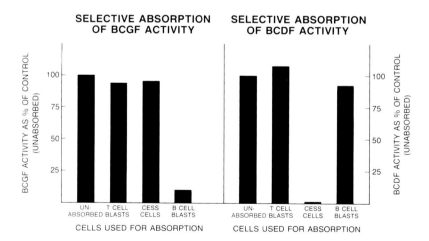

FIGURE 6. Selective absorption of B-cell growth factor (BCGF) and B-cell differentiation factor (BCDF) from 7D5 hybridoma supernatant. Using the absorption conditions described in the legend to Fig. 2, aliquots of 7D5 supernatant were absorbed with the following target cells: phytohemagglutinin-stimulated T-cell blasts, anti-μ-stimulated B-cell blasts, or CESS cells. Following absorption, supernatants were assayed for BCGF and BCDF activities.

Highly purified tonsillar B cells were separated on the basis of cell size by the use of countercurrent centrifugation elutriation. Subpopulations of small resting and large activated B cells were subjected to various combinations of anti-μ and monoclonal BCGF derived from $2B_{11}$ hybridoma supernatant (Table III) (Muraguchi et al., 1983). The small B-cell fractions required a surface Ig-mediated activation signal before they could proliferate in response to BCGF, similar to the proliferative response exhibited by the unfractioned B-cell population. In contrast, the large B cells were unresponsive to anti-μ and were able to proliferate in response to BCGF alone, suggesting that this B-cell subset was preactivated in vivo.

Next, the relationship between expression of a B-cell activation marker and response to anti-μ and BCGF was studied using the monoclonal antibody 4F2. This murine monoclonal antibody, developed in our laboratory by Haynes et al. (1981), recognizes a non-HLA, non-Ia cell surface antigen present on activated human lymphocytes; however, 4F2 does not recognize antigens on the surface of resting human lymphocytes. Additional studies performed by Kehrl et al. (1983) demonstrated that it is blast transformation (G_0 to early G_1 transition) that correlates with the expression of 4F2. In this regard, the 4F2 antibody did not react with surface antigens present on small resting B cells; however, when this B-cell subset was stimulated in vitro with anti-μ, surface antigens were expressed that reacted with 4F2, and the cells become responsive to BCGF.

Thus far, the study of human B-cell differentiation utilizing the anti-μ system as a model has been disappointing. In contrast to anti-μ-activated murine B cells, normal human B cells fail to differentiate in response to anti-μ and BCDF. On the other hand, studies by Falkoff et al. (1982b) demonstrate that human B cells activated by SAC readily respond to BCDF by differentiation into Ig-secreting cells. The absorption studies presented above demonstrate that anti-μ-activated B cells fail to absorb BCDF activity from 7D5 hybridoma supernatant, suggesting that these cells lack a high density of receptors for differentiation factors and are thus incapable of differentiating in response to BCDF.

TABLE III

Relationship between B-Cell Size and Response to Anti-μ and Monoclonal BCGF

Unfractionated B cells		
Medium control	205 ± 30	3,428 ± 215
Anti-μ	183 ± 30	17,550 ± 1,630
Small B cells		
Medium control	408 ± 86	382 ± 66
Anti-μ	832 ± 203	21,409 ± 2,886
Large B cells		
Medium control	1,832 ± 216	8,820 ± 520
Anti-μ	550 ± 303	8,250 ± 415

It is uncertain at present whether the B cells that will ultimately respond by differentiation to BCDF belong to a different subset than those that are triggered by anti-μ or these anti-μ-triggered cells need an additional signal(s) to become responsive to BCDF.

VII. Summary and Conclusions

In this chapter, we have described the development of two functional human T-cell hybridomas. One clone, $2B_{11}$, secreted high quantities of BCGF activity, while supernatant from the second hybrid clone, 7D5, was found to contain both BCGF and BCDF activities. No IL-2 or interferon was secreted by either hybridoma. Subsequent experiments utilizing these active supernatants delineated some of the biochemical properties of BCGF and BCDF. Finally, these hybridoma-derived lymphokines were used to identify the human B-cell subsets responsive to BCGF and BCDF, adding valuable information to our understanding of B-cell immunoregulation.

Although the production of functional human T-cell hybridomas is a recent development, this technique offers great promise as an immunologic tool. Yet, additional information regarding the biology of T-cell hybridomas is needed before the potential of this technology is realized. Studies directed toward achieving this goal include the establishment of new HAT-sensitive human T-cell lines with improved fusion characteristics and the development of more efficient techniques for selecting normal T-cell fusion partners that are genetically programmed to secrete the desired lymphokine. Growth characteristics of T-cell hybridomas may be improved through the use of alternative selection media, such as emetine and actinomycin D (Kobayashi et al., 1982) or azaserine and hypoxanthine (Foung et al., 1982). These media have proved to be less inhibitory to T-cell replication and may offer significant advantages over the traditional HAT media. In addition, improved methods of hybridoma cloning are being studied, including the use of accessory cell feeder layers and clonal selection in serum-free media.

These and other studies should delineate the optimal conditions for the production of human T-cell hybridomas, facilitating the development of additional hybrid cell lines secreting a variety of lymphokines. It is hoped that the application of these powerful tools to basic and clinical research will increase our understanding of both normal and aberrant human immunoregulation.

References

Butler, J. L., Muraguchi, A., Lane, H. C., and Fauci, A. S., 1983, Development of a human T–T cell hybridoma secreting B cell growth factor, *J. Exp. Med.* **157**:60.

Butler, J. L., Ambrus, J. L., and Fauci, A. S., 1984a, Characterization of monoclonal B cell growth factor (BCGF) produced by a human T–T hybridoma, *J. Immunol.* **135**:251.

Butler, J. L., Falkoff, R. J. M., and Fauci, A. S., 1984b, Development of a human T cell hybridoma secreting separate B cell growth and differentiation factors, *Proc. Natl. Acad. Sci. USA* **81**:2475.

Falkoff, R. M., Peters, M., and Fauci, A. S., 1982a, T cell enrichment and depletion of human peripheral blood mononuclear cell preparations. Unexpected findings in the study of the functional activities of the separated populations, *J. Immunol. Meth.* **50**:39.

Falkoff, R. J. M., Zhu, L. P., and Fauci, A. S., 1982b, Separate signals for human B cell proliferation and differentiation in response to *Staphylococcus aureus*: Evidence for a two-signal model of B cell activation, *J. Immunol.* **129**:97.

Foung, S. K. H., Sasaki, D. T., Grumet, F. C., and Engleman, E. G., 1982, Production of functional human T–T hybridomas in selection medium lacking aminopterin and thymidine, *Proc. Natl. Acad. Sci. USA* **79**:7484.

Grillot-Courvalin, C., and Brouet, J. C., 1981, Establishment of a human T-cell hybrid line with suppressive activity, *Nature* **292**:844.

Harwell, L., Skidmore, B., Marrack, P., and Kappler, J., 1980, Concanavalin A-inducible interleukin-2-producing T cell hybridoma, *J. Exp. Med.* **152**:893.

Haynes, B. F., Hemler, M. E., Mann, D. L., Eisenbarth, G. S., Shelhamer, J., Mostowski, H. S., Thomas, C. A., and Fauci, A. S., 1981, Characterization of a monoclonal antibody (4F2) which binds to human monocytes and to a subset of activated lymphocytes, *J. Immunol.* **126**:1409.

Irigoyen, O., Rizzolo, P. V., Thomas, Y., Rogozinski, L., and Chess, L., 1981, Generation of functional human T cell hybrids, *J. Exp. Med.* **154**:1827.

Kasahara, T., Oppenheim, J. J., Muraguchi, A., and Fauci, A. S., 1983, Biochemical characterization of human B cell growth factor (BCGF), in: *Interleukins, Lymphokines, and Cytokines* (S. Cohen and J. J. Oppenheim, eds.), Academic Press, New York, p. 211.

Kehrl, J. H., Muraguchi, A., and Fauci, A. S., 1984, Human B cell activation and cell cycle progression: Stimulation with anti-μ and *Staphylococcus aureus* Cowan strain I, *Eur. J. Immunol.* **14**:115.

Kobayashi, Y., Asada, M., Higuchi, M., and Osawa, T., 1982, Human T cell hybridomas producing lymphokines. I. Establishment and characterization of human T cell hybridomas producing lymphotoxin and migration inhibitory factor, *J. Immunol.* **128**:2714.

Köhler, G., and Milstein, C., 1975, Continuous cultures of fused cells secreting antibody of predefined specificity, *Nature* **256**:495.

Maizel, A., Sahasrabuddhe, C., Mehta, S., Morgan, J., Lachman, L., and Ford, R., 1982, Biochemical separation of a human B cell mitogenic factor, *Proc. Natl. Acad. Sci. USA* **79**:5998.

Muraguchi, A., and Fauci, A. S., 1982, Proliferative responses of normal human B lympocytes. Development of an assay system for B cell growth factor (BCGF), *J. Immunol.* **129**:1104.

Muraguchi, A., Kishimoto, T., Miki, Y., Kuritani, T., Kaieda, T., Yoshizaki, K., and Yamamura, Y., 1981, T cell-replacing factor (TRF) induced IgG secretion in a human B blastoid cell line and demonstration of acceptors for TRF, *J. Immunol.* **127**:412.

Muraguchi, A., Kasahara, T., Oppenheim, J. J., and Fauci, A. S., 1982, B cell growth factor and T cell growth factor produced by mitogen-stimulated normal human peripheral blood T lymphocytes are distinct molecules, *J. Immunol.* **129**:2486.

Muraguchi, A., Butler, J. L., Kehrl, J. H., and Fauci, A. S., 1983, Differential sensitivity of human B cell subsets to activation signals delivered by anti-μ antibody and proliferative signals delivered by a monoclonal B cell growth factor, *J. Exp. Med.* **157**:530.

Okada, M., Yoshimura, N., Kaieda, T., Yamamura, Y., and Kishimoto, T., 1981, Establishment and characterization of human T hybrid cells secreting immunoregulatory molecules, *Proc. Natl. Acad. Sci. USA* **78**:7717.

Okada, M., Sakaguchi, N., Yoshimura, N., Hara, H., Shimizu, K., Yoshida, N., Yoshizaki, K., Kishimoto, S., Yamamura, Y., and Kishimoto, T., 1983, B cell growth factors and B cell differentiation factor from human T hybridomas. Two distinct kinds of B cell growth factor and their synergism in B cell proliferation, *J. Exp. Med.* **157**:583.

Yoshizaki, K., Nakagawa, T., Kaieda, T., Muraguchi, A., Yamamura, Y., and Kishimoto, T., 1982, Induction of proliferation and Ig production in human B leukemic cells by anti-immunoglobulins and T cell factors, *J. Immunol.* **128:**1296.
Yoshizaki, K., Nakagawa, T., Fukunaga, K., Kaieda, T., Maruyama, S., Kishimoto, S., Yamamura, Y., and Kishimoto, T., 1983, Characterization of human B cell growth factor (BCGF) from cloned T cells or mitogen-stimulated T cells, *J. Immunol.* **130:**1241.

21

Generation and Characterization of Human T-Cell Hybridomas That Constitutively Produce Immune Interferon

JUNMING LE, JAN VILČEK, AND WOLF PRENSKY

I. Introduction

Regulation of immune responses by T lymphocytes is mediated mainly by the release of soluble factors, which can be either specific (Lonai et al., 1981; Sorensen et al., 1983) or nonspecific (Pick, 1980; Pierce and Kapp, 1980). Studies on the structure and function of these important mediators have been hampered by the great heterogeneity of crude preparations from lymphoid cell cultures induced with mitogens or antigens, and by the insufficient amounts of material available for characterization in such preparations. Construction of T-cell hybridomas by somatic cell hybridization techniques has allowed us to overcome these obstacles.

A number of functional T-cell hybridomas have been established recently in both the murine and human systems. Murine AKR T-cell thymoma BW5147 was widely used as a parental line to yield various mouse hybridomas secreting specific helper or suppressor factors (Apte et al., 1981; Minami et al.,

JUNMING LE AND JAN VILČEK • Department of Microbiology, New York University School of Medicine, New York, New York 10016. WOLF PRENSKY • Department of Hematology-Oncology, Hahnemann University Hospital, Philadelphia, Pennsylvania 19102.

1981), and nonspecific lymphokines (Howard *et al.*, 1979; Harwell *et al.*, 1980; Jones *et al.*, 1981; Pure *et al.*, 1981; Pace *et al.*, 1983). In contrast, the use of miscellaneous parental tumor lines of T-cell origin for the construction of functional human T-cell hybridomas appears to be less successful, although it has been possible to establish human T-cell hybridoma lines with antigen-specific functions (DeFreitas *et al.*, 1982; Lakow *et al.*, 1983) and with the ability to produce lymphokines, such as suppressive factor (Grillot-Courvalin *et al.*, 1981; Greene *et al.*, 1982), T-cell growth factor (TCGF) (Okada *et al.*, 1981; Foung *et al.*, 1982), and B-cell growth factor (BCGF) (Mayer *et al.*, 1982; Butler *et al.*, 1983).

In this chapter, we describe an experimental system generating human T-cell hybridomas by fusion of concanavalin A (Con A)-stimulated human peripheral blood lymphocytes with a hypoxanthine phosphoribosyltransferase (HPRT)-deficient mutant cell line, designated SH9. Constitutive production of human interferon γ (IFN-γ) and other lymphokines was obtained in these hybridoma cultures. Such hybrid cell lines should prove useful for structure–function studies of lymphokines and as sources of specific messenger RNAs for their genetic cloning.

II. Isolation of a Parent Cell Line Deficient in Hypoxanthine Phosphoribosyltransferase

To ensure the selective growth of human T-cell hybridomas in a medium containing hypoxanthine–aminopterin–thymidine (HAT) (Littlefield, 1964), it is essential to prepare a mutant tumor line of human T-cell origin deficient in hypoxanthine phosphoribosyltransferase (HPRT). A cloned human T-lymphoblast line, HUT102-B2, established previously from neoplastic lymph node cells of a male patient with mycosis fungoides (Gazdar *et al.*, 1980), was chosen as the original line. Because of the low frequency of the desirable mutation, it is critical to use a clonable original cell line for this purpose. Mutation was induced by irradiation of 1×10^8 HUT102-B2 cells in the exponential phase of growth with γ rays from a ^{137}Cs source at 110 rad for 1 min. The cells were cultured in RPMI 1640 medium with 5% fetal bovine serum (FBS) for 6 days with frequent medium changes; 6-thioguanine was then added at a final concentration of 5 µg/ml. On day 18, the cells were pelleted and resuspended in 20 ml of medium and then fractionated on a Ficoll/Metrizoate (1.077 g/ml) gradient. Live cells from the interphase were washed and cultured with 6-thioguanine at 5 µg/ml. The concentration of 6-thioguanine was gradually increased to 20 µg/ml, and about 30 mutants were cloned in the presence of 6-thioguanine at 20 µg/ml by limiting dilution. One of the clones, designated SH9, was used as the parent cell line to generate T-cell hybridomas because of its following characteristics.

First, the SH9 cell line, which showed a high growth rate with a doubling time around 17 hr, survived 6-thioguanine and 8-azaguanine treatment, and died off completely in HAT medium (Le *et al.*, 1983a). Determination of intracellular activity of purine-metabolizing enzymes (Yip and Balis, 1976) showed that SH9 cells are deficient in HPRT, but intact in adenine phosphoribosyltransferase (APRT) as compared to HUT102-B2 cells (Table I). The lack of HPRT appears to be a stable characteristic of the SH9 line, since no revertant of SH9 cells surviving in HAT medium has yet been detected. This might reflect an irreversible deletion of the *HPRT* locus in the HUT102-B2 line resulting from irradiation (Le *et al.*, 1982b).

Second, the SH9 line is a T-lymphoblast line suitable for generating human T-cell hybridomas for lymphokine studies because it was found that SH9 cells spontaneously secrete only a few detectable lymphokines at levels lower than produced by the HUT102-B2 line. For instance, whereas no IFN production was observed in SH9 cell cultures, HUT102-B2 cells synthesized trace amounts of IFN spontaneously after prolonged incubation (Le *et al.*, 1982a). This property ensured that lymphokine production of hybridomas formed by fusion with SH9 cells would not be likely to result from the expression of a genetically dominant character of the SH9 line, which possessed a diploid or hypodiploid karyotype with an average of 40 (34–48) chromosomes.

Third, cell-surface phenotype analysis of SH9 cells showed a helper T-cell pattern: OKT1$^+$, OKT3$^-$, OKT4$^+$, OKT8$^-$, OKT10$^-$, OKT11$^-$, Ia$^+$, and Ig$^-$. The absence of two pan-T antigens, OKT3 and OKT11, from SH9 cell line has proved valuable for identifying established hybridoma cells (Le *et al.*, 1982b, 1983a,b).

TABLE I

Intracellular Activity of Purine-Metabolizing Enzymes in HUT102-B2 and SH9 Cells

Cell[a]	Enzyme activity (nmol/mg protein per min)	
	HPRTase	APRTase
HUT102-B2	15.21	15.41
SH9	<0.01	15.50

[a]Approximately 5×10^5 cells/ml were incubated in growth medium for 48 hr. The cells were washed three times and intracellular hypoxanthine phosphoribosyltransferase (HPRTase) and adenine phosphoribosyltransferase (APRTase) activities were determined according to Yip and Balis (1976).

III. Derivation and Characterization of Human T-Cell Hybridomas

Activated T lymphocytes were prepared by stimulation of peripheral blood lymphocytes (PBLs) at approximately 2×10^6 cells/ml with 3–4 µg/ml of Con A (Sigma) at 37°C for 2–3 days. The PBLs were isolated by fractionation of a 1:5 diluted buffy coat preparation from healthy donors on Ficoll/ Metrizoate gradients, and washed PBLs were cultured in growth medium consisting of RPMI 1640 medium, 10% FBS, 0.1 mM nonessential amino acids, 1 mM sodium pyruvate, 2 mM L-glutamine, 100 U/ml penicillin, and 100 µg/ml streptomycin.

Construction of T-cell hybridomas can be carried out efficiently on a solid phase (Le *et al.*, 1982b, 1983a). Since Con A is known to bind to cell surface glycoproteins, various cells adhere readily to Con A-coated plastic petri dishes. When a very crowded cell culture is formed as a monolayer on such dishes, fusion takes place between adjacent cells in the presence of polyethylene glycol (PEG). To prepare Con A-coated dishes, 1 ml each of 15 mg/ml of Con A and 50 mg/ml of 1-(3-dimethylaminopropyl)-3-ethylcarbodiimide·HCl (Aldrich Chemical Co.) in 0.1 M sodium acetate buffer, pH 4.8, was added to a 60-mm tissue culture dish. The dishes were left at room temperature with intermittent shaking for 1 hr, and were then rinsed five times with phosphate-buffered saline (PBS). These Con A-coated dishes can be used for at least 6 weeks when stored at -20°C.

Con A-stimulated PBLs (about 16×10^6 cells) mixed with SH9 cells at a 3:1 or 2:1 ratio in 3 ml of growth medium were added to each Con A-coated dish. The dishes were incubated at 37°C for 20 min to allow the cells to attach to the dishes tightly. The adherent cells were then rinsed once with serum-free medium before fusion. Fusion was induced at room temperature by gently adding to each dish 3 ml of 50% PEG 6000 or PEG 1000 in RPMI 1640 medium, pH 7.5. PEG 1000 usually shows greater toxicity to the cells than PEG 6000, but yields a higher fusion frequency. Fusion was terminated 1 min later by adding 5 ml of growth medium, and the dishes were rinsed three times to remove PEG and then incubated overnight with the growth medium containing 30% of conditioned medium from SH9 cultures, which apparently helps to increase the viability of the fused cells.

The cells were dislodged on the next day by mechanical pipetting, suspended in HAT-containing growth medium, and distributed in 24-well plates at $(1–2) \times 10^5$/ml, based on the count of SH9 cells. The cultures were continued for at least 4 weeks in HAT medium, then 1 week in HT medium, and thereafter maintained in normal growth medium with one-half volume of the medium changed weekly. Under these experimental conditions it usually takes 2–3 months to obtain established hybridoma cultures with a frequency ranging from 5×10^{-6} to 2×10^{-5}, based on SH9 cell input. Once established, the hybridomas grew rapidly, with a doubling time around 24–48 hr. In contrast, no live cells could be detected when SH9 cells were fused with each other and cultured in HAT medium (Le et al., 1982b, 1983a). The established T-cell hybridomas can be cloned in 96-well plates by the limiting dilution method. The presence of normal allogeneic PBLs at $(0.6–1.0) \times 10^5$ per well, which had been irradiated with γ rays (2000 rad) to prevent the occurrence of a mixed lymphocyte reaction, remarkably increased the cloning efficiency. Apparently, monocytes/macrophages play a major part as feeder cells to support the early growth of the hybridomas (Brodin et al., 1983).

Several methods have been used to characterize these T-cell hybridomas (Le et al., 1983a,b). Karyotype analysis showed that, in comparison with SH9 cells, which had a diploid or hypodiploid karyotype, T-cell hybridomas regularly possessed a hypotetraploid karyotype (Le et al., 1982b, 1983b). When PBLs used as fusion partners were donated by a female, three X and one Y chromosomes could be observed in the hybrids because the SH9 cell line was derived originally from a male patient (Gazdar et al., 1980; Le et al., 1982b).

Recent studies have shown that restriction fragment length polymorphism (RFLP) of human DNA from the D14S1 gene of chromosome 14 is a useful marker in genetic linkage analysis (Wyman and White, 1980; De Martinville et al., 1982). We took advantage of this highly polymorphic locus to document the hybrid nature of the established cell lines (Le et al., 1983a,b). High-molecular weight DNA was purified from the cells, and digested with EcoRI restriction endonuclease (BRL). The resulting DNA fragments were subjected to electrophoresis in 0.6% agarose gels, denatured, and then hybridized to DNA probe pAW 101, kindly provided by Dr. R. White, University of Utah Medical School. The lengths of EcoRI-digested D14S1 DNA from SH9 and hybridoma cells were compared with each other. For instance, hybridization with probe pAW 101 showed that hybridomas L38-B and L38-D had four readily recognizable D14S1 bands (Fig. 1). Since only two of these (bands 2 and 3) were found in SH9-cell DNA, the DNA in bands 1 and 4 must have been acquired from a genome other than SH9. This result clearly indicates the hybrid nature of L38-B and L38-D cell lines (Le et al., 1983b).

Analysis of cell-surface antigen expression by immunofluorescence showed that all of the hybridomas tested had a phenotype OKT1$^+$, OKT3$^-$, OKT4$^+$, OKT8$^-$, as did SH9. However, the hybridomas uniformly expressed OKT11 antigen, which was absent on SH9 cells, suggesting the hybridomas were formed between SH9 cells and T lymphocytes (Le et al., 1982b, 1983a,b). The notion that these hybrid cells are indeed T–T hybridomas was further strengthened by the observations that the hybridomas did show a transient expression of OKT3 antigen on their surface during the early stage of growth (T. W. Chang, personal communication), and that these

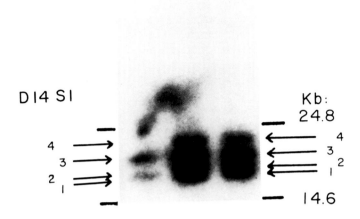

FIGURE 1. Autoradiographic pattern of D14S1 DNA in SH9 and hybridoma cells. High-molecular weight DNA purified from the cells was digested with *Eco*RI restriction endonuclease. The resulting DNA fragments were fractionated by electrophoresis in 0.6% agarose gels, and were hybridized with ^{32}P-labeled probe, pAW 101 DNA. (a) DNA from SH9 cells; (b) DNA of hybridoma L38-B; (c) DNA of hybridoma L38-D. Two additional bands were observed in the hybridoma DNA.

hybridomas expressed neither B-cell (surface immunoglobulin) nor monocyte (OKM1) markers (Le *et al.*, 1982b, 1983b).

IV. *Production of Immune Interferon by Hybridomas*

Extensive screening of hybridoma culture supernatants has resulted in detection of a number of lymphokines, among which are immune interferon (IFN-γ) (Le *et al.*, 1982b, 1983a,b), T-cell growth factor (TCGF, IL-2), macrophage growth factor (MGF) (Le *et al.*, 1983a), B-cell growth factor (BCGF), macrophage migration inhibitory factor (MIF), and lymphotoxin (LT) (J. M. Le, unpublished data). In this chapter we will focus on the production of IFN-γ by T-cell hybridomas and their potential application.

Typical results of screening for IFN-γ production by the hybridomas and their subclones are presented in Table II. While no significant activity was detected in the culture supernatant of HUT102-B2, SH9, or a majority of hybridoma cell lines, a few hybridomas, including L265, produced substantial quantities of IFN-γ spontaneously. By limiting dilution technique, numerous clones were obtained from the L265 culture, some of which yielded higher

TABLE II

Production of IFN by T-Cell Hybridomas and Their Subclones[a]

Hybridoma	IFN (U/ml)	First clone	IFN (U/ml)	Seocnd clone	IFN (U/ml)
HUT102-B2	<20	HUT102-B2	<20	HUT102-B2	<20
SH9	<20	SH9	<20	SH9	<20
L241	<20	L265-E	130	L265-K2	670
L243	<20	L265-H	30	L265-K3	670
L248	<20	L265-I	250	L265-K6	330
L252	100	L265-J	250	L265-K7	250
L255	<20	L265-K	250	L265-K8	1330
L256	<20	L265-L	30	L265-K9	250
L259	<20	L265-M	60	L265-O3	670
L263	<20	L265-O	500	L265-O4	330
L264	<20	L265-P	<20	L265-O5	1330
L265	200	L265-Q	30		
L279	<20	L265-R	<20		
L280	<20	L265-S	60		

[a]Approximately 8×10^5 cells/ml of growth medium were incubated for 48–72 hr, and the supernatants were tested for IFN activity according to Yip *et al.* (1982).

levels of IFN-γ. A further increment of spontaneous IFN-γ secretion was observed after subcloning of the L265-K and L265-O lines (Le *et al.*, 1982b).

The increased production of IFN-γ after subcloning might reflect instability of the hybridoma cells due to chromosome exclusion. However, chromosome exclusion appears to occur only in the early stage after establishment of hybridomas, since the subclones of L265-K and L265-O have been secreting substantial quantities of IFN-γ without further cloning. To date, spontaneous synthesis of IFN-γ by these T-cell hybridomas has continued for 25 months. In contrast, the production of TCGF by T-cell hybridomas was found to be unstable in this experimental system (Le *et al.*, 1983a). The instability of functional activities of human T-cell hybridomas was also reported by Irigoyen *et al.* (1981), Greene *et al.* (1982), and Butler *et al.* (1983).

Identification of the IFN produced by human T-cell hybridomas as IFN-γ was carried out by studies showing that the IFN preparation showed high antiviral activity in human FS-7 fibroblasts but exerted no protective effect on bovine EBTr cells, that it was unstable on dialysis against pH 2 buffer, and that its activity was completely neutralized by a specific antiserum to purified human IFN-γ (Le *et al.*, 1982b, 1983a). Availability of a neutralizing monoclonal antibody directed against human IFN-γ (Le *et al.*, 1984a,b) has made possible a conclusive identification of the IFN secreted by various cloned T-cell hybridoma lines. Table III shows that all of the IFN activity in hybridoma culture supernatants was abolished by treatment with monoclonal

TABLE III
*Identification of IFN-γ Produced
by T-Cell Hybridomas*

Hybridoma	IFN activity[a] (U/ml)	
	Without B3	With B3
L38-B	384	<4
L105-V	36	<4
L265-K8	192	<4
L265-O2	144	<4
L415-C	6	<4

[a]Approximately 5×10^5 cells/ml of growth medium were cultured for 48 hr. The supernatants were incubated with or without 1% of B3 hybridoma ascites for 1 hr at 37°C, and residual IFN activities were determined.

antibody B3, indicating that IFN-γ is the sole type of IFN produced by these hybridomas.

It is known that the phorbol ester 12-O-tetradecanoylphorbol 13-acetate (TPA) and T-cell mitogen phytohemagglutinin (PHA) induce high levels of IFN-γ in human lymphocytes (Vilček *et al.*, 1980; Yip *et al.*, 1982). The inducing effect of TPA and PHA at concentrations previously shown to be optimal for IFN-γ production (Yip *et al.*, 1982) was therefore examined in hybridomas L265-K and L265-O. An 8- to 16-fold enhancement of IFN production was obtained by treatment of the hybridomas with TPA (20 ng/ml). Neither spontaneous nor TPA-induced IFN secretion was significantly affected by the addition of PHA (Le *et al.*, 1982b). A study with specific antiserum to purified human IFN-γ showed that IFN-γ was the only type of IFN detectable in the hybridoma cultures induced with TPA (Le *et al.*, 1982b). In contrast, no IFN was produced by SH9 cells, either spontaneously or upon induction with TPA. Interestingly, the addition of TPA to the HUT102-B2 line from which the SH9 line was derived resulted in the synthesis of a mixture of IFN-α and IFN-γ in approximately equal amounts in terms of antiviral activity (Le *et al.*, 1982a). The fact that only IFN-γ, but not IFN-α, was produced by the T-cell hybridomas therefore suggested that in the hybrids the genetic control of IFN-γ synthesis might derive from Con A-activated T lymphocytes and not from the SH9 cells.

Establishment of T-cell hybridomas also makes it possible to answer the question of whether an activated T lymphocyte produces only one kind of lymphokine. Determination of various lymphokine activities in hybridoma supernatants revealed multiple lymphokine production by single cloned human T-cell hybridomas. For instance, hybridoma L265-K and L265-O lines were found to secrete LT and colony-stimulating factor I (CSF I) in addition

TABLE IV
Simultaneous Production of IFN-γ,
Lymphotoxin, and Colony-Stimulating
Factor I by T-Cell Hybridomas

Cell line	Lymphokine titer[a] (U/ml)		
	IFN-γ	LT	CSF I
SH9	<4	48	0
L265-D	64	ND	380
L265-K	256	512	300
L265-O	128	96	100

[a]Cells of each line were cultured at 6×10^5 cells/ml of growth medium for 48 hr, and the supernatants were tested for IFN-γ, lymphotoxin (LT), and colony-stimulating factor I (CSF I) by antiviral assay (Yip et al., 1982), cytotoxic assay (Stone-Wolff et al., 1984), and a radioreceptor assay (Das et al., 1980), respectively.

to IFN-γ (Table IV). In contrast, the SH9 cell line produced low levels of LT and no detectable IFN-γ or CSF I, the latter being identified by a radioreceptor assay (Das et al., 1980) as the protein responsible for the activity of MGF (Le et al., 1983a). This observation suggested that these cloned hybridomas are likely to have inherited the ability of simultaneously synthesizing IFN-γ and CSF I, if not LT, from their parental activated T lymphocytes. Different combinations of multiple lymphokine production were also observed in other cloned human T-cell hybridomas, suggesting that the production of more than one lymphokine is a characteristic common to activated human T lymphocytes (data not shown).

V. Application of Hybridomas to Structure–Function Studies of Immune Interferon

Most structural studies on human IFN-γ were carried out by using preparations from lymphocyte cultures induced with mitogens, e.g., TPA and PHA (Yip et al., 1982). It remained to be established if the mode by which IFN-γ production was induced affects the structural characteristics of natural IFN-γ. The availability of human T-cell hybridomas constitutively producing substantial quantities of IFN-γ makes it possible to perform structural studies on a natural form of human IFN-γ. Hybridoma L265-K2 was cultured in growth medium at 8×10^5 cells/ml for 3 days, and 1 liter of culture supernatant with

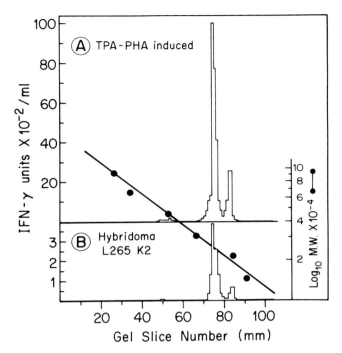

FIGURE 2. SDS–PAGE of human IFN-γ (A) induced with TPA and PHA in human peripheral blood lymphocytes or (B) spontaneously produced by hybridoma L265-K2 (from Yip *et al.*, 1983). Electrophoresis was carried out on a linear 10/16% acrylamide gradient slab gel. After electrophoresis the gel was cut into 1-mm slices, and each slice was eluted with MEM containing 5% FBS by incubation at 4°C overnight. Antiviral activity was assayed by inhibition of the cytopathic effect of encephalomyocarditis virus in human diploid fibroblasts.

a titer of 500 units IFN-γ/ml was harvested. This IFN-γ preparation, purified by a three-step protocol (Yip *et al.*, 1982), was analyzed by sodium dodecyl sulfate–polyacrylamide gel electrophoresis (SDS–PAGE). As can be seen in Fig. 2, the bulk of IFN-γ activity not destroyed by SDS treatment was recovered from two peaks with molecular weight 20,000 (20K) and 25,000 (25K) (Le *et al.*, 1983b), corresponding to the pure forms of IFN-γ prepared from human lymphocyte cultures induced by combined stimulation with TPA and PHA (Yip *et al.*, 1982). The similarities in molecular weights and in the ratio at which the 20K and 25K forms are made between the TPA–PHA-induced (Fig. 2a) and the hybridoma-derived IFN-γ (Fig. 2b) indicates that the 20K and 25K subspecies are natural forms of IFN-γ, rather than modified forms generated as a result of treatment with TPA and PHA (Le *et al.*, 1983b; Yip *et al.*, 1983).

Artificial modification of IFN-γ molecules could also occur during the process of isolation and purification. In order to look into this possibility, an experiment was performed in which hybridoma L265-K8 cells were cultured

Sorensen, C. M., Pierce, C. W., and Webb, D. R., 1983, Purification and characterization of an L-glutamic acid[60]-L-alanine[30]-L-tyrosine[10] (GAT)-specific suppressor factor from genetic responder mice, *J. Exp. Med.* **158:**1034–1047.

Stone-Wolff, D. S., Yip, Y. K., Kelker, H. C., Le, J. M., Henriksen-DeStefano, D., Rubin, B. Y., Rinderknecht, E., Aggarwal, B. B., and Vilček, J., 1984, Interrelationships of human interferon-gamma with lymphotoxin and monocyte cytotoxin, *J. Exp. Med.* **159:**828–843.

Vilček, J., Sulea, I. T., Volvovitz, F., and Yip, Y. K., 1980, Characteristics of interferons produced in cultures of human lymphocytes by stimulation with *Corynebacterium parvum* and phytohemagglutinin, in: *Biochemical Characterization of Lymphokines* (A. L. de Weck, F. Kristensen, and M. Landy, eds.), Academic Press, New York, pp. 323–329.

Wyman, A. R., and White, R., 1980, A highly polymorphic locus in human DNA, *Proc. Natl. Acad. Sci. USA* **77:**6754–6758.

Yip, L. C., and Balis, M. E., 1976, A rapid and simple radioassay for inosinic acid: Pyrophosphate phosphoribosyltransferase in the presence of xanthine oxidase and *vice versa, Anal. Biochem.* **71:**14–23.

Yip, Y. K., Barrowclough, B. S., Urban, C., and Vilček, J., 1982, Purification of two subspecies of human gamma (immune) interferon, *Proc. Natl. Acad. Sci. USA* **79:**1820–1824.

Yip, Y. K., Kelker, H. C., Le, J. M., Anderson, P., Barrowclough, B. S., Urban, C., and Vilček, J., 1983, The subunit structure of human interferon-gamma, in: *The Biology of the Interferon System 1983* (E. De Maeyer and H. Schellekens, eds.), Elsevier, Amsterdam, pp. 129–133.

22

Selection of Human T-Cell Hybridomas That Produce Inflammatory Lymphokines by the Emetine–Actinomycin D Method

TOSHIAKI OSAWA, YOSHIRO KOBAYASHI,
MAKOTO ASADA, MASAHIRO HIGUCHI,
AND SHU-ICHI TSUCHIYA

I. Introduction

T lymphocytes produce various physiologically active lymphokines upon stimulation with antigens or mitogens. These lymphokines can roughly be divided into two groups: cell regulatory lymphokines and inflammatory lymphokines. The lymphokines in the former group play roles in the effector mechanism of the immune response; interleukin 2, B-cell growth factor, and T-cell replacing factors belong to this group. Those in the latter group (Table I) react with macrophages and other inflammatory cells or with the vascular endothelium and are considered to be involved in the induction of delayed-type hypersensitivity. However, since activated lymphocytes produce a mixture of many inflammatory lymphokines in very tiny amounts (possibly ~1–10 ng from 10^6

TOSHIAKI OSAWA, YOSHIRO KOBAYASHI, MAKOTO ASADA, MASAHIRO HIGUCHI, AND SHU-ICHI TSUCHIYA • Division of Chemical Toxicology and Immunochemistry, Faculty of Pharmaceutical Sciences, University of Tokyo, Tokyo 113, Japan.

TABLE I
Representative Inflammatory Lymphokines

	Abbreviation	Major lymphokine effects
Macrophage migration-inhibitory factor	MIF	Inhibition of spontaneous motility of macrophages
Macrophage-activating factor	MAF	Increases of glucose oxidation, O_2^- production, microbicidal capacity, and tumor cell cytotoxicity of macrophages
Macrophage chemotactic factor	MCF	Accumulation of macrophages at the sites of delayed-type skin lesions
Vascular permeability factor	VPF	Vascular change at the sites of the immune reaction
Skin-reactive factor	SRF	Local inflammation at the sites of delayed-type skin lesions
Lymphotoxin	LT	Cell lysis
Colony-stimulating factor	CSF	Growth of monocyte and granulocyte colonies

activated lymphocytes), it has been very difficult to prove directly their participation in the development of various diseases related to delayed hypersensitivity, although some of these lymphokines have actually been detected in tissues or fluids of patients or lesion-bearing experimental animals (Honda and Hayashi, 1982; Cohen and Yoshida, 1983). Furthermore, this limited availability of inflammatory lymphokines has hampered their biochemical characterization and presented several controversial problems concerning the molecular identity between lymphokines. For example, migration-inhibitory factor (MIF) and macrophage-activating factor (MAF), and MAF and immune interferon (IFN-γ), have been assumed to represent identical molecular species, respectively, and skin-reactive factor has been considered to be not a single entity, but a mixture of various lymphokines, including MIF, macrophage chemotactic factor, and vascular permeability factor.

To solve these problems and to facilitate medical application of these physiologically very interesting substances, effective methods for their large-scale production and purification need to be devised, because the multiple biological activities in the culture supernatants of activated lymphocytes or semipurified lymphokine preparations have made it difficult to assign discrete biological functions to each lymphokine. Since the possibility of obtaining monoclonal lymphokines in unlimited amounts had been provided by the introduction of the cell hybridization technique to immunology by Köhler and Milstein (1975), we attempted to establish human T-cell hybridomas secreting inflammatory lymphokines by this technique.

II. Emetine-Actinomycin D Selection Method

The so-called hypoxanthine–aminopterin–thymidine (HAT) selection method has generally been used to produce human T-cell hybridomas. However, the growth rate of T-cell hybridomas is often low when they are selected in HAT medium, because thymidine in the medium effectively inhibits the growth of T cells (Kasahara and Shioiri-Nakano, 1976; Fox *et al.*, 1980). To avoid the inhibitory effect of thymidine, azaserine, which binds irreversibly to various L-glutamine amidotransferases that are necessary in *de novo* purine synthesis and therefore inhibits only the *de novo* syntheses of purine nucleotides, was used by Foung *et al.* (1982) instead of aminopterin, which blocks *de novo* syntheses of both purine and pyrimidine nucleotides.

We devised an alternative selection method (Kobayashi *et al.*, 1982) using the metabolic inhibitors emetine and actinomycin D. Since emetine inhibits the movement of ribosomes along the mRNA strand and the breakdown of polyribosomes into single ribosomes (Grollman, 1968), and since actinomycin D inhibits rRNA synthesis (Perry, 1963), the number of ribosomes available in a cell may be greatly decreased after emetine–actinomycin D treatment. Thus, the fusion of emetine- and actinomycin D-treated leukemia cells with human peripheral blood lymphocytes (PBLs) activated with a T-cell mitogen (PHA-P or Con A) under the optimum conditions for the production of inflammatory lymphokines resulted in the formation of human T-cell hybridomas secreting inflammatory lymphokines. Typical procedures for the emetine–actinomycin D treatment and hybridization were as follows.

Human acute lymphatic leukemia cells (CEM) were suspended in RPMI 1640 containing 20 mM HEPES at a cell density of 2×10^6/ml and treated with 5×10^{-5} M emetine hydrochloride and 0.25 µg/ml of actinomycin D at 37°C for 2 hr. These concentrations of emetine hydrochloride and actinomycin D inhibited proliferation of CEM cells completely. The cells were washed four times with 10 mM sodium phosphate buffer (pH 7.2) containing 0.15 M NaCl (PBS) in order to remove free emetine and actinomycin D.

These emetine–actinomycin D-treated CEM cells were then fused with mitogen-activated peripheral blood lymphocytes (PBLs). Mitogen (PHA-P or Con A)-activated PBLs were centrifuged and incubated with 0.1 M haptenic sugar (N-acetyl-D-galactosamine or methyl α-D-mannoside) solution at 37°C for 20 min to remove the cell-bound mitogen. Microscopic observation revealed only a few cell aggregates, confirming nearly complete removal of the cell-bound mitogen. The cells were centrifuged, suspended in Eagle's Essential Medium (MEM) containing 25 mM HEPES (pH 7.2), and mixed with the emetine- and actinomycin D-treated CEM cells in a ratio of 10:1. The mixed suspension was centrifuged. To the pellet was added 0.5 ml of prewarmed MEM containing 46% polyethylene glycol (PEG 1540; Wako Chemical Co.), 15% dimethylsulfoxide, and 5 µg/ml of poly-L-arginine (molecular weight 60,000; Sigma). This mixture was gently mixed at 37°C for 45 sec. The suspension was then gradually diluted to 10 ml with MEM containing 25 mM HEPES. The mixture was centrifuged. The pellet was then gently suspended in RPMI 1640 containing 60 mg/liter of kanamycin, 2 mM glutamine, 5 × 10^{-5} M 2-mercaptoethanol, and 10% fetal calf serum (enriched medium) at a concentration of 5 × 10^5 cells/ml. To the fused cells (6.0 × 10^6) was added 1.2 × 10^6 mitomycin C-treated CEM cells. The mixture was subcultured in 96 × 0.2-ml culture wells (Falcon microplate no. 3042). During the first week, 100 μl of the medium in each well was replaced by 100 μl of fresh enriched medium every day. The hybrid cell lines showed good growth in all of the wells within 2 weeks after fusion. However, in the control wells to which emetine–actinomycin D-pretreated CEM cells or mitomycin C-pretreated CEM cells were added, no cell growth was observed.

It should be noted here that the optimum concentrations of emetine and actinomycin D for the treatment of leukemia cells vary depending on the nature of the leukemia cell lines and should be determined for each individual cell line. However, the greatest advantage of our method is that we can obtain a much higher growth rate of T-cell hybridomas compared with previous methods, including the HAT selection method. Thus, one hybrid cell can be obtained from approximately ten CEM cells with our selection method (M. Higuchi, N. Nakamura, and T. Osawa, unpublished results), while it has been reported that only one hybrid cell can be obtained from 10^5 T-lymphoblastoid cells with the HAT selection method (Irigoyen *et al.*, 1981).

Recently, the emetine–actinomycin D selection method was successfully applied to a human plasmacytoma line, RPMI-8226, to produce human B-cell hybridomas (M. Terashima, H. Komatsu, and T. Osawa, unpublished results).

III. Migration-Inhibitory Factor and Macrophage-Activating Factor Activities in Culture Supernatants of Hybridomas

The possibility that MIF and MAF activities are exerted by the same molecule was first reported by Churchill *et al.* (1975) based on the fact that a culture supernatant of antigen-stimulated lymph node lymphocytes of guinea pigs previously sensitized with the same antigen exerted both MIF and MAF activities. More recently, Onozaki *et al.* (1981) reported that a guinea pig MIF sample bound to an immunoadsorbent column prepared by coupling polyclonal anti-MIF antibody to Sepharose G-200 showed MAF activity when assayed by measurement of the stimulation of glucose consumption of guinea pig peritoneal exudate cells, suggesting that MIF and MAF were identical. On the other hand, Kniep *et al.* (1981) demonstrated that mouse MIF in the culture supernatant of Con A-activated mouse spleen cells could be separated by isoelectric focusing and gel filtration from mouse MAF as judged by measurement of the induction of cytotoxicity of mouse macrophages toward tumor cells. Based on these results, they concluded that MIF and MAF activities were borne by distinct molecular species. Furthermore, Erickson *et al.* (1982) obtained a murine T-cell hybridoma whose culture supernatants were shown to contain MAF activity when assayed by determination of the tumoricidal activation of macrophages but not MIF, colony-stimulating factor (CSF), or interferon activities. However, there is a possibility that this discrepancy in their results may be due to the different assay systems used for MAF.

To study the relationship of factors that affect macrophage functions, we examined MIF activity in the culture supernatants of human T-cell hybridomas constructed by the emetine–actinomycin D method, using the agarose-droplet method (Harrington and Stastny, 1973) with oil-induced mouse peritoneal exudate cells as target cells, and measured MAF activity in the culture supernatants with the following three assay systems: (1) glucose consumption of oil-induced peritoneal exudate cells of guinea pigs measured by the method of Onozaki *et al.* (1981) (MAF-G activity), (2) cellular superoxide anion formation of a human macrophage-like cell line, U-937, after triggering with phorbol myristic acetate measured by the reduction of nitroblue tetrazolium according to the method of Henry (1981) (MAF-O activity), and (3) cytotoxicity toward tumor cells of human macrophages obtained by 6-day culture of human peripheral blood monocytes, evaluated by the method of Cameron and Churchill (1980) using an ^{3}H-labeled human erythroblastoid cell line, K-562, as target cells (MAF-C activity). If MIF activity and some of the MAF activities are borne by distinct molecular species, these activities can be expected to vary independently of one another when supernatants from a variety of clones are assayed.

As shown in Table II, the culture supernatant of PBLs (10^6 cells/ml) stimulated with 12.5 μg/ml of PHA-P (PHA-sup) showed strong MAF-O activity, weak MAF-G activity, and almost undetectable MIF activity, suggesting that these three activities are expressed by distinct molecular species.

To verify this point, we studied MIF-, MAF-G-, and MAF-O-producing activities of hybridomas. Figure 1 shows MIF-, MAF-G-, and MAF-O-producing activities of hybrid cell lines. In supernatants of some hybridomas, we detected MIF and MAF-G activities with little MAF-O activity, while other hybridomas produced mostly MAF-O and MAF-G with little MIF activity. Furthermore, in the supernatants of yet other hybridomas, we detected mainly MAF-G. We then cloned a high MIF producer, H-D4, and a high MAF-O producer, H-E4, by limited dilution (0.5 cell/well) using mitomycin C-treated CEM cells as feeder cells. MIF, MAF-G, and MAF-O activities in the culture supernatants of seven clones of H-D4 and ten clones of H-E4 were assayed at the same time (Fig. 1, Table II). In the culture supernatant of clone H-D4-2, for example, MIF, MAF-G, and low MAF-O activities were detected, while for H-E4-3, MAF-O, MAF-G, and low MIF activities were found, and in the

TABLE II

*MIF, MAF-G, and MAF-O Activities in Culture Supernatants
of Hybridomas and Their Parent Cells[a]*

Sample	Activity[b] (%)		
	MIF[c]	MAF-G[d]	MAF-O[e]
PHA sup	0	5.0	88.0 ± 1.0
CEM 11	4.7	25.2	8.1 ± 4.5
H-D4-2	25.7 (<0.01)	17.7 (<0.1)	3.3 ± 0.4 (>0.2)
H-E4-3	7.9 (>0.2)	21.4 (>0.2)	36.5 ± 1.9 (<0.01)
H-E4-9	40.2 (<0.001)	2.9 (<0.01)	48.4 ± 5.4 (<0.1)

[a]Higuchi *et al.* (1983).
[b]The results were compared with those obtained for a CEM 11 cell line by Student's *t*-test.
[c]MIF, % inhibition = (1 − migration distance in test sample/migration distance in control sample) × 100.
[d]MAF-G, % consumption = (1 − % glucose remaining in test sample/% glucose remaining in control sample) × 100.
[e]MAF-O, % nitroblue tetrazolium (NBT)-positive cells = (number of NBT-positive cells/number of U-937 cells) × 100.

culture supernatant of H-E4-9 cells, we detected large amounts of MIF and MAF-O and very low MAF-G activity. It is unlikely that these results can be explained on the basis that only one molecule expresses all three activities.

In order to clarify whether or not one or more of MIF, MAF-G, and MAF-O can exert MAF-C activity, we constructed strong MAF-C-producing human T-cell hybridomas and assayed MAF-C, MAF-G, MAF-O, and MIF activities in the culture supernatants of cloned sublines. As shown in Table III a cloned subline, H2-E3-5, produced strong MAF-C and MAF-G activities with relatively weak MAF-O and essentially no MIF activities. After precipitation of the MAF activities in the culture supernatant of H2-E3-5 with ammonium sulfate (80% saturation), the precipitates were fractionated by high-performance anion exchange chromatography (fast protein liquid chromatography) on a column of Mono Q. As shown in Fig. 2, MAF-C and MAF-O activities were clearly separated from each other, but MAF-C and MAF-G activities were found in the same fractions. However, when the ammonium sulfate precipitates of the culture supernatant of a MAF-G-producing cell line (CEM 11; the parent cell line of H2-E3-5) that does not excrete MAF-C were subjected to the anion exchange chromatography under the same conditions, MAF-G activity was eluted at exactly the same elution position as in the case of H2-E3-5, but this MAF-G fraction did not show MAF-C activity. These results indicate that MAF-C activity is apparently expressed by a distinct molecular species from MIF, MAF-G, and MAF-O.

In the MAF-C assays described above, we used human monocyte-derived macrophages as effector cells. We established a different assay system using

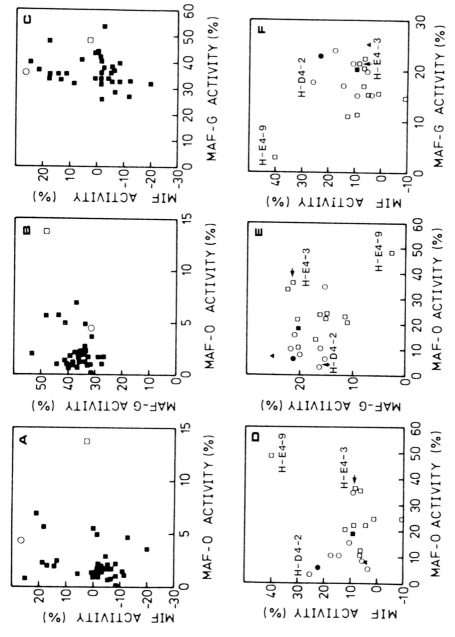

FIGURE 1. The MIF, MAF-G, and MAF-O activities in the culture supernatants of (A–C) 34 hybrid lines and (D–F) those of the cloned sublines derived from (○) H-D4 and (□) H-E4. [From Higuchi et al. (1983).]

TABLE III

MAF-C, MIF, MAF-G, and MAF-O Activities in Culture Supernatants of Hybridomas[a]

Sample	Activity (%)			
	MAF-C[b]	MIF	MAF-G	MAF-O
Control	0	0	0	2.8 ± 0.9
H2-D11-1	12.1 ± 1.2	1.4 ± 1.5	18.1 ± 0.1	8.1 ± 1.5
H2-D11-11	19.1 ± 1.0	15.2 ± 0.9	15.0 ± 1.8	7.1 ± 2.2
H2-E3-5	26.6 ± 2.2	0 ± 1.6	17.9 ± 1.6	12.1 ± 2.5
H2-E4-9	15.2 ± 1.0	40.0 ± 1.2	2.9 ± 0.2	40.4 ± 5.4

[a]Higuchi *et al.*(1984). Culture supernatants of hybridomas were obtained and diluted to a final concentration of 10% with appropriate culture medium, and then MIF, MAF-G, and MAF-O activities were calculated as described in the footnotes to Table II.

[b]MAF-C (%) = [(radioactivity released − radioactivity released spontaneously)/(total releasable radioactivity − radioactivity released spontaneously)] × 100.

human monocytes activated by a test sample for 24 hr as effector cells [MAF-C (monocyte) activity] and found that PHA sup could activate both monocytes and monoctye-derived macrophages, while H2-E3-5 sup and LPS could activate only monocyte-derived macrophages (Table IV). Thus, MAF-C derived from H2-E3-5 was found to activate tumor cell killing of only differentiated macrophages. However, it is not certain whether or not a single molecular species in the PHA sup is active toward two kinds of cells. The current investigation has revealed that two signals are required to generate tumoricidal activity in mouse macrophages, and mouse MAF is generally considered to be the first signal, which primes the macrophages for triggering by a second signal (Weinberg *et al.*, 1978; Hammerstrøm, 1979; Meltzer, 1981; Ratliff *et al.*, 1982a; Schreiber *et al.*, 1982). Hammerstrøm (1979) reported that LPS activation of tumoricidal activity of human monocytes occurred at a very low level, but gradually increased during an *in vitro* culture, and suggested that the *in vitro* culture acts as a priming signal and LPS as a triggering signal. Our results suggest that human MAF-C derived from H2-E3-5 may function as a triggering signal.

We constructed a new series of human T-cell hybridomas and assayed MAF-C (monocyte) activity in the culture supernatants of cloned sublines using K-562 cells as target cells. Among the hybridomas assayed, H3-E9-6 showed the strongest MAF-C (monocyte) activity. As shown in Table V, the MAF-C in the culture supernatant of H3-E9-6 can also activate human monocyte-derived macrophages and even proteose–peptone elicited mouse peritoneal exudate cells. Furthermore, we found that the tumoricidal activation of mouse macrophages by the H3-E9-6 sup was remarkably enhanced by the addition of culture supernatants of PHA-activated mouse spleen cells, but the

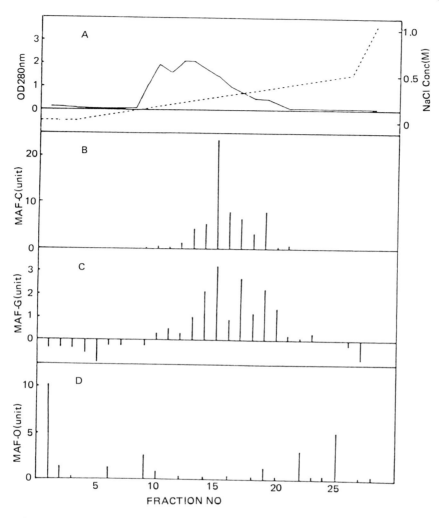

Figure 2. Mono Q column anion exchange chromatography of ammonium sulfate precipitates of H2-E3-5 culture supernatant. (A) (– – –) NaCl concentration and (—) OD_{280}. (B) MAF-G activity in each fraction. (C) MAF-G activity in each fraction. (D) MAF-O activity in each fraction. [From Higuchi *et al.* (1984).]

addition of LPS was found to have no effect (Table V). These results suggest that the MAF-C (monocyte) in the H3-E9-6 sup is a triggering signal at least toward mouse macrophages and the PHA sup contains certain priming signals.

The molecular identity between IFN-γ and MAF has recently been the subject of intensive investigation. Nathan *et al.* (1983) recently reported that human recombinant immune interferon (IFN-γ) stimulated H_2O_2 production

TABLE IV

Tumor Cytotoxicity by Activated Monocytes and Monocyte-Derived Macrophages

Effector cells	Activity[a] (%)			
	PHA sup (50%)	PHA sup (10%)	H2-E3-5 conc. sup (10%)	LPS (10 μg/ml)
Monocyte				
Expt. 1	17.8 ± 1.3	10.2 ± 0.4	2.7 ± 0.7	—
Expt. 2	8.7 ± 1.2	—	—	1.0 ± 0.9
Monocyte-derived macrophages				
Expt. 1	36.2 ± 1.9	26.2 ± 1.9	29.0 ± 2.8	—
Expt. 2	15.0 ± 1.9	—	—	40.5 ± 2.3

[a]All activities assayed as described in the footnotes to Tables II and III. Values in parentheses give final concentration in culture medium.

TABLE V

MAF-C Activity in the Culture Supernatant of H3-E9-6[a]

Sample[b]	Activity (%)		
	MAF-C (monocytes)	MAF-C (monocyte-derived macrophages)	MAF-C (mouse macrophages)
H3-E9-6 sup (0.5%)	37.2 ± 8.7	—	—
(1%)	—	27.8 ± 1.2	—
(5%)	43.0 ± 6.0	—	—
(10%)	—	—	10.9[c]
PHA sup (0.5%)	18.6 ± 1.3	—	—
(10%)	—	61.7 ± 13.7	—
Mouse PHA sup (50%)	—	—	−2.5[c]
LPS (10 ng/ml)	—	—	3.4[c]
Mouse PHA sup (50%) + LPS (10 ng/ml)	—	—	73.3[c]
Mouse PHA sup (50%) + H3-E9-6 sup (10%)	—	—	52.5[c]
LPS (10 mg/ml) + H3-E9-6 sup (10%)	—	—	10.5[c]

[a]M. Higuchi and T. Osawa, unpublished results. All activities were assayed as described in the footnotes to Tables II and III.
[b]Values in parentheses give final concentration in culture medium.
[c]Average values for duplicate determinations.

of human monocyte-derived macrophages and enhanced their ability to kill an intracellular microbial pathogen. Pace *et al.* (1983) reported that mouse IFN-γ produced by recombinant DNA technology can induce the priming step in macrophage activation for tumor cell killing. Schreiber *et al.* (1983) also reported that MAF-C produced by mouse T-cell hybridomas was indistinguishable from mouse IFN-γ by a variety of biochemical and functional criteria. Furthermore, Le *et al.* (1983) established human T-cell hybridomas that secrete a lymphokine with the ability to enhance the cytotoxicity of human peripheral blood monocytes toward human colon adenocarcinoma cells, and they demonstrated that this activity in the culture supernatants of the hybridomas was completely neutralized by antiserum of human IFN-γ.

On the other hand, Ratliff *et al.* (1982b) obtained a mouse T-cell hybridoma that produced MAF-C after stimulation with either Con A or PHA but no IFN-γ. We also could not detect any antiviral activity in the culture supernatants of the five MAF-producing cloned sublines (H-E4-9, H-E4-3, H-D4-2, H2-E3-5, and H3-E9-6). These results seem to suggest that at least MAF-G, MAF-O, and MAF-C produced by our human T-cell hybridomas are distinct from IFN-γ. However, Svedersky *et al.* (1984) have reported recently that a tiny amount of murine recombinant IFN-γ, less than what is detectable in antiviral assays, can exert potent macrophage activation activity if a second signal (LPS) is present. Since the MAF-C obtained from either H2-E3-5 or H3-E9-6 acts as a triggering signal in the tumoricidal activation of macrophages, the possibility that these MAF-C molecules and IFN-γ are the same molecular species is remote. However, to verify our assumption further, a neutralization test with an antibody raised against the purified preparation of human IFN-γ may be necessary.

Furthermore, although Wing *et al.* (1982) found that antitumor activity of mouse colony-stimulating factor (CSF) derived from L-cell conditioned medium against P815 tumor cells was mediated by macrophages, the culture supernatant of H2-E3-5 did not show CSF activity. Moreover, the culture supernatants of the cloned sublines in Table II that are MIF-, MAF-G-, or MAF-O-producers also did not contain CSF activity. These results indicate that MIF, MAF-G, MAF-O, and MAF-C produced by human T-cell hybridomas in our study are distinct molecular species from CSF.

IV. Functional Stability of Human T-Cell Hybridomas

Some cloned sublines of the human T-cell hybridomas E-10-20 selected by the emetine–actinomycin D method produced as much as 6000 times MIF activity as that secreted by Con A-activated human peripheral blood lymphocytes per cell immediately after cloning by limiting dilution. However, when assayed 30 weeks after cloning, these cloned sublines were found to secrete much less MIF. Furthermore, karyotype analysis of these MIF-producing hybridomas revealed that they had around 95 chromosomes per cell 8–9 weeks after fusion, whereas the parent cell line (CEM 11) had around 85 chromosomes, indicating rapid loss of chromosomes. Loss of secretion of lymphokines with concomitant deletion of chromosomes is a common occurrence in T–T hybridomas. In the case described above, the loss of the chromosome bearing the functional gene may be at least one of the causes of the functional instability, because careful cloning after fusion did not prevent the loss of the secretion of MIF. However, Irigoyen *et al.* (1981) reported that sublines carefully derived from human helper T-cell hybridomas gave rise to progeny with stable functional activity despite significant loss of chromosomes after continuous culture. Mayer *et al.* (1982) also found that their human helper T-cell hybridomas were not functionally stable in continuous culture, but repeated subcloning could maintain their functional stability.

However, we have recently established a human T-cell hybridoma (D6-18) by the emetine–actinomycin D selection method that stably produces a strong macrophage chemotactic factor of low molecular weight (~700–800) even in serum-free medium (S. Tsuchiya, Y. Kobayashi, and T. Osawa, unpublished results).

Clearly, the preservation of functionally stable human T-cell hybridomas and their culture in serum-free medium is of vital importance for the large-scale preparation of human lymphokines and their possible medical application.

References

Cameron, D. J., and Churchill, W. H., 1980, Cytotoxicity of human macrophages for tumor cells: Enhancement by bacterial lipopolysaccharides (LPS), *J. Immunol.* **124:**708–712.

Churchill, W. H., Jr., Piessens, W. F., Sulis, C. A., and David, J. R., 1975, Macrophages activated as suspension cultures with lymphocyte mediators devoid of antigen become cytotoxic for tumor cells, *J. Immunol.* **115:**781–786.

Cohen, S., and Yoshida, T., 1983, Physiological and pathological roles of lymphokines, in: *Humoral Factors in Host Defence* (Y. Yamamura, H. Hayashi, T. Honjo, T. Kishimoto, M. Muramatsu, and T. Osawa, eds.), Academic Press, New York, pp. 245–256.

Erickson, K. L., Cicurel, L., Gruys, E., and Fidler, I. J., 1982, Murine T-cell hybridomas that produce lymphokine with macrophage-activating factor activity as a constitutive product, *Cell. Immunol.* **72:**195–201.

Foung, S. K. H., Sasaki, D. T., Grumet, F. C., and Engleman, E. G., 1982, Production of functional human T–T hybridomas in selection medium lacking aminopterin and thymidine, *Proc. Natl. Acad. Sci. USA* **79:**7484–7488.

Fox, R. M., Tripp, E. H., and Tattersall, M. H. N., 1980, Mechanism of deoxycytidine rescue of thymidine toxicity in human T-leukemic lymphocytes, *Cancer Res.* **40:**1718–1721.

Grollman, A. P., 1968, Inhibitors of protein biosynthesis. V. Effects of emetine on protein and nucleic acid biosynthesis in HeLa cells, *J. Biol. Chem.* **243:**4089–4094.

Hammerstrøm, J., 1979, *In vitro* influence of endotoxin on human mononuclear phagocyte structure and function. 2. Enhancement of the expression of cytostatic and cytolytic activity of normal and lymphokine-activated monocytes, *Acta Pathol. Microbiol. Immunol. Scand. C* **87:**391–399.

Harrington, J. R., Jr., and Stastny, P., 1973, Macrophage migration from an agarose droplet: Development of a micromethod for assay of delayed hypersensitivity, *J. Immunol.* **110**:752–759.

Henry, W. M., 1981, Interaction of *Leishmania* with a macrophage cell line. Correlation between intracellular killing and the generation of oxygen intermediates, *J. Exp. Med.* **153**:1690–1695.

Higuchi, M., Asada, M., Kobayashi, Y., and Osawa, T., 1983, Human T cell hybridomas producing migration inhibitory factor and macrophage activating factors, *Cell. Immunol.* **78**:236–248.

Higuchi, M., Nakamura, N., Tsuchiya, S., Kobayashi, Y., and Osawa, T., 1984, Macrophage activating factor for cytotoxicity produced by a human T cell hybridoma, *Cell. Immunol.* **87**:626–636.

Honda, M., and Hayashi, H., 1982, Characterization of three macrophage chemotactic factors from PPD-induced delayed hypersensitivity reaction sites in guinea pigs, with special reference to a chemotactic lymphokine, *Am. J. Pathol.* **108**:171–183.

Irigoyen, O., Rizzolo, P. V., Thomas, Y., Rogozinski, L., and Chess, L., 1981, Generation of functional human T cell hybrids, *J. Exp. Med.* **154**:1827–1837.

Kasahara, T., and Shioiri-Nakano, K., 1976, Splenic suppressing factor: Purification and characterization of a factor suppressing thymidine incorporation into activated lymphocytes, *J. Immunol.* **116**:1251–1256.

Kniep, E. M., Domzig, W., Lohmann-Matthes, M.-L., and Kickhöfen, B., 1981, Partial purification and chemical characterization of macrophage cytotoxicity factor (MCF, MAF) and its separation from migration inhibitory factor (MIF), *J. Immunol.* **127**:417–422.

Kobayashi, Y., Asada, M., Higuchi, M., and Osawa, T., 1982, Human T cell hybridomas producing lymphokine. I. Establishment and characterization of human T-cell hybridomas producing lymphotoxin and migration inhibitory factor, *J. Immunol.* **128**:2714–2718.

Köhler, G., and Milstein, C., 1975, Continuous cultures of fused cells secreting antibody of predefined specificity, *Nature* **256**:495–497.

Le, J., Prensky, W., Yip, Y. K., Chang, Z., Hoffman, T., Stevenson, H. C., Balazs, I., Sadlik, J. R., and Vilček, J., 1983, Activation of human monocyte cytotoxicity by natural and recombinant immune interferon, *J. Immunol.* **131**:2821–2826.

Mayer, L., Fu, S. M., and Kunkell, H. G., 1982, Human T cell hybridomas secreting factors for IgA-specific help, polyclonal B cell activation, and B cell proliferation, *J. Exp. Med.* **156**:1860–1865.

Meltzer, M. S., 1981, Tumor cytotoxicity by lymphokine-activated macrophages: Development of macrophage tumoricidal activity requires a sequence of reactions, *Lymphokines* **3**:319–343.

Nathan, C. F., Murray, H. W., Wiebe, M. E., and Rubin, B. Y., 1983, Identification of interferon-γ as the lymphokine that activates human macrophage oxidative metabolism and antimicrobial activity, *J. Exp. Med.* **158**:670–689.

Onozaki, K., Haga, S., Ichikawa, M., Homma, Y., Miura, K., and Hashimoto, T., 1981, Production of an antibody against guinea pig MIF. III. Biological activity of MIF recovered from immunadsorbent column chromatography, *Cell Immunol.* **61**:165–175.

Pace, J. L., Russell, S. W., Torres, B. A., Johnson, H. M., and Gray, P. W., 1983, Recombinant mouse γ interferon induces the priming step in macrophage activation for tumor cell killing, *J. Immunol.* **130**:2011–2013.

Perry, R. P., 1963, Selective effects of actinomycin D on the intracellular distribution of RNA synthesis in tissue culture cells, *Exp. Cell Res.* **29**:400–406.

Ratliff, T. L., Thomasson, D. L., McCool, R. E., and Catalona, W. J., 1982a, Production of macrophage activation factor by a T-cell hybridoma, *Cell. Immunol.* **68**:311–321.

Ratliff, T. L., Thomasson, D. L., McCool, R. E., and Catalona, W. J., 1982b, T-cell hybridoma production of macrophage activation factor (MAF). 1. Separation of MAF from interferon gamma, *J. Reticuloendothel. Soc.* **31**:393–397.

Schreiber, R. D., Altman, A., and Katz, D. H., 1982, Identification of a T cell hybridoma that produces large quantities of macrophage activating factor, *J. Exp. Med.* **156**:677–689.

Schreiber, R. D., Pace, J. L., Russell, S. W., Altman, A., and Katz, D. H., 1983, Macrophage-activating factor produced by a T cell hybridoma: Physiochemical and biosynthetic resemblance to γ-interferon, *J. Immunol.* **131:**826–832.

Svedersky, L. P., Benton, C. V., Berger, W. H., Rinderknecht, E., Harkins, R. N., and Palladino, M. A., 1984, Biological and antigenic similarities of murine interferon-γ and macrophage-activating factor, *J. Exp. Med.* **159:**812–827.

Weinberg, J. B., Chapman, H. A., Jr., and Hibbs, J. B., Jr., 1978, Characterization of the effects of endotoxin on macrophage tumor cell killing, *J. Immunol.* **121:**72–80.

Wing, E. J., Waheed, A., Shadduck, K., Nagle, L. S., and Stephenson, K., 1982, Effect of colony stimulating factor on murine macrophages. Induction of antitumor activity, *J. Clin. Invest.* **69:**270–276.

23

Human T–T Hybridomas Specific for Epstein–Barr Virus
Generation and Function

Mary A. Valentine and Dennis A. Carson

I. Introduction

Two technologies currently exist to obtain clonal expression of human T cells. One relies on interleukin 2 (IL-2) to expand single-cell cultures. This creates lines of T cells whose maintenance remains totally dependent on the presence of the lymphokine. The second approach, somatic cell hybridization, generates clonal populations of T cells capable of autonomous growth. Successful hybridization is crucially dependent on the phenotype, functional properties, and growth characteristics of the parental cell lines. By appropriate matching of an immortal malignant T-cell line with a normal T cell prior to fusion, a hybrid can be created that expresses a specific molecule or activity in an antigen-specific or -nonspecific manner. The technique has its limitations, but it has resulted in initial successes.

The first human T–T hybridoma, reported by Grillot-Courvalin *et al.* (1981), derived from the fusion of mitogen-stimulated human peripheral blood T cells with the KE37 malignant T-cell line. The hybrid clones constitutively secreted a suppressor of mitogen-induced B-cell differentiation. Following this initial work, several other laboratories used a similar methodology to produce human T–T hybridomas that released lymphokines ei-

Mary A. Valentine and Dennis A. Carson • Scripps Clinic and Research Foundation, La Jolla, California 92037.

ther constitutively or after nonspecific stimulation. The results of these experiments are summarized in Table I.

The construction of human T-cell hybrids with functional expression of
antigen-specific receptors has been reported from two laboratories (DeFreitas
et al., 1982; Lakow *et al.*, 1983; Valentine *et al.*, 1983). In both cases, one of the
parental cells was a mutant strain of the JM (also known as Jurkat) malignant
T-cell line (Schwenk and Schneider, 1975). The following sections will discuss
briefly our own experience in the preparation of Epstein–Barr virus-specific
hybridomas, with emphasis on the methodology used and its rationale.

II. Choice and Construction of the Malignant T Lymphoblast

Two malignant T-cell lines, KE37 and CEM, had been used to generate
antigen-nonspecific human T-cell hybridomas (Table I). Neither cell line intrinsically expresses the functions of mature T cells, such as the synthesis and
release of IL-2 or interferon γ. In heterokaryons derived by fusion of immature to mature cells of a common lineage, the undifferentiated phenotype is
frequently dominant. We therefore reasoned that a more ideal cell line for
creation of antigen-specific T-cell hybrids would have the capacity to undergo
a biochemical or immunologic event that also occurs when normal T cells are
induced by antigen. In addition, the cell line should demonstrate vigorous
growth, a short doubling time, and have a high efficiency of fusion and
cloning. Among available human T-cell lines, the JM leukemia lymphoma
most closely met these requirements.

The JM cell line will release IL-2 on stimulation with T-cell mitogens
(Gillis and Watson, 1980). It was reasoned that this capability would impart
two advantages to hybrid cells: (1) the IL-2 released into the medium might
offer a growth advantage to the hybrids at a critical early stage postfusion, and
(2) IL-2 production could provide a facile biological assay for antigenic specificity. Indeed, an identical strategy had proven successful in the murine
hybridomas developed by Kappler *et al.* (1981). Accordingly, experiments
were initiated to produce mutants of the JM line suitable for fusion, as well as
to determine the optimal medium for the efficient selection of hybridomas.

In principle, the creation of a JM mutant deficient in hypoxanthine-
guanine phosphoribosyltransferase (HGPRT) would permit selection of
clones in standard HAT (hypoxanthine–aminopterin–thymidine) medium.
Aminopterin blocks the *de novo* synthesis of purines and of thymidylate. To
survive in HAT medium, cells must contain the purine salvage enzyme
HGPRT (Fig. 1) and the pyrimidine salvage enzyme thymidine kinase. However, thymidine can itself inhibit cell growth (Schachtschabel *et al.*, 1966;
Carson *et al.*, 1978). Previous experiments from this and other laboratories
had shown that immature T lymphoblasts are extraordinarily sensitive to
thymidine toxicity when compared to other cell types. For this reason, HAT

TABLE I

Human T-Cell Hybridomas

Parental T-cell line	Percent PEG (molecular weight)	Medium[a]	Activity	Reference
KE37	33 (4000)	HAT	Suppressive	Grillot-Courvalin et al. (1981)
CEM	50 (1000)	HAT	Helper	Irigoyen et al. (1981)
CEM	45 (6000)	HAT	IL-2	Okada et al. (1981)
CEM	46 (1546)	Not used	IL-2, LT	Kobayashi et al. (1982)
CEM	33 (1000) or 50 (4000)	HAT	Suppressive	Greene et al. (1982)
JM	50 (1500)	HAT	Antigen-specific IL-2	DeFreitas et al. (1982)
JM(CEM)	50 (1500)	HA	IL-2	Foung et al. (1982)
JM, KE37	? (1000)	HAT	Helper	Mayer et al. (1982)
CEM	50 (1500)	HAT	BCGF	Butler et al. (1983)
JM	33 (3350)	HAO	Antigen-specific IL-2	Lakow et al. (1983)
HUT 102	50 (6000)	HAT	IL-2, IFN, MGF	Le et al. (1983)
CEM	46 (1546)	Not used	MAF, LT	Asada et al. (1983)
JM	50 (4000)	HAO	Antigen-specific IL-2	Valentine et al. (1983)
MOLT-4	46 (1500)	HAT	—	Gallagher and Stimson (1983)
MOLT-4	38 (—)	HAT	(IFN)	Vervliet et al. (1983)
CEM	— (4000)	—	IgE binding factor	Huff and Ishizaka (1984)
CEM		HAT	MIF	Weiser et al. (1984)
—	—	—	Ig suppression	Murakami and Cathcart (1984)
CEM	—	—	LMIF	Theodore et al. (1984)
JM or MOLT-4	—	HAT	Suppresion	Platsoucas et al. (1984)

[a]HAT, hypoxanthine–aminopterin–thymidine selective medium; HAO, hypoxanthine–azaserine–ouabain; HA, hypoxanthine–azaserine.

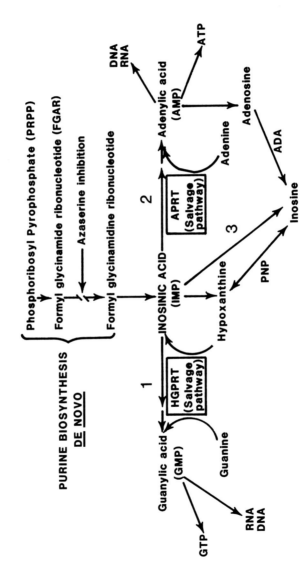

Figure 1. A simplified diagram of the purine biosynthetic pathways. (1) Inosine monophosphate dehydrogenase; (2) adenylosuccinate synthetase; HGPRT, hypoxanthine-guanine phorphoribosyltransferase.

medium is not ideal for the selection of T–T hybridomas from an HGPRT-deficient parental cell line.

Thymidine toxicity can be avoided by substituting the toxic glutamine analogue azaserine for aminopterin plus thymidine in the selective medium. Azaserine is an alkylating agent that irreversibly binds L-glutamine aminotransferases, thereby blocking *de novo* purine synthesis at two points (Fig. 1). Notably, it has no effect on thymidylate synthesis. Growth in selective medium containing azaserine–hypoxanthine (HA) medium is dependent upon the activity of HGPRT, but not thymidine kinase.

Cells able to survive a fusion between HGPRT-deficient JM lymphoblasts and normal peripheral blood T cells would be (1) hybrids with HGPRT acquired from the normal T-cell parent and (2) normal, IL-2-responsive T cells. To eliminate unfused normal T cells and increase the selection pressure for hybrid survival, it was therefore necessary to include a ouabain marker as well as HGPRT deficiency in the mutant JM lymphoma cell line. Ouabain kills cells by inhibition of the Na^+/K^+ ATPase on the outer cell membrane. Its toxicity toward human cells is quickly manifest and it is effective at low concentrations (Thompson and Baker, 1973). Hybrids generated between ouabain-sensitive and -resistant cells maintain the resistant phenotype.

HGPRT-deficient, ouabain-resistant "double" mutants were selected from wild-type JM cells using well-established methods. Briefly, JM cells in logarithmic growth were incubated with 2 µg/ml ethylmethane sulfonate. After 48 hr exposure to the mutagen, the cells were washed and grown for several days in standard medium, to allow for phenotypic expression. These cells were treated with gradually increasing concentrations of 8-azaguanine (8-Az), an antimetabolite whose toxicity depends upon the presence of HGPRT. By 4 weeks of culture, a population resistant to 25 µM 8-Az emerged. These cells were cloned by limiting dilution in 96-well microtiter plates. Several clones were chosen randomly and analyzed for HGPRT by a radiochemical method. One of the HGPRT-deficient clones was expanded in bulk culture and then was incubated with gradually increasing concentrations of ouabain from 0.01 to 10 µM. Eventually, an HGPRT-deficient, ouabain-resistant JM double mutant was isolated, expanded, and frozen. Notably, this cell line, like the parental JM cells, released IL-2 following stimulation. However, we have found that periodic subcloning of the JM cells is essential for continued maintenance of IL-2-producing ability.

III. Selection and Preparation of Epstein–Barr Virus-Specific Normal T-Cell Parent

The Epstein–Barr virus (EBV) is the causative agent of infectious mononucleosis in humans and has been implicated in the pathogenesis of several diseases (Epstein and Achong, 1977). Initially, we screened the blood of normal donors for antibody to the EBV viral capsid antigen (VSA). Lymphocytes were isolated from the heparinized peripheral blood of VCA antibody-positive subjects. Alternatively, blood was obtained from patients with documented EVB-induced mononucleosis. Two protocols were used to enrich the frequency of EBV-reactive T cells, depending upon the donor specimen. One protocol involved *in vitro* stimulation with autologous EBV-infected B lymphoblasts. The other consisted of selective *in vitro* expansion in IL-2-containing medium of activated T cells that developed after *in vivo* exposure to virus.

The first series of antigen-specific hybrids derived from the peripheral blood mononuclear cells of an EBV immune adult. These cells were incubated *in vitro* for 9 days with irradiated (6000 rad) autologous EBV-transformed B lymphoblasts prepared by prior infection of the patient's B cells with EBV derived from the B95-8 cell line. In previous experiments, this same strategy was shown to induce the expansion of EBV-specific T lymphocytes (Tsoukas *et al.,* 1981). Following initial stimulation, the surviving cells were either fused directly or were exposed to EBV-transformed B lymphoblasts for another 10 days prior to fusion.

A second series of antigen-specific hybrids was constructed from peripheral blood mononuclear cells obtained from a patient during the acute phase of infectious mononucleosis. IL-2 stimulates the proliferation of previously activated T lymphocytes (Ruscetti and Gallo, 1981), but has no direct affect on resting cells that lack the receptor for the lymphokine. We reasoned that brief cultivation of peripheral blood mononuclear cells in IL-2-conditioned medium, in the absence of exogenous antigen, would expand selectively those T cells activated previously *in vivo*. Heparinized blood was collected from a patient (MV) during the acute phase of mononucleosis. The cells were separated over Ficoll–Hypaque gradients, washed, and frozen in liquid nitrogen. As controls, cells from the same and other patients were collected at varying times before and after EBV infection. In preparation for fusion, the acute phase cells were thawed and dispersed into flat-bottom microtiter plates at a density of 10^5/ml. They were maintained in standard RPMI 1640 medium supplemented with 10% fetal calf serum and human IL-2-conditioned medium. The cells were fed weekly by half removal of the spent medium and exchange with fresh IL-2-supplemented medium. After 19 days culture, the viable cells were pooled and washed in preparation for fusion. At this time, the surface phenotype of the IL-2-expanded cells identified the population as exclusively T lymphocytes (Table II).

IV. Hybridization

Two weeks before fusion, the double mutant JM was carried for 1 week in 10 μM azaguanine to eliminate any possible HGPRT-positive revertants. The cells were then transferred back to standard medium (RPMI 1640 supplemented with L-glutamine, pyruvate, antibiotics, and 10% fetal calf serum).

TABLE II

Surface Phenotypic Markers of EBV-Specific T-Cell Hybrids[a]

Cell	Percent positive cells				
	OKT3	OKT4	OKT8	Leu 7	SC-2
JM-dm	90	90	0	0	0
MV-acute	100	4	47	15	ND
Hybrids					
A	96	78	4	8	20
B	94	95	3	8	1
C	96	83	0	0	1
D	95	80	0	1	0
E	95	90	0	2	0
F	64	90	1	1	0
G	90	85	0	0	0
H	81	89	0	0	0

[a]Valentine *et al.* (1984). Surface phenotype was determined microscopically by indirect immunofluorescence. ND, Not determined.

The cells were maintained thereafter in logarithmic growth phase at a density of $(0.2–1) \times 10^6$ cells/ml.

The malignant lymphoblasts and the normal T cells were washed separately in serum-free medium. Approximately 10^7 peripheral blood T lymphoblasts and 5×10^6 JM cells were pelleted, and all the supernatant removed. The cells were gently resuspended in 0.2–0.5 ml of a 50% (w/v) polyethylene glycol (PEG) solution. Our experience has indicated that the least toxicity and maximum fusion efficiency was obtained with Merck PEG with a molecular weight of 4000, a finding in agreement with other reports (Greene *et al.*, 1983). The PEG was dissolved in a calcium-free balanced salt solution, pH 7.3 (CBSS) (Klebe and Mancuso, 1981). Cell suspensions were then incubated for 3 min at 37°C and centrifuged for 30 sec at $250 \times g$ to increase cell–cell contact, and the supernatant PEG was carefully removed. Twenty milliliters of calcium-free CBSS was added dropwise during an approximately 10-min period and the cells incubated for another 30–60 min.

After addition of another 15–20 ml of plain RPMI, the cells were centrifuged ($250 \times g$, 5 min), the supernatants were removed, and about 25 ml of an IL-2-supplemented standard medium was added. After overnight incubation to allow for stabilization of the fusion products, the cells were adjusted to a density of 10^5/ml in the same medium supplemented with 100 μM hypoxanthine, 1 μM azaserine, and 10 μg/ml ouabain (HAO medium). One-milliliter aliquots were dispersed into 24-well plates. The cultures were fed weekly with half exchange of fresh IL-2-containing selective medium for 3 weeks. At the end of this period, fresh nonselective medium was used for feeding. This was done to release *de novo* purine synthesis and encourage more vigorous growth. Cultures became dense at about 7–8 weeks postfusion.

V. Proof of Hybridization

Having expanded growing cells, two essential characteristics of the fused cells had to be established: (1) that the fusion products were indeed hybrids, and (2) that the hybrids expressed functional receptors for the EVB. We selected three stringent criteria to demonstrate that the cells were true hybridomas: (1) survival in selective medium, (2) karyotype revealing chromosomal complement greater than the parental JM cells, and (3) phenotypic evidence for the acquisition of new surface antigens.

Figure 2 shows typical growth curves for the JM wild-type, double mutant, and hybrids in selective medium. Neither of the JM cell lines proliferated in HAO medium. Under the same conditions the T-cell hybrids grew normally.

Table III summarizes the karyotypic evidence for successful hybridiza-

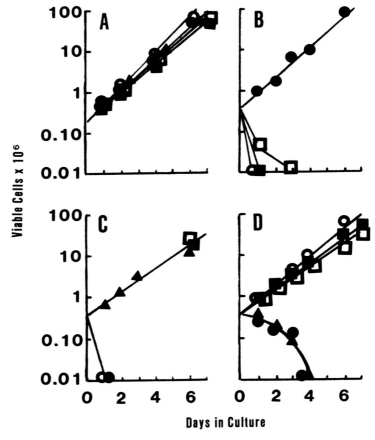

FIGURE 2. Growth of cell lines in (A) standard medium, (B) medium supplemented with 10 μM 8-Az, (C) 3 μM ouabain, and (D) HA medium. (○) JM, wild-type; (●) JM, HGPRT-deficient; (▲) JM, HGPRT-deficient, ouabain-resistant; (□, ■) hybrids. (Reprinted from E. Lakow *et al.*, 1983).

TABLE III
Chromosome Number of EBV-Reactive T-Cell Hybridomas

Cell	Chromosome number (number of metaphases counted)						
A	46 (5)	47 (7)	48 (4)	49 (1)	59 (1)	90 (2)	140 (1)
B	44 (1)	45 (2)	47 (6)	53 (1)	62 (1)	78 (1)	82 (1)
	100 (1)	124 (1)					
C	45 (1)	49 (1)	57 (3)	71 (1)	86 (1)	91 (1)	117 (1)
D	47 (6)	48 (9)	49 (8)	65 (1)	73 (1)		
E	47 (6)	48 (3)	72 (1)	75 (2)	83 (1)	87 (1)	95 (1)
F	44 (1)	51 (4)	76 (2)	77 (1)	86 (1)	>100 (5)	
G	44 (2)	46 (2)	47 (3)	49 (7)	51 (1)	52 (1)	58 (2)
H	44 (1)	47 (6)	48 (9)	59 (1)			
JM	44 (5)	46 (9)	48 (2)				
PBL	46 (10)						

tion. These analyses were undertaken approximately 12–14 weeks postfusion. Modal chromosome numbers in the hybrid cell lines varied over a wide range, but were always greater than diploid. Repeat analyses performed 2 months later revealed an ongoing attrition of chromosomes. This is a problem inherent to human T-cell hybridization. Other studies have indicated that chromosome deletion begins soon after fusion and is progressive (Greene *et al.*, 1983; Osawa *et al.*, 1983).

The hybridization was further documented using a series of monoclonal antibodies specific for surface molecules on T cells. The antibodies selected were: OKT3, a pan-T-cell marker; OKT4, reactive with helper/inducer-type cells; OKT8, associated with cytotoxic/suppressor-type cells; Leu 7, directed against NK cells; and SC2, recognizing a monomorphic determinant on human Ia molecules. Table II summarizes representative data for the staining of parental cells and eight antigen-reactive uncloned hybrids. After 19 days of maintenance in IL-2-supplemented medium, viable lymphocytes from the patient with acute phase mononucleosis had a predominantly T-cell phenotype. About half of the cells stained with the monoclonal antibody OKT8, while 15% stained with Leu 7. Following hybridization, the dominant phenotype was that of the JM parent. Nonetheless, in almost every hybrid cell line, a variable fraction of the T cells displayed antigens lacking in JM, but present on the normal parental cell. Five of the eight EBV-specific hybrids expressed either OKT8 of Leu 7 on a minor proportion of cells. One of the hybrids (A) initially stained intensely for the Ia molecule. This expression was unstable and was lost after 2 months of further culture, coincident with an ongoing chromosomal loss.

VI. Testing for Antigen Specificity

The JM cell line releases IL-2 into the supernatant medium only after stimulation. Therefore, if (1) a hybrid cell expressed an antigen-specific molecule on its surface, and (2) if the acquired receptor was functionally linked to the production of IL-2, then one could use IL-2 release as a measure of antigen reactivity. For our purposes, the IL-2 assay of Gillis *et al.* (1978) proved sensitive and convenient for screening the hybridoma clones. In this method, DNA synthesis by the murine cell line CTLL-2 is related in a dose-dependent way to the amount of IL-2 in the test supernatants.

In a typical experiment, 1×10^6 hybridoma cells were incubated with an equivalent number of irradiated (6000 rad) stimulator cells in 0.5 ml of medium in 12×17 mm, round-bottom plastic tubes for 48 hr and then were centrifuged for 15 min at $1000 \times g$. The supernatants were collected and immediately tested for IL-2 content as described (Gillis *et al.*, 1978). Briefly, 0.1-ml aliquots of murine CTLL-2 cells at a density of 10^5 cells/ml in medium lacking IL-2 were dispersed among the wells of a microtiter tray. An equal volume of each hybridoma supernatant was added to triplicate wells. After overnight incubation at 37°C, [^{3}H]thymidine incorporation into DNA was assessed.

Initially, all hybrid cultures with vigorous growth were screened by this procedure to determine the presence of functional receptors. Subsequently, those hybrid cell cultures that grew continuously in selective medium, had increased chromosome numbers, and had functionally active receptors as defined by IL-2 release were cloned by limiting dilution. The hybrids had an average cloning efficiency of approximately 25% in the presence of IL-2-supplemented medium.

Once the hybrid clones were expanded, they were further characterized, and multiple aliquots were frozen. A major problem with human T–T hybridomas, as mentioned earlier, is chromosomal instability. For this reason, early storage of cells in an active state is essential. Although the hybrid T cells are larger and more fragile than most human lymphoblastoid cell lines, they can be frozen and recovered successfully if the cells are processed with care. In our laboratory, the hybrids are first expanded in standard medium and kept for several days in logarithmic growth phase. The lymphoblasts are then pelleted and gently resuspended by dropwise addition of a cold freezing solution consisting of 95% fetal bovine serum and 5% dimethylsulfoxide. Final cell density is 10^7/ml. Freezing ampoules each receive 1 ml of cell suspension. After cooling at -60°C overnight, the ampoules are transferred to liquid nitrogen storage. Cells are recovered by rapid thawing in a 37°C water bath, followed by immediate suspension in fresh medium, and centrifugation to remove residual dimethylsulfoxide. Cells processed in this manner should be 60–80% viable initially as measured by dye exclusion.

VII. HLA-DR Restriction of Recognition

The experiments summarized in the previous sections proved that the fused cells were indeed hybrids. They also described stimulation assays employed to assess antigen specificity. A panel of irradiated EBV-infected or noninfected B-cell lines with diverse HLA-A, -B, and -DR types, was used to stimulate the hybrids. Additionally, the hybrids were exposed to normal B cells from both autologous and allogeneic sources. In some experiments, the non-B-cell lines K562 and CEM were used as stimulators. As shown in Figs. 3 and 4, the induction of the hybrids was dependent upon the presence of EBV-related antigens in the context of an appropriate HLA-DR molecule. The

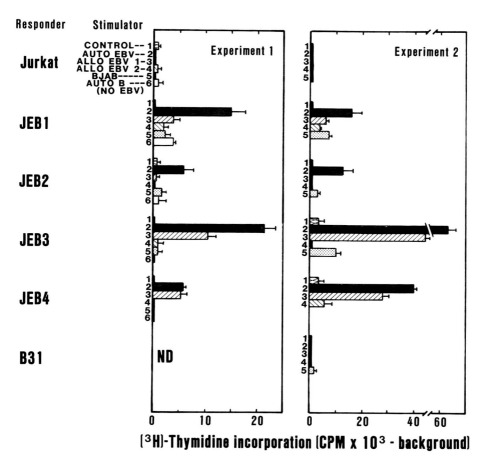

FIGURE 3. Reactivity of JM–T-cell hybridomas. The JM cell line and five hybrid cell lines were incubated *in vitro* as described with JM cells (control), autologous EBV-transformed B cells (AUTO EBV), two allogeneic EBV-transformed B-cell lines (ALLO EBV 1, ALLO EBV 2), BJAB, and autologous nontransformed peripheral blood B lymphocytes (AUTO B, NO EBV). Two days later, the supernatants were assayed for the presence of IL-2. The results show the mean thymidine uptake of triplicate CTLL-2 cultures ±SD. The HLA phenotypes of the EBV-transformed B cells were as follows: AUTO EBV: HLA-A2,28, B14,w39, DR2,7, MT3; ALLO EBV1: HLA-A3,9, B7, DR2,7, MT1,3; ALLO EBV2: HLA-A1,29, B15,w44, DR1,7, MT1,2. [From Lakow *et al.* (1983), by permission.]

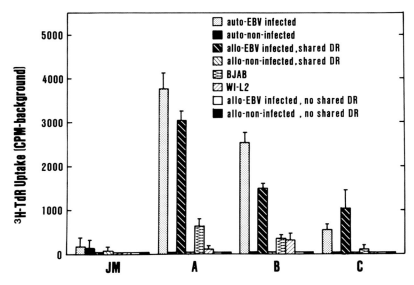

FIGURE 4. EBV- and HLA-DR-restricted reactivity of JM–T-cell hybridomas. The JM parent cell and three representative hybrids derived from the blood of a patient with infectious mononucleosis were incubated with autologous EBV-transformed B cells (auto-EBV infected), autologous noninfected B lymphocytes (auto-non-infected), allogeneic EBV-transformed B cells with one shared DR (allo-EBV infected, shared DR), nontransformed allogeneic B cells with one shared DR (allo-non-infected, shared DR), the B-cell lines BJAB and WI-L2, allogeneic EBV-transformed B cells with no shared DR (allo-EBV infected, no shared DR), and nontransformed allogeneic B cells with no shared DR (allo-non-infected, no shared DR). Three days later supernatants were assayed for the presence of IL-2. Results show the mean thymidine uptake of triplicate CTLL-2 cultures ±SD. The DR phenotypes of these cells are: autologous cells, DR 2,6; allogeneic cells with one shared DR, DR2,7; BJAB, DR 2,7; and WI-L2, DR 4,7; allogeneic cells with no shared DR, DR 7,8. In other experiments, EBV-transformed cells with HLA-DR phenotypes 4,4 did not trigger IL-2 release by hybrids. (Valentine et al., 1984).

parental JM mutant was incapable of IL-2 release following exposure to any of the panel of stimulator cells. In contrast, the selected hybridomas released IL-2 into the supernatant after stimulation with autologous EBV-transformed B lymphocytes or with allogeneic EBV-transformed lymphocytes sharing both HLA-DR antigens. Incubation of the same T-cell hybridomas with (1) non-EBV-infected autologous or allogeneic peripheral blood B lymphocytes, (2) allogeneic EBV-infected B cells sharing no HLA-DR antigens, or (3) EBV-negative B-lymphoblastoid cell lines, did not induce IL-2 production.

Similar results were obtained with the T–T hybrids derived from the peripheral blood T cells of an infectious mononucleosis patient (Fig. 4). It should be reemphasized that in this case, the normal T cells were not stimulated in vitro with EBV. Nevertheless, hybrid recognition of EBV-infected cells was clearly restricted by the HLA-DR locus of the donor. We interpret these

24

Factors Generated by Human T-Cell Hybridomas Regulate B-Cell Activation, Polyclonal Differentiation, and Isotype Expression

Lloyd Mayer

I. Introduction

The interactions between B and T lymphocytes appear to be mediated in large part by factors secreted by activated T cells (Schimpl and Wecker, 1972; Marrack *et al.*, 1982; Yoshizaki *et al.*, 1982). These factors in turn act on various B-cell subpopulations (to induce activation and/or differentiation), other T cells (as a recruitment effort), and monocytes, to effect an immune response. This system of interactions is enormously complex and difficult to characterize, especially since most studies employ either heterogeneous cell populations or cells that secrete multiple factors. This has been a major problem in the study of T–B collaboration. The source of factors is either lectin- or antigen (Ag)-stimulated T cells or T-cell lines, frequently requiring lectin for secretion. Contaminating mitogens can activate the residual T cells in most B-cell preparations and the multiple factors can interact with several different B-cell subpopulations (as well as contaminating T cells), making data in-

Lloyd Mayer • Department of Medicine, Division of Gastroenterology, Mount Sinai Medical Center, New York, New York 10029.

terpretation even more complex. Obviously, a monoclonal system as well as constitutive secretion of solitary factors would aid in dissecting specific stages of B-cell activation and differentiation.

The advent of cell fusion techniques has given us a tool to do just that. Murine hybridomas secreting monoclonal antibodies have resulted in tremendous growth in the field of immunology. Human hybridomas have been quite promising, although, especially in the case of T-cell hybridomas, chromosomal instability with subsequent loss of activity has been a major problem (Irigoyen *et al.*, 1981). In addition, the selection medium used is toxic to normal cells as well as the mutagenized parent lines (Foung *et al.*, 1982). Several different fusion partners have been tested in an effort to achieve better stability, but no long-term successes have been reported. Still, the availability of human T-cell hybrids has allowed for better characterization of B-cell differentiation as well as for the description of novel lymphokines mediating T–B interactions.

In this chapter, lymphokines derived from human T-cell hybrids, including class-specific and nonspecific differentiation factors, will be described. First we deal with the methodologies employed to generate these hybrids and the variations involved in an attempt to generate more stable human hybrids.

II. Methodology for Human T-Cell Hybridomas

Three different methods for generating human T-cell hybridomas have been employed, all with successful fusion and lymphokine secretion, but all with their inherent problems. The key for a successful fusion is the same for all methods, however: that is, log phase growth of the parent line and good blastogenic response to antigen or mitogen by the donor T cells. It has been quite difficult to fuse resting T cells, due, presumably, to the lack of membrane fluidity that is noted in activated cells.

HAT Selection Method (Fig. 1)

1. HGPRT-Deficient Mutant T-Cell Lines

In order to render T-cell lines sensitive to aminopterin, they must be mutagenized to become hypoxanthine-guanosine phosphoribosyltransferase (HGPRT)-deficient. This is accomplished by growing T-cell lines in ethylmethane sulfonate (EMS; 200 μg/ml in culture medium; Eastman Kodak, Rochester, New York) for 20 hr (Epstein *et al.*, 1977). After this period, 80–90% of the cells are dead, and are removed by Ficoll–Hypaque density gradient, and the remaining viable cells are grown in the presence of 6-thioguanine (6TG; 30–50 μg/ml; Sigma Chemicals, St. Louis, Missouri). HGPRT-

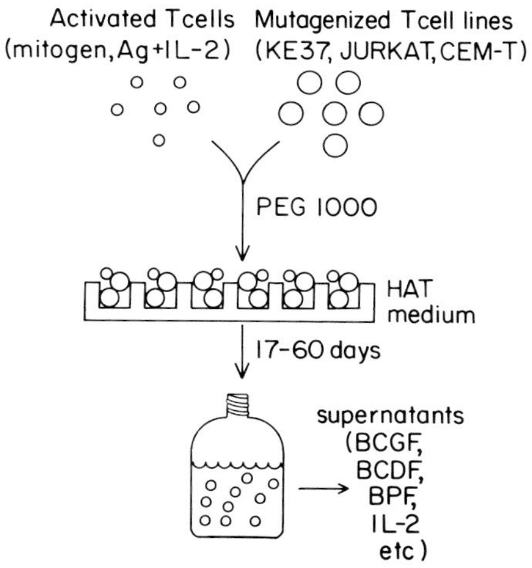

FIGURE 1. HAT selection method for generation of human T-cell hybridomas. Mutagenized human T-cell lines (HGPRT-deficient) are fused with either antigen- or lectin-stimulated T cells and cultured at 1×10^5 mutant cells/well in HAT medium. Growth-positive wells are expanded and screened for activities of interest.

deficient mutants resistant to 6TG are expanded in culture and cloned on soft agar (containing 6TG) using 6TG-resistant fibroblasts (Gm 1362; Human Genetic Cell Repository, Camden, New Jersey) as a feeder layer. Clones are picked, expanded in culture with 6TG, and screened for aminopterin sensitivity by serial dilutions in microwell plates (dose range 10^{-7}–10^{-9}M). Those lines demonstrating good cloning efficiency as well as a distinct cutoff of aminopterin sensitivity are used as fusion partners. HGPRT-deficient T-cell clones are continuously grown in medium containing 6TG to prevent revertants from growing out.

2. Fusion Procedure

Three different mutagenized T-cell lines have been used for fusion: Jurkat 3, a T-cell lymphoma line, and KE37 3.2 and 3671 1.1, human T-cell ALL lines. Twenty million antigen- or lectin-stimulated (48–72 hr) T cells are washed free of contaminating serum in RPMI 1640 and pelleted with 10×10^6 mutagenized T-cell-cloned cells at $200 \times g$. Medium is completely aspirated and the pellet is gently resuspended. Polyethylene glycol (35% in RPMI–PEG 1000, Sigma) is added slowly, dropwise, to a volume of 0.5 ml. The mixed cells are repelleted at $200 \times g$ for 4–5 min at 22°C. After cells have been exposed to PEG for 8 min, the PEG is aspirated and the pellet is gently resuspended. RPMI 1640 is added dropwise to 10 ml, stopping the reaction. The cells are repelleted at $200 \times g$ for 5 min and resuspended in RPMI 1640, 20% FCS, 1% penicillin–streptomycin, 2 mM glutamine, hypoxanthine (10^{-4}M), and thymidine (1.6×10^{-5}M) to 10 ml. The cells are then plated out 0.1 ml/well (1×10^5 mutant cells/well) and incubated for 24 hr at 37°C with 5% CO_2. After 24 hr, aminopterin, 3×10^{-8}M, is added in 0.1 ml to achieve a final concentration of 1.5×10^{-8}M. This level, however is dependent upon the sensitivity of the specific HGPRT-deficient line and may vary by several dilutions. Microwells are fed every 3 days by aspiration and replacement with fresh hypoxanthine–aminopterin–thymidine (HAT)-containing medium. Nonfused control wells (HGPRT-deficient mutants cocultured with activated T blasts) are also maintained in HAT medium. These controls are usually nonviable by day 14–17. Growth-positive fusion wells are transferred to flat-bottom macrowell plates and maintained in HAT until there is sufficient growth to transfer cells to 25-cm² flasks. At this point cells are maintained in complete medium (CM). Cell-free supernatants are obtained from cultures grown at 2×10^5/ml for 48 hr, at which time the cells are pelleted at $300 \times g$ and supernatants filtered with 0.45μ Millex filters. Supernatants are stored at 4°C or frozen until use.

Selection by Surface Marker(s) (Figs. 2 and 3)

It has been well documented that aminopterin and thymidine are inherently toxic to even normal cells (Foung *et al.*, 1982). Thus the slow growth of HAT-selected hybrids and, possibly, the chromosomal instability may in part relate to growth in these harsh conditions. Therefore a system whereby fusions are grown in normal culture medium in conditions that are optimal for both parent and donor cells might increase the yield and stability of T-cell hybrids. To this end we established two methods (Figs. 2 and 3) to isolate fusion products by the presence of a selectable surface marker.

The actual fusion procedure remains the same for all methods, but the ratio of donor to parent cells varies. In the first case (Fig. 2), lectin-stimulated

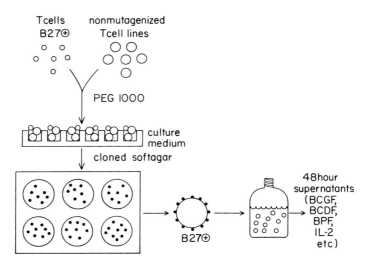

FIGURE 2. Selection of human T-cell hybridomas by surface marker. Fusion procedure is the same as the HAT method except that nonmutagenized T-cell lines are used as parents. Selection is performed by cloning on soft agar and staining for the presence of the specific surface marker.

TABLE VI
Induction of IgA Plaque-Forming Cells from Isolated Human B Cells by Supernatant from T–T Hybridoma J1.3 [a]

Cells	Medium control			Hybrid J1.3 sup			+T cells or +T cells + PWM		
	IgG	IgA	IgM	IgG	IgA	IgM	IgG	IgA	IgM
Tonsil B	0	0	100	200	700	0	0[b]	100[b]	800[b]
Tonsil B	0	300	0	0	2400	0		—	
Peripheral blood non-T	0	0	0	100	700	0	3420[c]	880[c]	1220[c]
Peripheral blood non-T	20	50	0	10	420	0		—	
Peripheral blood MNC	0	0	0	0	500	0		—	

[a] Values are PFC/10[6] cells by reverse hemolytic plaque assay.
[b] +T cells.
[c] +T cells + PWM.

2. Isotype-Specific BCDFs

The common thread of the heterogeneous BCDFs described above is that they all induced secretion of all isotypes. In marked contrast is the hybrid J1.3, which, when added to peripheral blood or tonsil B cells, resulted in the secretion of IgA (Mayer *et al.*, 1982). In general, the level of IgA secretion was low; however, the effect is indeed selective for IgA, in that IgG and/or IgM responses were not seen (Table VI). There is good evidence that the IgA response is under strict T-cell regulation (Clough *et al.*, 1971; Crewther and Warner, 1972) and that this regulatory control can occur either in the pre-switch, IgA-uncommitted (Kawanishi *et al.*, 1983a,b) or post-switch, IgA-committed (Kiyono *et al.*, 1984) B cell. The finding that supernatant from hybrid J1.3 induced virtually complete differentiation of B cells from a sIgA$^+$ B-cell leukemia (Mayer *et al.*, 1982) suggested that J1.3 acted on an already isotype-committed cell. This was further evaluated in the experiment depicted in Table VII. Depletion of sIgA$^+$ cells completely abrogated the IgA response to J1.3 supernatant. In addition, when J1.3 was added to cultures of sIgM$^+$ B cells devoid of IgG- and IgA-bearing cells, no IgA secretion was noted. Subsequent to the description of the J1.3 hybridoma, Kiyono and co-workers (1984) described an antigen-specific T-cell clone derived from murine Peyer's patches with similar activity. Their clone, however, is Fc α$^+$ and appears to secrete an IgA-binding factor that mediates its effect. In contrast, J1.3 is Fc μ$^+$ and, to date, no IgA-binding factors have been demonstrated. Thus, there is further evidence that even within isotype-specific BCDFs, there is considerable heterogeneity.

3. The Role of IL-2 in B-Cell Maturation

There has been considerable controversy in the literature regarding the role of IL-2 in normal human or murine B-cell differentiation (Howard *et al.*,

TABLE VII

Abrogation of the Effects of IgA-Specific Helper Factor (J1.3) Following the Depletion of sIgA-Bearing B Cells

Cells	PFC/well[a]								
	Medium			J1.3 sup			+T + PWM		
	IgG	IgA	IgM	IgG	IgA	IgM	IgG	IgA	IgM
Tonsil B	80	0	120	40	990	0	10120	2120	11680
sIgA-Depleted tonsil B[b]	110	0	150	80	40	110	9690	440	6280
sIgM + tonsil B[c]	20	0	80	60	0	210	5280	4180	7120

[a]As per Table III; reverse plaque assay performed with isotype-specific developing antiserum (Cappel, 1:100 dilution).
[b]sIgA + B cells depleted by direct rosetting technique using F(ab')₂ sheep anti-human IgA-coated ox RBCs (<0.4% sIgA + cells).
[c]sIgA + B cells negatively selected by directly rosetting out sIgG- and sIgA-bearing cells as above (<0.1% sIgA + <0.3% sIgG + cells).

1982; Parker, 1982; Marrack *et al.*, 1982). Initial reports demonstrating a positive role for IL-2 used preparations contaminated with other B-cell activating factors (Howard and Paul 1983). With the ability to synthesize IL-2 through recombinant DNA technology, this question of IL-2 regulation could again be addressed. Several groups have now reported that recombinant IL-2 acts as a proliferation and/or a differentiation signal (Jung *et al.*, 1984; Waldmann *et al.*, 1984). However, the number of units of recombinant IL-2 required to see an effect has been extraordinarily high, raising the question as to whether IL-2 has any physiological relevance in normal B-cell maturation.

There is little question that B cells can express the IL-2 receptor (Tsudo *et al.*, 1984; Jung *et al.*, 1984; Waldmann *et al.*, 1984), but it appears that the number of receptors is an order of magnitude lower than that found on T cells, and the affinity for IL-2 is lower on B cells as well (Tsudo *et al.*, 1984). Thus, although there may be some physiological role for IL-2 in B-cell maturation, it would not be likely to be a primary role. Using our BCDF preparations, we attempted to evaluate IL-2 as a second or synergistic signal. As shown in Table VIII, the addition of increasing doses of recombinant IL-2 to vigorously T-depleted peripheral blood B-cell populations did not result in any significant increase in [³H]thymidine incorporation or differentiation. However, when IL-2 was added to cultures stimulated with various BCDF preparations, there was a 10- to 100-fold increase in the PFC response. This was evident even when the IL-2 was added up to day 3 (Table IX). This synergy was especially marked in cultures of monoclonal leukemic B cells and, interestingly, if the leukemic B cells expressed the Tac antigen at the onset of culture (data not shown). Despite the increase in PFC response, there was no increase in [³H]thymidine incorporation. This may have been due to the fact

TABLE VIII
Effect of IL-2 on B-Cell Differentiation

Target[a]	IL-2 (U/culture)	BCDF[b]	[3H]Thymidine incorporation[c] (cpm)	PFC/well[d]
Peripheral blood				
Non-T	—	—	226	60
Non-T	1000	—	342	40
Non-T	—	+ (MOPIL)	484	1,840
Non-T	1000	+	364	22,360
Non-T	500	+	120	21,680
Non-T	100	+	427	26,280
Non-T	50	+	633	34,860
Non-T	5	+	169	12,340
Non-T	0.5	+	303	3,170
Non-T	—	+ (MTP7)	—	780
Non-T	50	+	—	54,220
Non-T	—	+ (MOW10)	—	4,230
Non-T	50	+	—	64,370

[a]Peripheral blood non-T cells were depleted of residual T cells (<0.1%) by rosetting twice with neuraminidase-treated SRBCs.
[b]Added 1% (v/v) at onset of culture.
[c]Result is mean of triplicate cultures. [3H]Thymidine was added to cultures at 72 hr and harvested 18 hr later.
[d]As per Table III.

TABLE IX
Kinetics of IL-2 Effect on B-Cell Differentiation

Target	Day IL-2 added[a]	BCDF	PFC/culture
Non-T	—	—	160
Non-T	—	+	2,120
Non-T	0	+	34,320
Non-T	1	+	30,690
Non-T	2	+	24,230
Non-T	3	+	37,170
Non-T	4	+	3,030
Non-T	5	+	1,384
Non-T	0	—	65

[a]Recombinant IL-2 (5OU) was added to cultures of non-T cells ± BCDF on the specified day of culture. A reverse plaque assay was performed on day 6.

that the initial stimulus was a differentiation signal. The synergy was noted with as little as 5 U of IL-2, certainly within the physiological range. Thus, although IL-2 may not be a primary differentiation signal, it may certainly play a role in augmenting B-cell responses.

IV. Model of B-Cell Maturation

Based on the description of factors in this chapter as well as numerous factors described by others, one can now generate a complex model of B-cell activation and differentiation. Figure 6 depicts such a hypothetical model. *In vivo,* antigen activates clones of B cells to enlarge and express receptor for BCGF. Antigen can also activate T cells to secrete nonspecific factors concomitantly (BCPF) that polyclonally stimulate B cells to enlarge and possibly express receptors for BCGF of go on to proliferate independently. After proliferation of specific and nonspecific B-cell clones, receptors for various BCDFs might be expressed. The response to BCDFs might be a cascade pattern, possibly including those regulating isotype switching. Depending on the antigen and/or location of the immune response, there might be a selective advantage for a particular isotype(s). In this case, isotype-specific factors might augment a particular isotypic response. In conjunction with these factors, other nonspecific augmenting agents, such as IL-2 and possibly IFN-γ, might play a role. The enormous complexity of this pathway can be appreciated by the myriad of factors described; however, only with the actual isola-

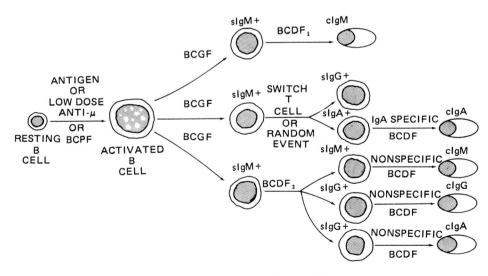

FIGURE 6. Model for normal B-cell differentiation.

tion and purification of these factors will it be possible to come to some reasonable understanding of the immune response.

References

Clough, J. D., Mims, L. H., and Strober, W., 1971, Deficient IgA antibody responses to arsenilic acid–bovine serum albumin (BSA) in neonatally thymectomized rabbits, *J. Immunol.* **106:**1624.

Crewther, P., and Warner, N. L., 1972, Serum immunoglobulins and antibodies in congenitally athymic (nude) mice, *Aust. J. Biol. Med. Sci.* **50:**625.

DeFranco, A. L., Ashwell, J. D., Schwartz, R. H., and Paul, W. E., 1984, Polyclonal stimulation of resting B cells by antigen-specific T cells, *J. Exp. Med.* **159:**861.

Epstein, J., Leyva, A., Kelley, W. N., and Littlefield, J. W., 1977, Mutagen-induced diploid human lymphoblast variants containing altered hypoxanthine guanine phosphoribosyl transferase, *Somat. Cell Genet.* **3:**135.

Foung, S. K. H., Sasaki, D. T., Grumet, F. C., and Engleman, E. G., 1982, Production of functional human T–T hybridomas in selection medium lacking aminopterin and thymidine, *Proc. Natl. Acad. Sci. USA* **79:**7484.

Geha, R. S., Schneeberger, E., Merler, E., and Rosen, F. S., 1974, Heterogeneity of "acquired" or common variable agammaglobulinemia, *N. Engl. J. Med.* **291:**1.

Haynes, B. F., Hemler, M. E., Mann, D. L., Eisenbarth, G. S., Schelhamer, J., Mostowski, H. S., Thomas, C. A., Strominger, J. L., and Fauci, A. S., 1981, Characterization of a monoclonal antibody (4F2) that binds to human monocytes and to a subset of activated lymphocytes, *J. Immunol.* **126:**1409.

Howard, M., and Paul, W. E., 1983, Regulation of B cell growth and differentiation by soluble factors, *Annu. Rev. Immunol.* **1:**307.

Howard, M., Farrar, J., Hilfiker, M., Johnson, B., Takatsu, K., Hamaoka, T., Paul, W. E., 1982, Identification of a T cell derived B cell growth factor distinct from interleukin 2, *J. Exp. Med.* **155:**914.

Irigoyen, O., Rizzolo, P. V., Thomas, Y., Rogozinski, L., and Chess, L., 1981, Generation of functional human T cell hybrids, *J. Exp. Med.* **154:**1827.

Isakson, P. C., Pure, E., Vitetta, E. S., and Krammer, P. V., 1982, T cell derived B cell differentiation factor(s). Effect on the isotype switch of murine B cells, *J. Exp. Med.* **155:**734.

Jung, L. K. L., Hara, T., and Fu, S. M., 1984, Detection and functional studies of p60–65 (Tac antigen) in activated B cells, *J. Exp. Med.* **160:**1597.

Kawanishi, H., Saltzman, L., and Strober, W., 1983a, Mechanisms regulating IgA-class specific Ig production in murine gut-associated lymphoid tissues. I. T cells derived from Peyer's patches which switch sIgM B-cells to sIgA B cells *in vitro*, *J. Exp. Med.* **157:**433.

Kawanishi, H., Saltzman, L., and Strober, W., 1983b, Mechanisms regulating IgA-class specific Ig production in murine gut-associated lymphoid tissues. II. Terminal differentiation of post switch sIgA bearing Peyer's patch B cells, *J. Exp. Med.* **158:**649.

Kiyono, H., Cooper, M. D., Kearney, J. F., Mosteller, L. M., Michalek, S. M., Koopman, W. J., and McGhee, J. R., 1984, Isotype specificity of helper T cell clones. Peyer's patch Th cells preferentially collaborate with mature IgA B cells for IgA responses, *J. Exp. Med.* **159:**798.

Marrack, P., Graham, Jr., S. D., Kushnir, E., Liebson, H. J., and Marrack, J., 1982, Nonspecific factors in B cell responses, *Immunol. Rev.* **63:**33.

Mayer, L., Fu, S. M., and Kunkel, H. G., 1982, Human T cell hybridomas secreting factors for IgA specific help, polyclonal B cell activation and B cell proliferation, *J. Exp. Med.* **156:**1860.

Mayer, L., Fu, S. M., and Kunkel, H. G., 1984a, Regulation of B cell activation and differentiation with factors generated by human T cell hybridomas, *Immunol. Rev.* **78:**119.

Mayer, L., and Kunkel, H. G., 1984b, Heterogeneity of B cell growth and differentiation factors, *Lymphokine Res.* **3:**107.

Mayer, L., Fu, S. M., Cunningham-Rundles, C. C., and Kunkel, H. G., 1984c, Polyclonal immunoglobulin secretion in patients with common variable immunodeficiency using monoclonal B cell differentiation factors, *J. Clin Invest.* **74:**2115.

Muraguchi, A., and Fauci, A. S., 1982, Proliferative responses of normal human B lymphocytes. Development of an assay system for human B cell growth factor (BCGF), *J. Immunol.* **129:**1104.

Muraguchi, A., Butler, J. L., Kehrl, J. H., and Fauci, A. S., 1983, Differential sensitivity of human B cell subsets to activation signals delivered by anti-u antibody and proliferative signals delivered by a monoclonal B cell growth factor, *J. Exp. Med.* **157:**530.

Parker, D. C., Separable helper factors support B cell proliferation and maturation Co Ig secretion, *J. Immunol.* **129:**469.

Nakanishi, K., Howard, M., Muraguchi, A., Farrar, J., Takatsu, K., Hamaoka, T., Paul, W. E., 1983, Soluble factors involved in B cell differentiation: Identification of two distinct T cell-replacing factors (TRF), *J. Immunol.* **130:**2219.

Schimpl, A., and Wecker, E., 1972, Replacement of T cell function by a T cell product, *Nature* **237:**15.

Sell, S., and Gell, P. G. H., 1965, Studies on rabbit lymphocytes *in vitro.* 1. Stimulation of blast transformation with an anti-allotype serum, *J. Exp. Med.* **122:**923.

Swain, S. L., Howard, M., Kappler, J., Marrack, P., Watson, J., Booth, R., Wetzel, G. D., Dutton, R. W., 1983, Evidence for two distinct classes of murine B cell growth factor with activities in different functional assays, *J. Exp. Med.* **158:**822.

Tsudo, M., Uchiyama, T., and Uchino, H., 1984, Expression of Tac antigen on activated normal human B cells, *J. Exp. Med.* **160:**612.

Waldmann, T. A., Durm, M., Broder, S., Blackman, M., Blaese, R. H., and Strober, W., 1974, Role of suppressor cells in pathogenesis of common variable hypogammaglobulinemia, *Lancet* **ii:**609–613.

Waldmann, T. A., Goldman, C. K., Robb, R. J., Depper, J. M., Leonard, W. J., Sharrow, S. O., Bongiovanni, K. F., Korsmeyer, S. J., and Greene, W. C., 1984, Expression of interleukin-2 receptors on activated human B cells, *J. Exp. Med.* **160:**1450.

Wu, L., Lawton, A. R., and Cooper, M. D., 1973, Differentiation capacity of cultured B lymphocytes from immunodeficient patients, *J. Clin. Invest.* **52:**3180.

Yoshizaki, K., Nakagawa, T., Kaieda, A., Muraguchi, A., Yamamura, Y., and Kishimoto, T., 1982, Induction of proliferation and Ig production on human B leukemic cells by anti-immunoglobulins and T cell factors, *J. Immunol.* **128:**1296.

APPENDIX

1

Human T- and B-Cell Lines

JAMES W. LARRICK AND STEVEN K. H. FOUNG

Many of the T- and B-cell lines used to make hybridomas are available from the investigators. A few are now available from the ATCC* or the Camden Cell Repository.† Table I presents a list of human B-lineage cell lines that have been reported to make successful hybridomas. Table II presents a list of human T-lineage cell lines that have successfully produced human hybridomas.

The best medium for growth of human T- and B-cell lines is Iscove's Dulbecco's Modified Eagle's Medium (DMEM) with high glucose (4.5 g/liter) or RPMI 1640. RPMI 1640 can also be supplemented with up to 4.5 g/liter of glucose to improve growth at high cell densities. Most of the cell lines are maintained in stationary suspension cultures at concentrations of 10^5-10^6/ml. To obtain maximum fusion efficiency, it has been repeatedly found that cells in log phase growth work best. Most of the cell lines can be seeded at 10^5/ml and will have maximal growth rates at $(3-5) \times 10^5$/ml. However, growth curves should be determined on each line prior to fusion. Several serum-free media are now available. We have found HB101 and HB104 (HANA Biologicals, Emeryville, California) and HL-1 (Ventrex Laboratories, Portland, Maine) to be useful (McHugh *et al.*, 1983).

---

*American Type Culture Collection, 12301 Parklawn Drive, Rockville, Maryland 20852 (301 881-2600).

†Human Genetic Mutant Cell Repository, Institute for Medical Research, Capewood and Doris Streets, Camden, New Jersey 08103 (609 966-7377).

JAMES W. LARRICK • Cetus Immune Research Laboratories, Palo Alto, California 94303. STEVEN K. H. FOUNG • Department of Pathology, Stanford University School of Medicine, Stanford University Medical Center, Stanford, California 94305.

TABLE I
Currently Used Human Parent Cell Lines

Cell line	Secreted Ig	EBNA	Cell type	References
SKO-007	IgE(γ)	—	Myeloma	Olsson et al. (1983), Olsson and Kaplan (1980), Nilsson et al. (1970)
KARPAS 707	γ	—	Myeloma	Karpas et al. (1982)
RPMI-8226	γ	—	Myeloma	Matsuoka et al. (1967)
KMM1	γ	—	Myeloma	Togawa et al. (1982)
GM1500	IgG(κ)	+	LCL	Croce et al. (1980)
KR-4	IgG(κ)	+	LCL	Kozbor et al. (1982)
LIC-LON-HMy2	IgG(κ)	+	LCL	Cote et al. (1983), Edwards et al. (1982)
GM467	IgM(γ)	+	LCL	Sato et al. (1972)
LTR228	IgM(κ)	+	LCL	Larrick et al. (1983)
UC729-6	IgM(κ)	+	LCL	Glassy et al. (1983), Handley and Royson (1982)
UC729-HF2	IgM(κ)	+	LCL	Strike et al. (1984)
GM4672	IgG(κ)	+	LCL	Satoh et al. (1983)
H351.1	IgM(κ)	+	LCL	Chiorazzi et al. (1982)
MC/CAR	None	+	LCL	Ritts et al. (1983)
ARH-77	IgG(κ)	+	LCL	Burk et al. (1978)
LSM2-7	None	+	LCL	Schwaber et al. (1983)
H.S.Sultan	None	+	LCL	Lazarus et al. (1982)
GK-5	κ	+	LCL	Satoh et al. (1983)
HFB-1	None	+	LCL	Hunter et al. (1982)
RH-L4	None	?	Lymphoma	Olsson et al. (1983)
SBC-H20	None	—	Mouse–human hybrid myeloma	Foung et al. (1984)
KR12	IgG(γ,κ)	+	Human–human hybrid myeloma	Kozbor et al. (1984)
FU-266 neo^R	—	—	Human–mouse hybrid myeloma	Teng et al. (1983)

[a]LCL, EBV-transformed B lymphoblastoid cell line.

TABLE II
T-Cell Lines Used for the Generation of T–T Hybridomas

Cell line	Reference
CEM derivatives	Asada et al. (1983), Butler et al. (1983), Greene et al. (1982), Howell et al. (1982), Huff and Ishizaka (1984), Irigoyen et al. (1981), Kobayaski et al. (1982), Le et al. (1983), Okada et al. (1983), Okada et al. (1981), Theodore et al. (1984), Welser et al. (1984)
Jurkat derivatives	DeFreitas et al. (1982), Foung et al. (1982), Lakow et al. (1983), Platsoucas et al. (1984) Ritts et al. (1983), Valentine et al. (1983)
KE 37	Grillot-Courvalin et al. (1981, 1982), Laurence and Mayer (1984), Mayer (1982)
MOLT-4	Gallagher and Stimson (1983), Platsoucas et al. (1984), Vervliet et al. (1983)
HUT102-32	Le et al. (1982, 1983)

References

Asada, M., Higuichi, M., Kobayashi, Y., and Osawa, T., 1983, Human T-cell hybridomas producing lymphokines. 1. Enhancement of lymphotoxin secretion from human T-cell hybridomas by phorbol myristate acetate, *Cell. Immunol.* **77**:150–160.

Burk, K. M., Drewinko, B., Trujillo, J. M., and Ahearn, M. J., 1978, Establishment of a human plasma cell line *in vitro, Cancer Res.* **38**:1508–2513.

Butler, J. L., Muraguchi, A., Lane, H. C., and Fauci, A., 1983, Development of a human T–T cell hybridoma secreting B cell growth factor, *J. Exp. Med.* **157**:60–68.

Chiorazzi, N., Wasserman, R. L., and Kunkel, H. G., 1982, Use of Epstein–Barr virus transformed B cell lines for the generation of immunoglobulin-producing human B cell hybridomas, *J. Exp. Med.* **156**:930–935.

Cote, R. J., Morrissey, D. M., Houghton, A. N., Beattie, Jr., E. J., Oettgen, H. F., and Old, L. J., 1983, Generation of human monoclonal antibodies reactive with cellular antigens, *Proc. Natl. Acad. Sci. USA* **80**:2016–2030.

Croce, C. M., Linnenbach, A., Hall, W., Steplewski, Z., and Koprowski, H., 1980, Production of human hybridomas secreting antibodies to measles virus, *Nature* **288**:488–489.

DeFreitas, E. C., Valla, S., Linnenbach, A., Zmijewski, C., Koprowski, H., and Croce, C. M., 1982, Antigen-specific human T-cell hybridomas with helper activity, *Proc. Natl. Acad. Sci. USA* **79**:6646–6650.

Edwards, P. A. W., Smith, C. M., Neville, A. M., and O'Hare, M. J., 1982, A human/human hybridoma system based on a fast growing mutant of the ARH-77 plasma cell leukemia derived line, *Eur. J. Immunol.* **12**:641–648.

Foung, S. K. H., Sasaki, D., Grumet, F. C., and Engleman, E. G., 1982, Production of functional human T–T hybridomas in selection medium lacking aminopterin and thymidine, *Proc. Natl. Acad. Sci. USA* **79**:7484–7488.

Foung, S. K. H., Perkins, S., Raubitschek, A., Larrick, J., Lizak, G., Fishwild, D., Engleman, E. G., and Grumet, F. C., 1984, Rescue of human monoclonal antibody production from an EBV-transformed B cell line by fusion to a human–mouse hybridoma, *J. Immunol. Meth.* **70**:83–90.

Gallagher, G., and Stimson, W. H., 1983, Generation of human T-cell hybrids with the characteristics of human peripheral blood T-lymphocytes, *Immunol. Lett.* **6**:203–207.

Glassy, M. C., Handley, H. H., Hagiwara, H., and Royston, I., 1983, UC-729–6, a human lymphoblastoid B-cell line useful for generating antibody-secreting human/human hybridomas, *Proc. Natl. Acad. Sci. USA* **80**:6327–6331.

Greene, W. C., Fleisher, T. A., Nelson, D. L., and Waldman, T. A., 1982, Production of human suppressor T cell hybridomas, *J. Immunol.* **129**:1986–1991.

Grillot-Courvalin, C., Brouet, J., Berger, R., and Bernheim, A., 1981, Establishment of a human T-cell hybrid line with suppressive activity. *Nature* **292**:844–845.

Grillot-Courvalin, C., Dellagi, K., Chevalier, A., and Brouet, J. C., 1982, Characterization of a suppressive factor produced by a human T hybridoma, *J. Immunol.* **129**:1008–1011.

Handley, H. H., and Royston, I., 1982, A human lymphoblastoid B cell line useful for generating immunoglobulin secreting human hybridomas, in: *Hybridomas in Cancer Diagnosis and Treatment,* (M. S. Mitchell and H. F. Oettgen, eds.), Raven Press, New York, pp. 125–132.

Howell, D. N., Berger, A. E., and Cresswell, P., 1982, Human T–B lymphoblast hybrids express HLA-DR specificities not expressed by either parent, *Immunogenetics* **15**:199–206.

Huff, T. F., and Ishizaka, K., 1984, Formation of IgE-binding factors by human T-cell hybridomas, *Proc. Natl. Acad. Sci. USA* **81**:1514–1518.

Hunter, K. W., Jr., Fischer, G. W., Hemminy, V. G., Wilson, S. R., Hartzman, R. J., and Woody, J. N., 1982, Antibacterial activity of a human monoclonal antibody to *Haemophilus influenzae* type B capsular polysaccharide, *Lancet* **II**:798–799.

Irigoyen, O., Rizzolo, P. V., Thomas, Y., Hemmler, M. E., Shen, H. H., Friedman, S. M., Strominger, J. L., and Chess, L., 1981, Generation of functional human T cell hybrids, *J. Exp. Med.* **154**:1827–1837.

Karpas, A., Fischer, P., and Swirsky, D., 1982, Human myeloma cell lines carrying a Philadelphia chromosome, *Science* **216**:997–999.

Kobayashi, Y., Asada, M., Higuchi, M., and Osawa, T., 1982, Human T cell hybridomas producing lymphokines, *J. Immunol.* **128:**2714–2718.

Kozbor, D., Lagarde, A. E., and Roder, J. C., 1982, Human hybridomas constructed with antigen-specific EBV transformed lines, *Proc. Natl. Acad. Sci. USA* **79:**6651–6655.

Kozbor, D., Tripputi, P., Roder, J. C., and Croce, C. M., 1984, A human hybrid myeloma for production of human monoclonal antibody, *J. Immunol.* **133:**3001–3005.

Lakow, E., Tsoukas, C. D., Vaughan, J. H., Altman, A., and Carson, D. A., 1983, Human T cell hybridomas specific for Epstein–Barr virus-infected B lymphocytes, *J. Immunol.* **130:**169–172.

Larrick, J. W., Truitt, K. E., Raubitschek, A. A., Senyk, G. S., and Wang, J. C. N., 1983, Characterization of human hybridomas secreting antibody to tetanus toxoid, *Proc. Natl. Acad. Sci. USA* **80:**6376–6380.

Laurence, J., and Mayer, L., 1984, Immunoregulatory lymphokines of T hybridomas for AIDS patients: Constitutive and inducible suppressor factors, *Science* **225:**66–69.

Lazarus, H., Posner, M., Schlossman, S., and Schwaber, J., 1982, A human cell line capable of supporting monoclonal antibody secretion upon fusion with human immunocytes, *Fed. Proc.* **41:**1911 (abstract).

Le, J., Vilček, J., Saxinger, C., and Prensky, W., 1982, Human T cell hybridomas secreting immune interferon, *Proc. Natl. Acad. Sci. USA* **79:**7857–7861.

Le, J., Vilček, J., Sadlik, J. R., Cheung, M. K., Balazs, I., Sarngadharan, M. G., and Prensky, W., 1983, Lymphokine production by human T cell hybridomas, *J. Immunol.* **130:**1231–1235.

Mayer, L., Fu, S. M., and Kunkel, H. G., 1982, Human T cell hybridomas secreting factors for IgA-specific help, polyclonal B cell activation, and B cell proliferation, *J. Exp. Med.* **156:**1860–1865.

McHugh, Y. E., Walthau, B. J., and Steiner, K. S., 1983, Serum-free growth of murine and human lymphoid and hybridoma cell lines, *Biotechniques* **1:**72–77.

Matsuoka, Y., Moore, G. E., Yagi, Y., and Pressman, D., 1967, Production of free light chains of immunoglobulin by a haematopoietic cell line derived from a patient with multiple myeloma, *Proc. Soc. Exp. Biol. Med.* **125:**1246–1250.

Nilsson, K., Bennich, H., Johansson, S. G. O., and Pontén, J., 1970, Established immunoglobulin producing myeloma (IgE), *Clin. Exp. Immunol.* **7:**477–489.

Okada, M., Yoshimura, N., Kaieda, T., Yamamura, Y., and Kishimoto, T., 1981, Establishment and characterization of human T hybrid cells secreting immunoregulatory molecules, *Proc. Natl. Acad. Sci. USA* **78:**7717–7721.

Okada, M., Sakaguchi, N., Yoshimura, N., Hara, H., Shimizu, K., Yoshida, N., Yashizak, K., Kishimoto, S., Yamamura, Y., and Kishimoto, T., 1983, B cell growth factors and B cell differentiation factor from human T hybridomas, *J. Exp. Med.* **157:**583–590.

Olsson, L., and Kaplan, H. S., 1980, Human/human hybridomas producing monoclonal antibodies of predefined antigenic specificity, *Proc. Natl. Acad. Sci. USA* **77:**5429–5431.

Olsson, L., Kronstrom, H., Cambon-de Mouzon, A., Honsik, C., Brodin, T., and Kakobsen, B., 1983, Antibody producing human/human hybridomas. I. Technical aspects, *J. Immunol. Meth.* **61:**17–32.

Platsoucas, C, D., Calvelli, T. A., Kunicka, J. E., Lawless, B. D., and Higgins, J. A., 1984, Constitutive production of a suppressor factor by human T–T cell hybridomas, *Fed. Proc.* **43(6):**1605 (abstract).

Ritts, R. E., Jr., Ruiz Arguelles, A., Weyl, K. G., Bradley, A. L., Weihmeier, B., Jacobssen, D. J., and Strehlo, B. L., 1983, Establishment and characterization of a human non-secretory plasmacytoid cell line and its hybridization with human B cells, *Int. J. Cancer* **31:**133–141.

Sato, K., Sleskinski, R. S., and Littlefield, J. W., 1972, Chemical mutagenesis at the phosphoribosyltransferase locus in cultured human lymphoblasts, *Proc. Natl. Acad. Sci. USA* **69:**1244–1248.

Satoh, J., Prabhakar, B. S., Haspel, M. V., Ginsberg-Fellner, F., and Notkins, A. L., 1983, Human monoclonal autoantibodies that react with multiple endocrine organs, *N. Engl. J. Med.* **309:**217–220.

Schwaber, J., Molgaard, H., Orkin, S. H., Gould, H. J., and Rosen, F. S., 1983, Early pre-B cells from normal and X-linked agammaglobulinemia produce Cμ without an attached V_H region, *Nature* **304**:355–358.

Strike, L. E., Devens, B. H., and Lundak, R. L., 1984, Production of human/human hybridomas secreting antibody to sheep erythrocytes after *in vitro* immunization, *J. Immunol.* **132**:1798–1803.

Teng, N. N. H., Lam, K. S., Riera, C. and Kaplan, H. S., 1983, Construction and testing of mouse–human heteromyelomas for human monoclonal antibody production, *Proc. Natl. Acad. Sci. USA* **80**:7308–7312.

Theodore, A. C., Beer, D. J., Picarella, D. E., Rosenwasser, L. J., and Center, D. M., 1984, Production of lymphotactic lymphokines by human T–T cell hybridomas, *Fed. Proc.* **43**(6):1603 (abstract).

Togawa, A., Inoue, N., Miyamoto, K., Hyodo, H., and Namba, M., 1982, Establishment and characterization of a human myeloma cell line, *Int. J. Cancer* **29**:495–500.

Valentine, M. A., Lakow, E. S., Vaughan, J. H., and Carson, D. A., 1983, T cell hybridomas: A new approach for studying the functional properties of T cells in rheumatoid arthritis, *Arthritis Rheum.* **16**:545 (abstract).

Vervliet, G., Asma, G., Vossen, J., and Billiau, A., 1983, Isolation and characterization of a human HAT-sensitive T-cell line as a tool for the construction of human T-cell hybridomas, *Arch. Int. Physiol. Biochem.* **90**(A):B224–225.

Welser, W., Kawaguchi, T., David, J., and Remold, H., 1984, Generation of human hybridomas producing MIF and of murine hybridomas secreting monoclonal antibodies to these MIF species, *Fed. Proc.* **43**(6):1500 (abstract).

2
Preparation of Mutant Cell Lines

STEVEN K. H. FOUNG, SUSAN PERKINS, AND EDGAR G. ENGLEMAN

Materials

1. Complete medium with 10% FCS
   (See Human Hybridoma Fusion Protocol for composition of medium, Appendix, Chapter 8)
2. 6-Thioguanine (6TG)-containing medium:

   6TG stock (500 ×):
   a. Add 0.0334 g 6TG (Sigma) to 10 ml distilled water and dissolve by adding 1 N NaOH
   b. Adjust pH to 9–9.5
   c. Bring volume to 20 ml, sterile filter, and store in 1-ml aliquots at −20°C

3. Ethyl methanesulfonate (EMS)-containing medium:
   one hundred milligrams EMS (Eastman)/ml complete medium.

Methods

6TG-resistant mutants can be generated with irradiation- or EMS-induced mutagenesis. Cells must be in log phase growth before mutagenesis is

STEVEN K. H. FOUNG, SUSAN PERKINS, AND EDGAR G. ENGLEMAN • Department of Pathology, Stanford University School of Medicine, Stanford University Medical Center, Stanford, California 94305.

attempted. The entire process of procuring a HAT- or AH-sensitive cell line will take 2–4 months.

Irradiation-Induced Mutagenesis

Day 1:

1. Start with 10^8 cells in log phase growth.
2. Irradiate with 100 rad.
3. Plate in 24-well tray (Costar) at 10^6 cells/ml per well in complete medium.

Day 2:
Feed with 1 ml 6TG-containing medium that is further diluted 1:10 with complete medium. The medium should be changed every 2–3 days by aspirating and replacing with 1 ml.
~Day 14:
When macroscopic colonies become visible, start feeding with 6TG-containing medium diluted 1:5.
~Day 21:
Increase concentration of 6TG in feeding medium to 1:2.
Day 28:
Start feeding with undiluted 6TG-containing medium.
~Days 30–35:

1. When the cells are growing well in 6TG, obtain viable cells by Ficoll–Hypaque density gradient centrifugation.
2. Wash viable cells with complete medium and resuspend in undiluted 6TG-containing medium and place in a 25-ml flask.
3. Over the following 2 weeks gradually increase the 6TG concentration tenfold by twofold increment with each feeding (3- to 4-day intervals).

EMS-Induced Mutagenesis

Day 1:
Suspend 10^8 cells in EMS-containing medium at 10^6 cells/ml in several 75-ml flasks and place in a CO_2 humidified incubator at 37°C for 3 hr. Flasks should be maintained in a horizontal position. Harvest cells in 50-ml conicals, wash once, and resuspend cells in 25 ml of complete medium.
Day 4:
Feed cells with an additional 25 ml of medium.
Day 7:
Generally cells are growing vigorously at this point and 6TG selection can begin as stated above.

When cells are growing in $10 \times$ 6TG-containing medium, they can be tested for HAT or AH sensitivity by placing them in the selection medium. One hundred percent cell death should be observed by day 7 before the particular cell line should be used as a fusion partner.

References

Choy, W. N., Gopalakrishnan, T. V., and Littlefield, J. W., 1982, Techniques for using HAT selection in somatic cell genetics in: *Techniques in Somatic Cell Genetics* (J. W. Shay, ed.), New York, Plenum Press, pp. 11–21.

Sato, K., Slesinski, R. S., and Littlefield, J. W., 1972, Chemical mutagenesis at the phosphoribosyl-transferase locus in cultured human lymphoblasts, *Proc. Natl. Acad. Sci. USA* **69**:1244–1248.

3

Freezing Human Cell Lines

JAMES W. LARRICK

Cells can be stored in liquid nitrogen indefinitely and recovered in a healthy state if they are frozen properly.

1. Pellet cells from a healthy culture in mid-log-phase growth.
2. Resuspend the cells (at $10^6–10^7$/ml) in ice-cold fetal calf serum (95%) supplemented with DMSO (5%).
3. Place a 1-ml aliquot of the cells into 2-ml plastic freezing ampoules (e.g., Nunc).
4. Place ampoules in a styrofoam container or in a cardboard container rack in a $-70°C$ freezer overnight to provide a slow, uniform rate of freezing.
5. Move the cells to liquid nitrogen and record their location, viability, passage number, etc., on index cards or computer inventory (Franklin, 1982).
6. Thaw cells by immersion in a $37°C$ water bath and dilute with 10 ml of culture medium. An ampoule from each freeze should be test-thawed to check cell viability.

Reference

Franklin, R. M., 1982, Microcomputer inventory systems for stored cell lines, *J. Immunol. Meth.* **54**:141–157.

JAMES W. LARRICK • Cetus Immune Research Laboratories, Palo Alto, California 94303.

4
Mycoplasma Testing

JAMES W. LARRICK AND BRADLEY J. DYER

Principle

Spent culture medium from the cell ine in question is placed on a monolayer
of mycoplasma-free Swiss 3T3 cells. The cells are cultured for 5 days and the
cells are stained with a fluorescent DNA-binding dye (Chen, 1977). Mycoplasma can be readily identified in the large cytoplasm of these fibroblasts.

Materials

Setup

1. Confluent Swiss 3T3 cells (or other suitable fibroblast line)
2. Versene (1:5000 EDTA disodium salt in PBS) (GIBCO)
3. Trypsin: 0.25% in Tris-buffered saline (GIBCO)
4. RPMI 1640 supplemented with 10% FCS and 0.03% L-glutamine
   (GIBCO)
5. Sterile culture tubes and centrifuge tubes: 16 × 125 mm; 50 ml
6. Disposable culture tubes
7. Vital dye: 0.5% trypan blue
8. Two-chamber slides (Miles Laboratories, #4802)
9. Sterile PBS
10. Positive and negative controls: cell lines with and without my-
    coplasma infection

JAMES W. LARRICK AND BRADLEY J. DYER • Cetus Immune Research Laboratories, Palo Alto,
California 94303.

Staining

1. Forceps
2. PBS
3. Fixative: acetic acid–methanol 10:90
4. DNA stain H33258 (Calbiochem): 5 mg/ml dilution in PBS
5. Coplin jars
6. Kimwipes or paper towels
7. Cover slips for slides: 22 × 50 mm or 2-25 × 25 mm/slide
8. PBS–glycerol mixture 50:50
9. Clear nail polish
10. Fluorescent microscope

Mycoplasma Testing

Setup Protocol

1. Detach 3T3 cells from T75 flask with trypsin and resuspend in 10 ml cold RPMI with 10% FCS and glutamine in a 15-ml culture tube. Place the tube on ice.
2. Resuspend the cells; perform a viable count using trypan blue.
3. Dilute the cell suspension with growth medium (with serum and glutamine) to a density of 2.5×10^4 cells/ml. Use 2 ml of this suspension per two-chamber slide. Unused cell suspension may be diluted 1:3 and seeded into culture flasks at this time.
4. Add 1 ml cell suspension to each chamber and incubate until test cell suspensions are prepared, or until fibroblasts have attached to the slides.
5. Dilute test cells with sterile PBS.
6. Add one drop of test cell suspension to corresponding chamber, using a single plugged Pasteur pipette for each line.
7. Incubate in 5% CO_2 humidified incubator for 5 days.

Staining Protocol

1. On day 5, aspirate medium from each chamber with Pasteur pipette. *Never let slides dry!*
2. Rinse each chamber with 1–2 ml PBS and aspirate. Repeat twice.
3. Add 1 ml fixative (acetic acid–methanol) to each chamber for 5–10 min.

APPENDIX

4. Aspirate fixative and add 1 ml DNA stain (H33258, 1:1000 in PBS). Incubate for 15 min.
5. Aspirate DNA stain.
6. Remove chamber walls and rubber linings using forceps. Place slides in Coplin jar under cold, running tap water and rinse for 5 min.
7. Gently dry the slides on Kimwipes or paper towels.
8. Place one drop (22 × 22 mm coverslips) or three drops (122 × 50 mm coverslip) of PBS–glycerol (1:1) mixture on each slide. *Do not use mounting medium,* such as Permount, since this will decrease and diffuse fluorescence.
9. Seal edges of coverslips with clear nail polish and allow to dry before viewing.
10. Read results on fluorescent microscope.
11. The blue fluorescent *dots* or *threads* of mycoplasma infection should be evenly distributed throughout the field, with distinct fluorescence. Hazy or diffuse fluorescence is most likely due to the drying of 3T3 cytoplasm during staining.
12. The cytoplasm of the 3T3 cells is clear of any fluorescence, except possibly at the edges, which can appear faintly fluorescent. The bright spots in the 3T3 nuclei are normal.

Eradicating Mycoplasma Infection from Cell Cultures

Several methods have been described for curing mycoplasma-infected cell lines (McGarrity, 1976). These include:

1. Brief exposure of all infected lines to elevated temperature (41–42°C) (Hayflick, 1960).
2. Cocultivation of infected cell lines with macrophages in the presence of antibiotics (Schummelpfeng et al., 1980).
3. Exposure of infected cells to hypotonic solutions (Gori and Lee, 1964).
4. Exposure of infected cells to antibiotics (Gurney et al., 1981) or antibiotics and specific antibodies (Vogelsang and Compeer-Dekker, 1969).
5. Treatment of cultures with Tricine buffer (Spendlove et al., 1971) or sodium polyanethol sulfonate (Mardh, 1975).
6. Passage of cell lines through mice (Howell et al., 1982; Lombardo and Lauks, 1982).
7. Selective incorporation of 5-bromouracil into mycoplasma DNA with subsequent exposure to visible light (Marcus et al., 1980).

We have found the following technique particularly effective:

1. Infected cells are washed four times in culture medium.
2. Cells are then cultured overnight at 3×10^5/ml in culture medium containing:

    a. Tylocine (120 μg/ml) (GIBCO; Cat #600-5220)

    b. Spectinomycin sulfate tetrahydrate (1 mg/ml) (GIBCO; Cat #600–5610)

3. The following day cells are washed twice and resuspended in medium containing tylocine (60 μg/ml) and spectinonycin sulfate tetrahydrate (500 μl/ml).

4. Cells are then grown for 2 weeks in the presence of antibiotics. Cells are washed twice between each passage and transferred to new culture flasks.

5. After the 2-week antibiotic treatment, cells are washed once, transferred to medium without antibiotics, grown to confluency, and tested for the presence of mycoplasma.

6. Tests for mycoplasma in a culture grown in the absence of antibiotics are carried out for 6 weeks before a cell line is declared free of infection.

Notes

1. Mycoplasmas are commonly introduced into cell cultures through fetal calf sera and aerosolized nasal secretions. In recent years fetal calf sera have been screened for the presence of mycoplasma, and most infections are now initiated by poor laboratory technique. *The routine use of antibiotics in long-term cultures of cell lines should be strongly discouraged.* Obviously most aerosol particles containing mycoplasma will carry bacteria. Contamination of antibiotic-free cell cultures indicates an immediate source of potential mycoplasma (Mardh, 1975).

2. The routine prophylactic use of the above-mentioned antibiotics is *also to be deplored* because in a short time it will lead to resistant mycoplasma stains.

References

Chen, T. R., 1977, *In situ* detection of mycoplasma contamination in cell culture by fluorescent Hoechst 33258 stain, *Exp. Cell Res.* **104:**255–262.

Gori, G. B., and Lee, Y. D., 1964, A method for eradication of mycoplasma infections in cell cultures, *Proc. Soc. Exp. Biol. Med.* **117:**918–921.

Gurney, T., Woolf, M. J., Abplanalp, L. J., McKittrick, N. H., Dietz, J. N., and Cole, B. C., 1981, Elimination of *Mycoplasma hyorhinis* infection from four cell lines, *In Vitro* **17:**993–996.

Hayflick, L., 1960, Decontaminating tissue cultures infected with pleuropneumonia-like organisms, *Nature* **185:**783–784.

Howell, D. N., Machamer, C. E., and Cresswell, P., 1982, Elimination of mycoplasma from human B-lymphoblastoid cell lines, *Hum. Immunol.* **5:**233–238.

Lombardo, J. M., and Lauks, K. W., 1982, Elimination of *M. hyorhinis* from murine neuroblastoma cell lines by *in vivo* passage, *In Vitro* **18**:251–253.

Marcus, M., Lavi, U., Nattenburg, A., Rottem, S., and Markovitz, O., 1980, Selective killing of mycoplasmas from contaminated mammalian cells in cell cultures, *Nature* **285**:659–661.

Mardh, P. A., 1975, Elimination of mycoplasmas from cell cultures with sodium polyanethol sulphonate, *Nature* **254**:515–516.

McGarrity, G. J., 1976, Spread and control of mycoplasma infection of cell cultures, *In Vitro* **12**:643–648.

Schummelpfeng, L., Langenberg, V., and Hinrich, P. J., 1980, Macrophages overcome mycoplasma infections of cells *in vitro*, *Nature* **285**:661–662.

Spendlove, R. S., Crosbie, R. B., and Hayes, S. F., 1971, Tricine buffered tissue culture media for control of tissue culture contaminants, *Proc. Soc. Exp. Biol. Med.* **137**:258–263.

Vogelsang, A. A., and Compeer-Dekker, G., 1969, Elimination of mycoplasma from various cell cultures, *Antonie Van Leeuwenhoek* **35**:393–408.

5

Peripheral Blood Lymphocyte Separation from Whole Blood or Buffy Coats

STEVEN K. H. FOUNG, SUSAN PERKINS, AND EDGAR G. AND EDGAR G. ENGLEMAN

Materials

1. Buffy coat unit or whole blood drawn in heparin or acid citrate–dextrose anticoagulant solutions
2. Diluent/wash solutions:
   a. Hank's Balanced Salt Solution (GIBCO)
   b. RPMI 1640 (GIBCO)
   c. Phosphate-buffered saline, calcium- and magnesium-free (GIBCO). Four ml of heparin (1000 USP units/ml) is added to each 500 ml of solution.
3. Ficoll–Hypaque (FH, 1 liter):
   a. Ficoll (Sigma): 64 g
   b. Diatrizoate sodium (Sterling Drug, New York): 99 g
   c. NaCl: 0.7 g

Dissolve Ficoll and NaCl in 600 ml of distilled water using a stir bar rotor at low speed and then add diatrizoate sodium. After all substances are in solution, add more water to 1 liter.

STEVEN K. H. FOUNG, SUSAN PERKINS, AND EDGAR G. ENGLEMAN • Department of Pathology, Stanford University School of Medicine, Stanford University Medical Center, Stanford, California 94305.

Methods

1. Bring diluent/wash solution to room temperature.
2. Place blood to be separated in 50-ml conicals (Corning) using the following sterile technique: alcohol and flame openings of glass tubes; wipe exterior of plastic tubing with alcohol before entering a buffy coat unit.
3. Dilute blood (30 ml total per tube):
    Whole blood: one part blood/one part diluent
    Buffy coat: one part blood/four parts diluent
4. Mix with 10-ml pipette or by inverting the conical.
5. Underlayer with 10–14 ml FH solution gently by letting the solution flow out of a pipette by gravity.
6. Centrifuge at room temperature with no braking at $900 \times g$ for 30 min.
7. Harvest lymphocyte interface by removing most of the plasma and diluent by aspirating or removing it with a 10-ml pipette and harvesting the lymphocytes carefully with a Pasteur pipette.
8. Combine lymphocytes from two interfaces in one conical and wash by filling the conical to 50 ml with diluent.
9. Pool all lymphocytes in one conical and wash two more times before resuspending in medium needed for the work.

Reference

Boyum, A., 1968, Isolation of mononuclear cells and granulocytes from human blood, *Scand. J. Clin. Lab. Invest.* (Suppl.) **97**:77–87.

6

Separation of Human T and Non-T Lymphocytes from Peripheral Blood

STEVEN K. H. FOUNG, STEVEN COUTRE, AND EDGAR G. ENGLEMAN

The procedures used to separate T cells from non-T cells are based on differential binding to sheep erythrocytes (SRBC). Three separate methods can be employed: (1) rosetting utilizing SRBC-absorbed fetal calf serum (abs FCS); (2) rosetting with AET-treated sheep red blood cells (AET–SRBC); or (3) rosetting with neuraminidase-treated sheep cells (NSRBC).

Materials

1. Peripheral blood mononuclear leukocytes (PBL) obtained by Ficoll–Hypaque density gradient centrifugation of fresh defibrinated blood
2. Fresh sheep red blood cells in Alsever's solution
3. Dulbecco's phosphate-buffered saline (PBS), pH 7.0–7.2
4. RPMI 1640 with 10% fetal calf serum (RPMI–FCS)
5. Ficoll–Hypaque, specific gravity 1.077
6. Red-cell-lysing reagent (ACK)
   Dissolve 0.874 g NH_4Cl, 0.1 g $KHCO_3$, and 3.67 mg EDTA in a final

STEVEN K. H. FOUNG, STEVEN COUTRE, AND EDGAR G. ENGLEMAN • Department of Pathology, Stanford University School of Medicine, Stanford University Medical Center, Stanford, California 94305.

volume of 100 ml distilled water. Adjust pH to 7.4 with 1 N NaOH. Filter sterilize through a 0.2-μm filter and store at room temperature.

7.a. Neuraminidase stock

Dissolve lyophilized neuraminidase powder in PBS to a final concentration of 1 U/ml. Filter sterilize through a 0.2-μm filter. Store in 10-ml aliquots at −20°C.

b. AET stock

Dissolve 0.402 g 2-aminoethylisothiouronium bromide hydrobromide (AET) in 10 ml distilled water (0.14 M). Adjust pH to 8.4 with 10 N NaOH. Filter sterilize through a 0.2-μm filter. Prepare fresh before use.

c. 40% SRBC-absorbed FCS–PBS

Forty milliliters of SRBC-absorbed fetal calf serum (abs FCS) and 60 ml PBS.

Methods

Preparation of NSRBCs

1. Dilute SRBCs in PBS and centrifuge at $1000 \times g$ for 10 min. Remove buffy coat and aspirate the supernatant. Repeat twice more.
2. Resuspend packed cells in RPMI 1640 to a final concentration of 5% (v/v).
3. Add 0.2 ml neuraminidase stock to 1 ml 5% SRBC.
4. Incubate for 60 min at 37°C.
5. Dilute with RPMI and wash three times as before.
6. Resuspend in RPMI to a final concentration of 5% (v/v).
7. Store at 2–8°C.

Rosetting with NSRBCs

1. Count PBLs and adjust concentration to 5×10^6 cells/ml in RPMI.
2. Add 5% NSRBCs to PBLs at a 1:3 (v/v) ratio.
3. Divide into 20-ml aliquots in 50-ml conical tubes.
4. Underlay with 10 ml Ficoll–Hypaque and incubate for 2 hr at 2–8°C.
5. Centrifuge for 30 min at $1000 \times g$.
6. Aspirate all aqueous supernatant.
7. Remove cells from nonrosetted interface, pooling two interfaces into one tube.
8. Aspirate off remaining Ficoll–Hypaque layer.

9. Add 10 ml ACK to pellet and resuspend. Upon complete hemolysis (about 1 min) flood with RPMI–FCS.
10. Wash the rosetted and nonrosetted cells separately in RPMI.

Preparation of AET–SRBCs

1. Wash SRBCs three times in PBS as per NSRBC protocol.
2. Add AET solution to packed SRBCs at a 1:4 (v/v) ratio.
3. Incubate for 10–12 min at 37°C (suspension should darken).
4. Wash three times in PBS as before.
5. Resuspend in RPMI to final concentration of 2% (v/v).
6. Store at 2–8°C.

Rosetting with AET–SRBCs

1. Count PBLs and adjust concentration to 1×10^7 cells/ml in RPMI.
2. Add 2% AET–SRBCs to PBLs at a 1:2 (v/v) ratio.
3. Divide into 10-ml aliquots in 50-ml conical tubes.
4. Centrifuge at $100 \times g$ for 10 min.
5. Incubate in an ice-water bath for 1 hr.
6. Resuspend pellets gently.
7. Underlay with 10 ml Ficoll–Hypaque and centrifuge for 30 min at 2200 rpm.
8. Proceed as per NSRBC protocol.

Preparation of Absorbed FCS (abs FCS)

1. Heat-inactivate FCS by incubating for 60 min at 56°C.
2. Wash SRBCs as per NSRBC protocol.
3. Add packed SRBCs to the FCS at a 1:2 (v/v) ratio.
4. Incubate for 60 min at 37°C.
5. Refrigerate overnight.
6. Centrifuge at $1000 \times g$ for 10 min.
7. Filter sterilize the FCS supernatant through a 0.45-μm filter followed by a 0.2-μm filter.
8. Store in 40-ml aliquots at −20°C.

Rosetting with abs FCS

1. Count PBLs and adjust concentration to 5×10^6 cells/ml in 40% abs FCS–PBS.

2. Wash SRBCs three times in PBS as per NSRBC protocol.
3. Resuspend packed cells in 40% abs FCS–PBS to 3% (v/v) final concentration.
4. Mix equal volumes of PBLs and SRBCs.
5. Divide into 20-ml aliquots in 50-ml conical tubes.
6 Underlay with 10 ml Ficoll–Hypaque and incubate in an ice-water bath for 30 min.
7. Centrifuge for 30 minutes at 1000 × g.
8. Proceed as per NSRBC protocol.

References

Neuraminidase Rosetting

Weinger, M. D. S., Bianco, C., and Nussenzweig, V., 1973, Enhanced binding of neuraminidase-treated sheep erythrocytes to human T lymphocytes, *Blood* **42:**939–946.

AET Rosetting

Madsen, M., and Johnson, H. E., 1979, A methodological study of E-rosette formation using AET-treated sheep red blood cells, *J. Immunol. Meth.* **27:**61–74.
Saxon, A., Feldhaus, J., and Robins, R. A., 1976, Single step separation of human T and B cells using AET treated sheep red cells, *J. Immunol. Meth.* **12:**285–289.

Abs FCS Rosetting

Gmelig-Meyling, F., and Ballieux, R. E., 1977, Simplified procedure for the separation of human T and non-T cells, *Vox Sang.* **33:**5–8.

7

Panning for Human T-Lymphocyte Subpopulations

STEVEN COUTRE, CLAUDIA J. BENIKE, AND EDGAR G. ENGLEMAN

Human T-lymphocyte subpopulations can be isolated based upon the expression of specific cell surface antigens by a method known as panning. Human T cells, preincubated with monoclonal antibody, are added to petri dishes coated with goat anti-mouse immunoglobulins, and only those cells recognized by the specific monoclonal antibody bind to the dishes.

Materials

1. E-rosette-positive (T) cells obtained from human peripheral blood mononuclear leukocytes
2. Affinity-purified goat anti-mouse IgG
3. Murine monoclonal antibody to human T-cell subpopulation
4. 0.05 M Tris buffer, pH 9.5
5. Dulbecco's phosphate-buffered saline (PBS), pH 7.0–7.2, with either 5% (v/v) fetal calf serum (FCS) or 1% (v/v) FCS
6. Polystyrene bacteriological-grade petri dishes, 15 × 100 mm

STEVEN COUTRE, CLAUDIA J. BENIKE, AND EDGAR G. ENGLEMAN • Department of Pathology, Stanford University School of Medicine, Stanford University Medical Center, Stanford, California 94305.

441

Method

1. Dilute the goat anti-mouse IgG to 10 μg/ml in 0.05 M Tris buffer.
2. Add 10 ml of this antibody solution to each petri dish and incubate at room temperature for 40 min. Decant and wash dish three times with PBS to remove any unbound antibody and once with 1% FCS–PBS to protein coat any sites on the dish not already occupied by antibody.
3. Dilute monoclonal anti-T cell antibody to be used to 10 μg/ml in PBS.
4. Suspend (2–3) $\times$ 10^7 T lymphocytes in 20 μg (100 lambda volume) of monoclonal antibody in a 15-ml conical tube. Incubate at room temperature for 20 min before washing twice with 1ml PBS. After final wash resuspend (2–3) $\times$ 10^7 cells in 3 ml of 5% FCS–PBS and pour into one coated petri dish. Incubate for 70 min at 2–8°C.
5. Remove the nonadherent cells by swirling the dish and decanting the supernatant. Wash the dishes gently with 5–10 ml of 1% FCS–PBS. Pool four washes with the original decantant. This represents the negatively selected population.
6. Fill a 30-ml syringe with 15–20 ml of 1% FCS–PBS and then fit with a 25 gauge needle. Dislodge adherent cells from the plate with a steady stream of fluid from the syringe. Use an inverted microscope to check plate for any remaining cells and repeat procedure if necessary. This represents the positively selected population.

Notes

1. The concentration of specific monoclonal anti-T-cell antibody used will vary depending on the affinity of the antibody.
2. With subset antibodies such as anti-Leu 2 or anti-Leu 3 the purity of the positively selected cells should routinely be greater than 96%.

Reference

Engleman, E. G., Benike, C. J., Grumet, F. C., and Evans, R. L., 1981, Activation of human T lymphocyte subsets: Helper and suppressor/cytotoxic T cells recognize and respond to distinct histocompatibility antigens, *J. Immunol.* **127**:2124–2129.

8

Human Hybridoma Tube Fusion Protocol

STEVEN K. H. FOUNG, SUSAN PERKINS,
AND EDGAR G. ENGLEMAN

Materials

1. Human lymphocytes to be immortalized
2. Hypoxanthine–aminopterin–thymidine (HAT)- or azaserine–hypoxanthine (AH)-sensitive cell line
3. Complete medium composed of high-glucose Iscove's Modified Dulbecco's Medium (IMDM, GIBCO), L-glutamine, penicillin–streptomycin, 2-mercaptoethanol, FM, and 10–20% fetal calf serum (FCS):

   a. Penicillin–streptomycin 100 ×:
      Penicillin 10,000 U/ml (GIBCO)
      Streptomycin 10,000 µg/ml (GIBCO)
   b. L-Glutamine (100×):
      29.2 mg/ml (GIBCO)
   c. FM (100×):
      0.45 g sodium pyruvate (Sigma), store at 4°C
      0.1 g bovine insulin (Sigma), store at −20°C
      1.32 g cis-oxalacetic acid (Sigma), store at −20°C
      Dissolve in 100 ml distilled water at room temperature with stir bar (approximately 1 hr). Sterile filter and store in 5-ml aliquots at −20°C (freeze–thaw one time only).

STEVEN K. H. FOUNG, SUSAN PERKINS, AND EDGAR G. ENGLEMAN • Department of Pathology, Stanford University School of Medicine, Stanford University Medical Center, Stanford, California 94305.

d. 2-Mercaptoethanol (2-ME) stock (1000×, Biorad):
In a fume hood, dilute 0.5 ml of 2-ME into 6.6 ml distilled water
and add 5 ml of dilution to 95 ml distilled water. Sterile filter and
store at −20°C in 1–2 ml aliquots. Thaw once with subsequent
storage at 4°C.

4. HAT, HT, AH, and H media
Depending on the desired selection, the following supplement
should be added to complete medium with 15–20% fetal calf
serum:

a. HT (100×):
0.0776 g thymidine (Sigma)
0.2772 g hypoxanthine (Sigma)
Dissolve in 200 ml distilled water at 70°C. Sterile filter and store
in 5-ml aliquots at −20°C.

b. Aminopterin (1000×):
0.0176 g aminopterin (Sigma)
Dissolve in 5 ml 1 N NaOH and add 40 ml distilled water. Adjust
pH to 7.0–7.3 and bring volume to 50 ml. Store in 0.5-ml aliquots
at −20°C.

c. H (100×):
0.2772 g hypoxanthine (Sigma)
Dissolve in 200 ml distilled water at 70°C. Sterile filter and store
in 5-ml aliquots at −20°C.

d. Azaserine stock:
Depending on the cell line that is used in the production of
human hybrids, between 1 and 10 μg/ml final concentration is
needed for selection. Stock solution is generally 100 × and is
made up by dissolving in distilled water and storing at −20°C in
1-ml aliquot to be thawed only once.

5. Polyethylene glycol (PEG), molecular weight 1500 (BDH Chemicals,
Poole, England)
Autoclave PEG for 15 min in liquid cycle and store at room temper-
ature.

Methods

1. Dissolve PEG at 56°C.
2. In 15-ml conical, mix 45% PEG (v/v) in IMDM without serum and
adjust pH 7.0–7.2.
3. Place in 37°C water bath.
4. Wash cells to be fused in medium without serum three times in 50-ml
conical for total cell numbers greater than 10^7. Ratio of fusion partner to normal cells is between 1:1 and 10:1.
5. To cell pellet, add 1 ml PEG solution over 1 min with slow stirring of
pellet with pipette.

6. After an additional minute at room temperature add 1 ml IMDM without serum over 30 sec; follow with 5 ml over additional 30 sec.
7. Centrifuge at 350× g for 3 min.
8. At 8 min from the start of fusion suction off supernatant and add 1 ml of complete medium with slow stirring and then add 9 ml of complete medium.
9. Centrifuge at 150× g.
10. Suction off supernatant and resuspend cells to a concentration of 10^6 cells/ml in desired selection medium.
11. For both methods of selection it is recommended that the cells be placed in HT or H medium for 24 hr prior to the addition of aminopterin or azaserine. Selection medium is generally maintained for 2–3 weeks, at which point it is then switched to the corresponding medium without aminopterin or azaserine. Generally hybrids can be seen after 2–3 weeks for human B-cell hybridomas and 3–4 weeks for human T-cell hybridomas.

Fusion with EBV-Activated Lymphocytes

Fusing procedure is as described above, with the following exceptions:

Additional materials
Ouabain stock (1000× or 10^{-3} M):

1. Dissolve 0.0584 g ouabain (Sigma) in 100 ml IMDM and store at −20°C in 1-ml aliquots.
2. Dilute 1:1000 just prior to use. Ouabain is light-sensitive, so medium must be covered with aluminum foil.

Methods

Day 1:
   After fusion, a control well of unfused EBV transformed cells should be plated in the same tray with the fused cells.
Day 2:
   Feed with HAT–ouabain-containing medium of equal volume as on day 1.
Days 3,7:
   Change medium by aspirating one-half the volume and replacing it with more HAT–ouabain medium.
Day 10:
   If cells in the EBV control well are dead, aspirate one-half the medium and feed the cells from then on with HAT. Continue with HAT for 2–3 weeks as stated previously.

9

Plate Fusion Technique for Nonadherent Cells

JAMES W. LARRICK

We have found plate fusion to be a superior method for producing human hybridomas. This protocol uses nontoxic lectins to adhere cells together.

Materials

1. Fusion plates
   Costar 3506, six-well cluster plates, 35 mm well diameter.
2. HBSS−/+
   Hank's Balanced Saline Solution, Ca^{2+}-free, 2 mM $MgSO_4$ (Sigma). Filter sterilized.
3. PNA, peanut agglutinin (Sigma) stock solution
   One hundred μg/ml, in HBSS−/+, filter sterilized.
4. PEG fusion mixture
   Polyethylene glycol 4000 (BDH Chemicals, Poole, England), 40% (w/v); DMSO, 10% (v/v) in HBSS−/+. Prior to use, pH of solution is adjusted to between 7.5 and 8.0 with sterile NaOH solution.
5. Fusion dilution mixture (FDM)
   Five percent DMSO (v/v) in HBSS−/+. Filter sterilize.
6. Appropriately stimulated PBLs
   Mitogen- or antigen-induced blasts fuse best.
7. Immortal cell line.
   Drug-marked or otherwise prepared for hybrid selection.

JAMES W. LARRICK • Cetus Immune Research Laboratories, Palo Alto, California 94303.

Methods

1. Add 1 ml of HBSS$-$/+ and 50 µl of freshly thawed PNA stock to each fusion well. Allow plates to incubate at 37°C for at least 1 hr prior to fusion.
2. Each fusion well can accommodate 10–20 million cells. If the number of available cells is limited, smaller wells can be used. The optimum fusion ratio appears to be 1:1, stimulated PBLs to "immortal" cells. Cell-line cultures should be in log phase growth.
3. Wash cells twice in HBSS$-$/+ at room temperature.
4. Resuspend and combine cell populations in HBSS$-$/+ warmed to 37°C. Add 2 ml of the suspension (10–20 million cells) to each pretreated well. For best results, do not remove the PNA coating solution.
5. Spin cells onto the plate at 400–500 × g for 6 min. Centrifuge must be at room temperature or cells will not adhere.
6. Aspirate supernatant off the monolayer.
7. Add 2 ml of warmed PEG fusion mix, 37°C, down the side of the well. Swirl once or twice.
8. After 1 min, begin dilution with FDM, 37°C. Dilute at a rate of 2 ml/min (0.5 ml every 15 sec). Constantly swirl the plate to ensure optimal mixing. Continue for 3 min (or 6 ml). Now dilute at 4 ml/min until fusion well is full. Gently pipette (up and down) a few ml of the solution in the well to facilitate mixing. Aspirate the well.
9. Add FDM, 37°C, to the well at a rate of 2 ml/min for 2 min, Always swirl the plate.
10. Over a period of 15 sec, add 5 ml of 37°C HBSS$-$/+. Swirl. Aspirate.
11. Wash plate two times with 5–10 ml warm HBSS$-$/+.
12. Add 5 ml of normal serum-supplemented medium to fusion well. Incubate at 37°C for 18 hr.
13. Remove cells from fusion well by pipetting. Use of a rubber policeman is not recommended. If cells still stick to the plate bottom, incubate in the fusion well for another day.
14. Pellet fused cells, and resuspend in selective medium (100 mM hypoxanthine and 8 µg/ml azaserine in the case of HGPRT-negative parent lines).
15. Aliquot into 96-well, flat-bottom microtiter plates (Costar) at 10^5 cells/well. Feeder layer requirement, if any, will vary with cell lines.

Notes

1. Choice of lectins used to precoat the fusion plate may vary with needs of the particular experiment. Con A, PHA, and PNA all cause cells to

adhere quite nicely. Optimal coating concentrations may differ according to cell type.
2. During fusion, always add solutions down the side of the plate. Avoid disturbing the monolayer.
3. Best mixing results by swirling the plate when it is supported on a flat, horizontal surface.
4. Optimum exposure time of the "straight" PEG fusion mixture may be decreased for more sensitive cell lines.
5. This protocol has successfully produced hybrids with U266, Jurkat, U937, and various lymphoblastoid cell lines.

References

Brahe, C., and Serra, A., 1981, A simple method for fusing human lymphocytes with rodent cells in monolayer by polyethylene glycol, *Somat. Cell Genet.* **7**:109–115.

Davidson, R. L., and Gerald, P. S., 1976, Improved techniques for the induction of mammalian cell hybridization by polyethylene glycol, *Somat. Cell Genet.* **2**:165–176.

Norwood, T. H., Ziegler, C. J., and Martin, G. M., 1976, Dimethyl sulfoxide enhances polyethylene glycol-mediated somatic cell fusion, *Somat. Cell Genet.* **2**:263–170.

O'Malley, K., and Davidson, R. L., 1977, A new dimension in suspension fusion techniques with polyethylene glycol, *Somat. Cell Genet.* **3**:441–448.

Schneiderman, S., Farber, J. L., and Baserga, R., 1979, A simple method for decreasing the toxicity of polyethylene glycol in mammalian cell hybridization, *Somat. Cell Genet.* **5**:263–269.

Sharon, J., Morrison, S. L., and Kabat, E. A., 1980, Formation of hybridoma clones in soft agarose: Effect of pH and of medium, *Somat. Cell Genet.* **6**:435–441.

10

Identification of Human Chromosomes in Mouse– Human Lymphocyte Hybrids

JIM SCHRODER

Introduction

Because of the paucity of suitable human myelomas and the limitations in the use of human lymphoblastoid cell lines for human–human hybridomas, mouse–human hybridomas have become widely used for the production of human monoclonal antibodies. As is the case with all interspecies-specific cell hybrids, mouse–human hybridomas tend to be unstable, and progressively lose most, or all, of their human chromosomes. Extinction of human antibody secretion can also occur with the chromosomes responsible for human Ig production present, but in most cases is probably the consequence of chromosome segregation. Fast and reliable methods for the identification of human chromosomes from those of the mouse parental cell line are thus of considerable value.

Chromosome Banding Methods

G-11 Banding

The fastest method for screening mouse–human hybridomas for the presence of human chromosomes is the Giemsa-11 (G-11) banding method

JIM SCHRODER • Folkhalsan Institute of Genetics, Helsinki 10, Finland.

(Bobrow and Cross, 1974). By simply staining chromosome spreads from hybridomas in Giemsa at pH 11, most human chromosomes and the mouse centromeres will stain pale blue, while certain human chromosome regions and all mouse chromosomes (all except the centromere regions) will stain dark reddish blue.

Although the basic protocol is very simple, the G-11 banding is rather tricky, and the results are not very reproducible. I will describe two protocols for G-11 banding: first the basic protocol described by Bobrow *et al.* (1972), and then a modified protocol using Giemsa components rather than whole Giemsa stain (Wyandt *et al.*, 1976).

Protocol 1

Air-dried chromosome spreads are left at room temperature for about 1 week and then stained for 10–20 min in a 2% aqueous solution of Giemsa (Gurr; Merck; Harleco) at pH 11. The pH is adjusted with NaOH. Slides are then rinsed in phosphate buffer at pH 6.8 and dried, and are ready for examination.

Protocol 2

Slides prepared as above are stained for 5–10 min at 37°C in 50 ml of an alkaline phosphate buffer (pH 11.3–11.6) containing 0.6 ml of a 1% aqueous solution of azure B (Chroma-Gesellschaft; Schmid & Co.) and 0.5 ml of a 0.25% aqueous solution of eosin Y (Difco). After staining, the slides are rinsed as above and ready for examination.

After both protocols, slides can be destained in acetic acid–ethanol and rebanded for G- or Q-banding if necessary.

The method using Giemsa components seems to give more reproducible results, and is the method of choice in my laboratory.

Hoeschst 33258 Banding

A fast and very popular method for the identification of human chromosomes in mouse–human hybrid cells is Hoechst 33258 banding. The protocol is based on the staining of metaphase spreads with the fluorescent dye Hoechst 33258 and examining the slides under a fluorescence microscope with an exitation wavelength of 365 nm and an emission wavelength of 420 nm (Hilwig and Gropp, 1972).

With this protocol, the mouse chromosomes are very easily recognizable, with brightly fluorescent centromeric regions, while the human centromeres show moderate fluorescence. With this banding method, mouse and human chromosomes also show faint Q-like bands.

Protocol

Air-dried chromosome spreads are stained in a freshly prepared solution of 0.04 µg/ml of Hoechst 33258 stain in saline for 10 min, rinsed in distilled water, and mounted in glycerol. Slides can be analyzed immediately with a fluorescence microscope, or stored in a refrigerator for a few days. This staining procedure can be successfully preceded or followed by G-banding (Kozak *et al.*, 1977).

G-Banding

The G- and Q-banding methods are more laborious for distinguishing human from mouse chromosomes. These methods will not give different colors or totally different banding patterns in mouse and human chromosomes, but on the other hand, they will give very delicate bands that allow not only distinction of human chromosomes from mouse chromosomes, but also accurate identification of individual human and mouse chromosomes.

Protocol

Air-dried chromosome preparations are stored for approximately 1 week at room temperature, incubated for 30 min in a 2× SSC (saline–sodium citrate) solution at 60°C, and rinsed in distilled water. Slides are then incubated in a 0.05% trypsin solution (in Ca- and Mg-free saline) for 1–2 min, rinsed repeatedly in saline, and stained for 20–30 min in a 2% phosphate-buffered Giemsa solution (Seabright, 1971). After rinsing the slides under running tap water, they are air-dried and mounted in mounting medium, and are ready for examination.

Q-Banding

Protocol

Air-dried chromosome preparations are stained in an aqueous solution with 0.05 mg guinacrine mustard/ml for 20 min, rinsed, and mounted in a phosphate buffer (pH 6–7) or in buffered glycerol. Slides are examined with a fluorescence microscope with an excitation of 360 nm and an emission of 510–530 nm (Caspersson et al., 1970).

Discussion

Is there any value in karyotypic studies of mouse–human hybridomas, and if so, which of these different methods should one use? The first question should undoubtedly be answered positively. Chromosome number or DNA content alone is a poor indication of the chromosome retention in a hybrid cell line. As an example, the AKR thymoma cell line BW5147 consists of several clones with different chromosome numbers. One of the most predominant clones is almost tetraploid, and another almost diploid. These compete for growth in cultures, and even upon cloning, disturbances in cell divisions will cause reappearance of clones with different chromosome numbers. The BALB/c myelomas used for antibody production are more stable and generally have a chromosome number around 63, but karyotypic variation can often be found here as well. Thus, a high chromosome number or a high DNA content can often only reflect variability in the mouse parental line, and not indicate retention of human chromosomes.

As an answer to the second question, I would suggest using a fast, simple method like G-11 or Hoechst staining for the screening of the presence of human chromosomes. Of these, Hoechst staining is more reliable but requires a fluorescence microscope, while G-11 allows detection of small translocations between mouse and human chromosomes, which can be hard or impossible to detect with the other methods.

Since the human Ig genes are located on chromosomes 2 (κ), 14 (heavy chain cluster), and 22 (λ), it is often necessary to identify all individual human and mouse chromosomes. For this, G- or Q-banding is the method of choice.

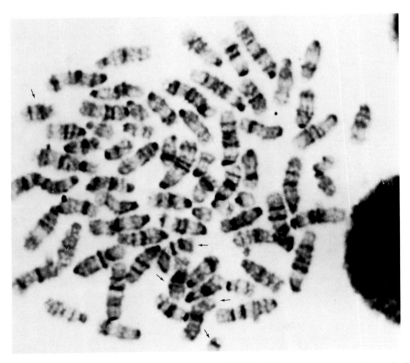

FIGURE 1. A G-banded mouse–human lymphocyte hybrid. Mouse centromeres show dark staining, while human centromeres stain lightly (arrows). (Photograph made by Dr. Heli A. Suomalainen.)

The standard technique in my laboratory is the G-banding method as described here, since it gives high-resolution banding of mouse and human chromosomes, and additionally stains the mouse, but not the human, centromeres strongly (Fig. 1).

References

Bobrow, M., and Cross, J., 1974, Differential staining of human and mouse chromosomes in interspecific cell hybrids, *Nature* **251**:77–79.

Bobrow, M., Madan, K., and Pearson, P. L., 1972, Staining of some specific regions of human chromosomes, particularly the secondary constriction of No. 9, *Nature New Biol.* **238**:122–124.

Caspersson, T., Zech, L., and Johansson, C., 1970, Differential binding of alkylating fluorochromes in human chromosomes, *Exp. Cell Res.* **60**:315–319.

Hilwig, I., and Gropp, A., 1972, Staining of constitutive heterochromatin in mammalian chromosomes with a new fluorochrome, *Exp. Cell Res.* **75**:122–126.

Kozak, C. A., Lawrence, J. B., and Ruddle, F. H., 1977, A sequential staining technique for the chromosomal analysis of interspecific mouse/hamster and mouse/human somatic cell hybrids, *Exp. Cell Res.* **105**:109–117.

Seabright, M., 1971, A rapid banding technique for human chromosomes, *Lancet* **2**:971–972.

Wyandt, H. E., Wysham, D. G., Minden, S. K., Anderson, R. S., and Hecht, F., 1976, Mechanisms of Giemsa banding of chromosomes. 1. G-11 banding with azure and eosin, *Exp. Cell Res.* **102**:85–94.

11

Epstein–Barr Virus Transformation

Andrew A. Raubitschek

Materials

1. AET–SRBC-purified B cells
2. B-958 supernatant: concentrate
   The B958 marmoset cell line produces active EBV in culture.

Preparation of EBV-Enriched Supernatant

The cell line B-958 was established by Miller *et al.* (1972) and is the most commonly used cell line to produce EBV. Supernatants are easily produced by growing the cells in T-75 flasks in 50 ml of Iscove's complete medium with 10% FCS starting at 2×10^5 cells/ml. Supernatant is harvested at 7 days and cells spun out at $200 \times g$. The supernatant is then filtered through a 0.45-μm filter and then spun at $13,000 \times g$ for 2 hr at 4°C. Supernatant is carefully aspirated and the small pellet (sometimes barely viable) containing the virus is resuspended in 1/100 of the original volume. The virus should be used immediately or frozen in liquid nitrogen; once thawed, it should be used or discarded.

Standard viral precautions should be taken, since EBV is infective for humans. In our laboratory, we do not let anyone who is seronegative work

Andrew A. Raubitschek • Cetus Immune Research Laboratories, Palo Alto, California 94303. *Present address:* Radiation Oncology Branch, National Cancer Institute, National Institutes of Health, Bethesda, Maryland 20205.

with the virus and we try to limit individuals from working with their own EBV transformants.

Transformation Method

1. PBLs are separated by standard Ficoll–Hypaque centrifugation.
2. For highest transformation efficiency, T cells are depleted by AET–SRBC rosetting.
3. After rosetting, the T-depleted population is cultured at 10^7/ml in Iscove's complete medium with 10% of EBV concentrate. Cultures are generally done in 15-ml tubes at 37°C in a water bath for 1 hr.
4. Cells are washed twice with Iscove's complete medium and then plated at 5000–50,000 cells/well in flat-bottom microtiter plates in Iscove's medium with 10% FCS.
5. Growing transformed colonies are readily visible after 1 week.

Reference

Miller, G., Shope, T., Lisro, H., Stitt, D., and Lipman, M., 1972, Epstein–Barr virus: Transformation, cytopathic changes, and viral antigens in squirrel, monkey, and marmoset leukocytes, *Proc. Natl. Acad. Sci. USA* **69**:383–387.

12

Growth of Human Cell Lines in Mice

JAMES W. LARRICK

Human–human hybridomas have been difficult to grow in mouse ascites (Truitt *et al.*, 1984; Ohlsson *et al.*, 1984). However, one group has reported that mouse–human heterohybrids grew well in nude mice (Abrams *et al.*, 1984). The lack of success probably reflects the recessive nature of genes required for true "tumorigenicity." EBV-transformed lymphoblastoid parents may have active "establishment" genes, but not true "transforming" genes. A successful, albeit laborious method to grow these cells as well as various heterohybridoma lines is described below.

Adaptation of Hybridoma Cells to Grow in Nude Mice

Five million hybridoma cells are injected subcutaneously (SC) into mice previously irradiated with a dose of 455 rad. By 4–6 weeks, solid tumors form. Mice are sacrificed, and the tumor cell mass is removed, suspended, and placed back into culture medium, supplemented with 0.1 mg/ml gentamicin sulfate (Sigma Chemical Co.).

After 2 weeks in culture, 2×10^7 SC-adapted hybridoma cells are injected intraperitoneally (ip) into irradiated (455 rad) mice that had been injected ip with 0.5 ml of pristane (tetramethylpentadecane; Aldrich, Milwaukee, Wisconsin) 2 weeks previously. Ascites fluid forms in 10–14 days and is withdrawn two or three times using a 21 gauge needle.

JAMES W. LARRICK • Cetus Immune Research Laboratories, Palo Alto, California 94303.

References

Abrams, P. G., Ochs, J. J., Giardina, S. L., Morgan, A. C., Wilburn, S. B., Wilt, A. R., Oldham, R. K., and Foon, K. A., 1984, Production of large quantities of human immunoglobulin in the ascites of athymic mice: Implication for the development of anti-human idiotype monoclonal antibodies, *J. Immunol.* **132**:1611–1613.

Ohlsson, L., Andreasen, B., Ost, A., Christensen, B., and Biberfield, P., 1984, Antibody-producing human/human hybridomas. II. Derivation and characterization of an antibody specific for human leukemia cells, *J. Exp. Med.* **159**:537–550.

Truitt, K. E., Larrick, J. W., Raubitschek, A. A., Buck, D. W., and Jacobson, S. W., 1984, Production of human monoclonal antibody in mouse ascites, *Hybridoma* **3**:195–199.

13

Methods of Large-Scale Tissue Culture

Wolf Hanisch and James W. Larrick

Introduction

There is a growing need to produce human cells and cell products in larger quantities for research and development and eventually for marketing of highly bioactive therapeutics. These products span the range from human monoclonal antibodies to lymphokines and enzymes. This chapter will outline some of the techniques available for mass culturing cells in a fashion compatible with scaleup to industrial processes, as well as for supplying the researcher sufficient quantities of cells and products for characterization of their biological properties.

A number of alternatives exist for large-scale cultivation of mammalian cells (Feder and Tolbert, 1983; Glacken *et al.*, 1983). Numerous excellent reviews cover the field (Kruse and Patterson, 1973; McLimans, 1979; Tolbert and Feder, 1983). The culture method of choice is dependent on cell characteristics and degree of sophistication desired.

Suspension Cultures

Cells that grow in suspension are perhaps the easiest to scale up. Human cells (Namalwa) are being grown in tanks as large as 4000 liters for the commercial production of human leukocyte interferons (Finter and Fantes, 1980).

Wolf Hanisch • Cetus Corporation, Emeryville, California 94608. James W. Larrick • Cetus Immune Research Laboratories, Palo Alto, California 94303.

Vessels in the range from 1 to several hundred liters are readily available for cell culture applications and numerous installations exist. The design of these installations reflects the fragility of cells and sensitivity to contamination (Acton et al., 1979; Pollard and Khosrovi, 1978; Lynn and Acton, 1975).

In concept, the cell growth reactor is no different than a standard microbial fermenter. It consists basically of a stainless steel tank, preferably electropolished (e.g., 316 SS), with an agitator to provide for mixing, mass transfer, and heat transfer and an aeration system. Variations exist where aeration alone is used for mixing and mass transfer (L. H. Engineering, U.K., air lift cell culture vessels). The air-lift design is being used successfully by Cell Tech for the commercial production of monoclonal antibodies.

In the design of these vessels, baffles are omitted and cells are agitated with propellers that set up a defined flow field which minimizes direct shear forces. Marine impellers appear to be preferred, although other designs are available. Instrumentation to regulate temperature, agitation, and gas flow control is essential. To obtain adequate scaleup data, pH, dissolved oxygen, redox, and dissolved CO_2 control will be necessary. Gas analysis for O_2 consumption/CO_2 production rates also provides valuable data. Conventional control systems are available through the suppliers of fermentation equipment (see Appendix to this chapter).

Continuous Culture

Suspension cultures readily lend themselves to operation on a continuous basis (Fazekas de St. Groth, 1983). Continuous cultivation is easily carried out by matching the nutrient input to cell growth rate and medium withdrawal rate. A complete harvest of product is obtained with every doubling of the cells over several weeks. Perhaps of greater benefit from the engineering viewpoint is that one is able to change single variables in steady state growth and evaluate their significance. It is then relatively trivial to optimize growth rate, medium, pH, dissolved oxygen, etc., in order to obtain the highest productivity.

The major drawback of suspension culture systems is that cell concentrations rarely exceed 2×10^6 cells/ml even on the richest media. Consequently, yields of product are low. For murine monoclonal antibodies, the yields are usually 10–100 μg immunoglobulin/ml, while human hybridomas generally have a yield an order of magnitude lower. Assuming that culture media often contain 1–5 mg protein/ml, this makes for significant purification problems. Perfusion culture systems avoid or minimize this problem since higher cell densities result in higher product concentration.

There are numerous variations of the perfusion technique. In concept it is simple continuously to add fresh nutrient medium while removing spent medium. The cells remain within the reactor system and perfusion culture is equally applicable to suspension and anchorage-dependent cell lines. Patterson (1976) gives a comprehensive listing of the literature on perfusion culture from its beginnings through the mid 1970s.

In its simplest configuration, the spent medium is continuously filtered out of the culture through an external filtration device such as a microporous membrane or ceramic filter (Lydersen *et al.*, 1983). This allows for removal of spent medium containing toxic metabolites, such as lactate and ammonium ions. This permits the cells to grow to higher densities (i.e., metabolite inhibition is minimized). In practice, concentrations of $(1-3) \times 10^7$ cells/ml are attainable. The yield of cells on serum also increases by a factor of up to four (Feder and Tolbert, 1983; Tolbert and Feder, 1983). There are numerous variations of perfusion systems, as follows.

Spin Filter

The spin filter system, as described by Himmelfarb *et al.* (1969) and Thayer (1973), consists of a rotating drum that is internal to the vessel and covered in a microporous filter membrane. Spent medium filters into the rotating drum and is continuously removed by a pump. The filter drum is mounted via a hollow, rotating seal arrangement and spins at a rate sufficient to remove cells from the membrane by the shear forces at the membrane surface. Tolbert *et al.* (1981; Feder and Tolbert, 1983) have scaled this system to a 40-liter vessel with full controls. Cell concentrations were around 10^7/ml with greater than 90% viability. Continuous monoclonal antibody production was demonstrated in filter perfusion systems (Lewis *et al.*, 1984).

Perfusion Culture Using Hollow Fibers

Hollow fibers have been used in cell culture in an effort to mimic normal tissue growth by supplying nutrients and removing wastes through "artificial capillaries" (Ehrlich *et al.*, 1978; Hopkinson, 1982; Knazek *et al.*, 1972; Quarles *et al.*, 1980). By forcing fresh medium through tube hollow fibers into the shell of a reactor, it is possible to continually renew the medium at a rate equal to the bleedoff of product. The hollow fiber concept is central to the cell culture method developed by Bioresponse, where fresh cow lymph fluid is perfused into a culture. Amicon Corporation is marketing a hollow fiber device (Vitafiber™) for use in cell culture. A wide variety of cell types have been grown in hollow fibers, including numerous human cells (both anchorage-dependent and suspension cultures).

The hollow fiber systems work best where the product is extracellular and has a molecular weight greater than the apparent molecular weight cutoff of the membrane. The product can then be harvested in a concentrated solution relatively uncontaminated by serum proteins.

There are, however, significant negative aspects to hollow fiber culture; it is extremely difficult to monitor, much less control, the environment within the hollow fiber reactor (Feder and Tolbert, 1983). This is an undesirable circumstance, especially where a large-scale unit needs to be on line production for weeks or months. These difficulties can be overcome by using the hollow fiber system as an adjunct to a conventional stirred reactor system (i.e., external to the reactor where culture conditions are monitored and controlled).

Hollow fiber cell culture technology is still very much in the research and development stage. Yet, it is not unlikely that future cell culture systems will rely heavily on hollow fibers.

Encapsulation

Damon Biotech has patented an elegant procedure for encapsulating a variety of mammalian cells in a poly L-lysine membrane (Jarvis and Grdina, 1983; Lim and Sun, 1980; Littlefield *et al.*, 1983). The capsules range in size from 100 to several hundred μm in diameter. The poly L-lysine membrane can be formed under conditions where the pore size is controlled to allow for diffusion of nutrients into the encapsulated cells while retaining product in the microcapsules. In essence, this is a microperfusion technique that lends itself extremely well to scaleup.

Encapsulated cells, including human–human hybridomas, grow extremely well and secrete their products into the capsules. The product can accumulate to levels of 10–50% of the total extracellular protein within the capsule. Purification of the product becomes relatively trivial at these concentrations. Of major significance is the claim that human–human hybridomas can produce monoclonals in the mg/ml range within the capsules, clearly a significant increase over conventional systems.

The encapsulation appears to work equally well on most cell types, irrespective of whether they are anchorage-dependent or not. This is a general phenomenom with perfusion culture systems.

Anchorage-Dependent Cells

The scaleup of anchorage-dependent cell cultures has, quite simply, been done by increasing the surface available for attachment of cells. A number of methods have been adopted, ranging from reactors containing multiple plates (Litwin, 1973) to bundles of tubes (Girard *et al.*, 1980). Experimental- through to production-scale equipment is commercially available. Recently, Corning developed a novel ceramic cartridge for culturing large quantities of cells in monolayer culture (Lydersen *et al.*, 1983). This system increases the available surface area for cell growth by several orders of magnitude over roller bottles in an equivalent total volume. The unit is now commercially available through K. C. Biologicals.

The majority of scaleup work of anchorage-dependent cells has been done using microcarriers. There is a vast body of literature in this field, perhaps best reviewed in a Pharmacia publication (Pharmacia, 1981). A wide variety of beads have been used as microcarriers for cell cultivation. Similarly, the list of cells grown on microcarriers is extensive. The apparent major factor affecting the success of cell cultivation in these systems is the surface chemistry of the beads (Reuveny *et al.*, 1983). Microcarriers are used extensively for large-scale production of vaccines, and special reactors have been designed for this application (Van Wezel and Van der Velden-de Groot, 1978).

The major drawback of microcarrier systems is the relatively low cell density achievable per unit culture volume (Thilly *et al.*, 1982). Microcarriers cannot be used at concentrations much above 5 mg/ml, due to excessive cell damage on impaction. Also, their size must be no less than 50 μm in diameter to facilitate adequate cell adhesion. With these constraints on the system, it is impossible to achieve much more than 2×10^6 cells/ml culture volume at confluence. The operational problems of trypsinization on a large scale, although hardly insurmountable, can be significant.

Since hybridomas can generally be coaxed into growing in suspension culture, anchorage-dependent cell cultivation systems have limited applicability to monoclonal antibody production.

Serum-Free Growth of Human Cells

The development of suitable culture media will be an important component of large-scale tissue culture. Defined, serum-free media will also be useful for reducing costs of purification. As more experience is gained with large-scale growth of mammalian cells, conventional media will undoubtedly be modified. Several widely used serum-free media for growth of human B and T cells are derived from the work of Iscove, Sato, and co-workers (Iscove and Melchers, 1978; Sato *et al.*, 1982; Uittenbogaart *et al.*, 1983; Murakami *et al.*, 1982; Kawamoto *et al.*, 1983). It is possible to purchase serum-free media tailor-made for various lymphoid cell lines from Hana Biologicals (McHugh *et al.*, 1983) and Ventrex Laboratories. The components of a serum-free medium used in our laboratories are listed in Table I. This medium supports the growth of mouse and human lymphoid cell lines and was modified from information from the literature (McHugh *et al.*, 1983; Murakami *et al.*, 1982; Chang *et al.*, 1980), as well as experience.

Appendix. Some Manufacturers of Cell Culture Equipment

Braun B. Melsungen AG, Carl Braun Strasse 1, Melsungen, Hesse D-3508, West Germany

Chemap AG, Alte Landstrasse 415, Maennedorf, Zurich 8708, Switzerland

Contact-Roesturijstaal, G. V. Ridderkerk, Holland (the Bilthoven-Unit System)

L. H. Engineering Co., Bells Hill, Stoke Poges, Bucks., England

TABLE I

Serum-Free Medium

1. Mix
   a. 500 ml RPMI 1640 (GIBCO #430-1800)
   b. 250 ml Dulbecco's Modified Engle's Medium (GIBCO #430-2100) or Iscove's DMEM
   c. 250 ml HAM's F1.2 (GIBCO #430-1700) Iscove's DMEM
2. Or use 1 l of Iscove's DMEM
3. Supplement with:
   2 mM L-glutamine
   0.01% sodium pyruvate
   15 mM HEPES (N-2-hydroxyethylpiperazine-N'-2-ethanesulfonic acid
   4 g/liter glucose
   2.2 g/liter sodium bicarbonate
   10 µg/ml human insulin
   10 µg/ml human transferrin
   10 µM 2-aminoethanol
   10 mM 2-mercaptoethanol
   1×10^{-9} M sodium selenite
   4 µg/ml oleic acid–HSA complex[a]

[a] 100 × stock prepared by adding at 25°C 20 µl of 20 mg/ml oleic acid in 100% ethanol to each ml of fatty acid-free human serum albumin (50 mg/ml in PBS, pH 7.4). Stirred overnight at 4°C, filtered, and protected from light.

L. S. L. Biolafitte, Zac des Coteaux du Belair, 78100 St. Germain en Laye, France

Marubishi Scientific Instruments, 6-6 Kitashinagawa, 3-Chome, Shinagawa, KU, Tokyo 140, Japan

New Brunswick, 44 Talmadge Road, Edison, New Jersey 08817

Versatec, 2805 Bowers Avenue, Santa Clara, California 95054

References

Acton, R. T., Barstad, P. A., and Zuerner, R. K., 1979, Propagation and scaling-up of suspension culture, *Meth. Enzymol.* **LVIII:**211–221.

Chang, T. H., Steplewski, Z., and Koprowski, H., 1980, Production of monoclonal antibodies in serum-free medium, *J. Immunol. Meth.* **39:**369–375.

Erhlich, K. C., Stewart E., and Klein, E., 1978, Artificial capillary perfusion cell culture: Metabolic studies, *In Vitro* **14:**443–450.

Fazekas de St. Groth, S., 1983, Automated production of monoclonal antibodies in a cytostat, *J. Immunol. Meth.* **57:**121–136.

Feder, J., and Tolbert, W. R., 1983, Large scale cultivation of mammalian cells, *Sci. Am.* **248:**36–43.

Finter, N. B., and Fantes, K. H., 1980, The purity and safety of interferons prepared for clinical use: The case for lymphoblastoid interferon, in: *Interferon II* (I. Gessor, ed.), Academic Press, New York, pp. 65–80.

Girard, H. C., Sutcu, M., Erden, H., and Gurhan, I., 1980, Monolayer cultures of animal cells with the cyrogen equipped with tubes, *Biotechnol. Bioeng.* **22:**477–493.

Glacken, M. W., Fleischaker, R. J., and Sinskey, A. J., 1983, Mammalian cell culture: Engineering principles and scale-up, *Trends Biotechnol.* **1:**102–108.

Himmelfarb, P., Thayer, P. S., and Martin, H. E., 1969, Spin filter culture: The propagation of mammalian cells in suspension, *Science* **164:**555–557.

Hopkinson, J., 1982, Hollow Fiber Cell Culture: A Sleeping Giant Awakening, Amicon Literature, Amicon Corp., Lexington, Massachusetts.

Iscove, N. N., and Melchers, 1978, Complete replacement of serum by albumin, transferrin, and soybean lipid in cultures of lipopolysaccharide-reactive B lymphocytes, *J. Exp. Med.* **147:**923–933.

Jarvis, A. P., and Grdina, T. A., 1983, Production of biologicals from microencapsulated living cells, *Bio Techniques* **1:**24–27.

Kawamoto, T., Sato, J. D., Lo, A., McClure, D. B., and Sato, G. H., 1983, Development of a serum-free medium for growth of NS-1 mouse myeloma cells and its application to the isolation of NS-1 hybridomas, *Anal. Biochem.* **130:**445–453.

Knazek, R. A., Gullino, P. M., Kohler, P. O., and Dedrick, R. L., 1972, Cell culture on artificial capillaries: An approach to tissue culture *in vitro*, *Science* **178:**65–67.

Kruse, P. F., Jr., and Patterson, M. K. Jr., (eds.), *Tissue Culture, Methods and Applications,* Volume XXVII, Academic Press, New York, pp. 283–363.

Lewis, C., Tolbert, W. R., and Feder, J., 1984, Large scale perfusion culture system for production of monoclonal antibodies, presented at Hybridoma Conference, San Diego, California.

Lim, F., and Sun, A., 1980, Microencapsulated islets of bioartificial endocrine pancreas, *Science* **210:**908–910.

Littlefield, S. G., Gilligan, K. J., and Jarvis, A. P., 1983, Growth and monoclonal antibody production from rat × mouse hybridomas: A comparison of microcapsule culture with conventional suspension culture, presented at Hybridoma Conference, San Diego, California.

Litwin, J., 1973, Titanium disks, in: *Tissue Culture Methods and Applications* (P. F. Kruse, Jr., and M. K. Patterson, Jr., eds.), Academic Press, New York, Chapter 5.

Lydersen, B. K., Pugh, G. G., Duncan, E. C., Overman, K. T., Johnson, D. M., and Sharma, B. P., 1983, Novel ceramic material for large scale cell culture, presented at Tissue Culture Association, 34th Annual Meeting, Orlando, Florida, June 12–16.

Lynn, J. D., and Acton, R. T., 1975, Design of a large scale mammalian cell suspension culture facility, *Biotechnol. Bioeng.* **XVII:**659–673.

McHugh, Y. E., Walthall, B. J., and Steimer, K. S., 1983, Serum-free growth of murine and human lymphoid and hybridoma cell lines, *Biotechniques* **1:**72–77.

McLimans, W. F., 1979, Mass culture of mammalian cells, *Meth. Enzymol.* **LVIII:**194–211.

Murakami, H., Masui, H., Sato, G. H., Sueoka, N., Chow, T. P., and Kano-Sueoka, T., 1982, Growth of hybridoma cells in serum-free medium: Ethanolamine is an essential component, *Proc. Natl. Acad. Sci. USA* **79:**1158–1162.

Patterson, N. K., Jr., 1976, Perfusion and mass culture systems, *Tiss. Culture Assoc. Manual* **4:**243–249.

Pharmacia, 1981, *Microcarrier Cell Culture: Principles and Methods,* Pharmacia Fine Chemicals AB, Uppsala, Sweden.

Pollard, R., and Khosrovi, B., 1978, Reactor design for fermentation of fragile tissue cells, *Process Biochem.* **1978:**31–37.

Quarles, J. M., Morris, N. G., and Leibovitz, A., 1980, Carcinoembryonic antigen production by human colorectal adenocarcinoma cells in matrix-perfusion culture, *In Vitro* **16:**113–118.

Reuveny, S., Mizrahi, A., Kotler, M., and Freeman, A., 1983, Factors affecting cell attachment, spreading and growth on derivatized microcarriers. I. Establishment of working system and effect of the type of the amino-charged groups, *Biotechnol. Bioeng.* **25:**469–480; Introduction of hydrophobic elements, *Biotechnol. Bioeng.* **25:**2969–2981.

Sato, G., Pardee, A. B., and Sirbasku, D. A. (eds.), 1982, *Growth of Cells in Hormonally Defined Media,* Parts A, B, Cold Spring Harbor Laboratory, Cold Spring Harbor, New York.

Thayer, P. S., 1973, Spin filter device for suspension cultures, in: *Tissue Culture, Methods and*

Applications (P. F. Kruse, Jr. and M. K. Patterson, Jr., eds.), Academic Press, New York, pp. 345–351.

Thilly, W. G., Barngrover, D., and Thomas, J. N., 1982, Microcarriers and the problem of high cell density culture, in: From Gene to Protein: Translation into Biotechnology (F. Ahmad, J. Schultz, E. E. Smith, and W. I. Whelan, eds.), Academic Press, New York, pp. 75–103.

Tolbert, W. R., and Feder, J., 1983, Large scale cell culture technology, *Annu. Rep. Fermentation Processes* **6:**35–74.

Tolbert, W. R., Feder, J., and Kimes, R. C., 1981, Large scale rotating filter perfusion systems for high density growth of mammalian suspension cultures, *In Vitro* **17:**885–890.

Uittenbogaart, C. H., Cantor, Y., and Fahey, J. L., 1983. Growth of human malignant lymphoid cell lines in serum-free medium, *In Vitro* **19:**67–72.

Van Wezel, A. L., and Van der Velden-de Groot, C. A. M., 1978, Large scale cultivation of animal cells in microcarrier culture, *Process Biochem.* **1978:**6–8.

14

In Vitro Stimulation of Human B Lymphocytes

MICHAEL K. HOFFMANN AND JOHN A. HIRST

Materials

Salt Solutions

1. Balanced salt solution (BSS)
   a. Stock 1 (10×):
      Add to 100 ml H_2O

      10 g dextrose
      0.6 g KH_2PO_4
      3.58 g $Na_2HPO_4 \cdot 7H_2O$
      20 ml 0.5% phenol red solution

   b. Stock 2 (10×):
      Add to 100 ml H_2O

      1.86 g $CaCl_2 \cdot 2H_2O$
      4.0 g KCl
      80.0 g NaCl
      1.04 g $MgCl_2$ anhydrous (or 1.0 g $MgCl_2 \cdot 6H_2O$)
      2.0 g $MgSO_4 \cdot 7H_2O$

   Prepare 1× solution by adding 100 ml stock 1 to 800 ml H_2O, add 100 ml stock 2. Use double-distilled water. Sterilize by membrane filtration.

MICHAEL K. HOFFMANN AND JOHN A. HIRST • Memorial Sloan-Kettering Cancer Center, New York, New York 10021.

2. Culture medium

> Eagle's Minimal Essential Medium (Microbiological Associates, MA, no. 12-126) or RPMI, 91 ml
> Glutamine, 200 mM (MA, no. 17-605F), 1 ml
> Nonessential amino acids 100× (MA, no. 13 -114), 1 ml
> Sodium pyruvate, 100 mM (MA, no. 13-115), 1 ml
> 2-Mercaptoethanol 5 mM (filter sterilized daily), 1 ml
> Fetal calf serum, 5 ml

3. Nutritional cocktail for daily feeding

> Essential amino acids 50× (MA, no. 13-606), 5 ml
> Nonessential amino acids (MA, no. 13-14), 2.5 ml
> Glutamine, 200 mM (MA, no. 17-605F), 2.5 ml
> Dextrose, 500 mg
> Fetal calf serum, 27.5 ml
> Minimal Essential Medium without $NaHCO_3$ (GIBCO, no. 109S), 35 ml

Sera

Fetal Calf Serum

Fetal calf serum (FCS) is commercially available from many companies. Originally Mishell and Dutton (1967) had found that 85% of the tested batches were unsatisfactory. The inclusion of 2-mercaptoethanol increased the frequency of FCS batches active in lymphocyte cultures. Presently, and with our culture system, we found that only 14% of tested batches were unsatisfactory, but pretesting is recommended to select the most active batches.

Human Serum

Batches of human serum (HS) may also vary in supportive activity and we recommend that HS be screened prior to use. Blood group type is irrelevant in our experience and we have not found heat inactivation necessary. Absorption of HS with SRBCs is important, however, to remove naturally occurring anti-SRBC antibody. This antibody can have two undesirable effects: (1) anti-SRBC antibody may inhibit immunization against SRBCs, and (2) anti-SRBC antibody can lead to the occurrence of pseudoplaques in the hemolytic plaque assay (Muchmore *et al.*, 1976). For absorption we mix 50 ml HS with 2 ml packed SRBCs, incubate for 10 min on ice, and spin for 10 min at 2500 rpm in a refrigerated centrifuge. It should be noted that absorbed HS contains immunogenic, solubilized SRBCs and is therefore unsuitable for control experiments in which SRBC specificity is tested.

Antigens and Mitogens

The culture system described here has been established with heterologous red blood cells as antigens. The system is suitable for *in vitro* antibody production to red blood cell-bound haptens such as the trinitrophenyl (TNP) group. We have also generated antibody to influenza virus (M. K. Hoffmann and J. A. Hirst, unpublished results) and others have successfully immunized PBM suspensions against tetanus toxoid (E. DeFreitas, personal communication) using this culture method.

We make it a practice to use blood from a single sheep, since this helps to avoid hazy plaques in the plaque assay.

Heat-inactivated, formalin-fixed *Staphylococcus aureus* Cowan I (SAC) strain bacteria [described to be exclusively a B-cell mitogen (24) are commercially available (Pansorbia, Calbiochem-Shering Corp., California, no. 507858).

Incubation Boxes

To establish an atmosphere of 7% O_2, 10% CO_2, and balance N_2, the culture dishes are placed in air-tight boxes and gassed with this mixture at low flow rate for 30 sec (Mishell and Dutton, 1967). Use of this gas mixture may not be essential, since other investigators have reported success using 5% CO_2 in air. Boxes made from Lucite are commercially available (Biotec, CH-4121, Shoenenbuch, Switzerland).

Procedures

Preparation of Human Lymphoid Cell Suspensions

Blood from human donors is collected in heparin (50 U/ml), diluted with an equal volume of balanced salt solution or serum-free culture medium, and layered over 15 ml of Ficoll–Hypaque (Lymphoprep, Nyegaard, Oslo, Norway) in 50-cm³ centrifuge tubes not exceeding a total volume of 45 cm³. Tubes are centrifuged for 30 min at 400 × *g* at room temperature. PBMs are collected from the interface, washed twice with serum-free culture medium, and resuspended in culture medium. Tonsil cells are prepared by cutting tonsils in half with a hot scalpel blade and teasing single-cell suspensions from the cut surface in serum-free medium. Spleen cells are prepared by mechanically dissociating sterile pieces of human spleen. It is helpful to isolate mononuclear tonsil and spleen cells by centrifugation over Ficoll–Hypaque.

References

Falkoff, R. J. M., Zhu, L. P., and Fauci, A. S., 1982, Separate signals for human B cell proliferation and differentiation in response to *Staphylococcus aureus:* Evidence for a two-signal model of B cell activation, *J. Immunol.* **129:**97–102.

Fauci, A. S., Lane, H. C., and Volkman, D. J., 1983, Activation and regulation of human immune responses: Implications in normal and diseased states, *Ann. Intern. Med.* **99:**61–75.

Lane, H. C., Volkman, D. J., Whalen, G., and Fauci, A. S., 1982, *In vitro* antigen-induced, antigen-specific antibody production in man, *J. Exp. Med.* **154:**1043–1057.

Misiti, J., and Waldmann, T. A., 1981, *In vitro* generation of antigen-specific hemolytic plaque-forming cells from human peripheral blood mononuclear cells, *J. Exp. Med.* **154:**1069–1078.

Stevens, R., Macy, E., Morrow, C., and Saxon, A., 1979, Characterization of a circulating subpopulation of spontaneous anti-tetanus toxoid antibody producing B cells following *in vivo* booster immunization, *J. Immunol.* **122:**1503–1508.

16
Soft Agar Cloning Protocol

JAMES W. LARRICK, ANDREW A. RAUBITSCHEK,
AND GEORGE SENYK

Materials

1. Sea Plaque agarose (FMC Corporation, Marine Colloids Division, Rockland, Maine 04841)
2. Costar or Falcon 60-mm tissue culture dishes
3. Cloning medium
   Iscove's Dulbecco's MEM with high glucose (4.5 g/liter) supplemented with:

   a. Glutamine (2mM) (freshly prepared)
   b. Ten percent NCTC 109 (Microbiological Associates)
   c. Twenty percent fetal bovine serum (prescreened for capacity to support clonal growth of various cell lines)

   d. OPI: Prepare oxaloacetate pyruvate insulin:
      0.15 mg/ml oxaloacetate acetate (Sigma)
      0.05 mg/ml pyruvate (Sigma)
      0.2 U/ml bovine insulin (Sigma) as a $50\times$ stock and store frozen in plastic bottles

   e. 2-Mercaptoethanol: final concentration, 5×10^{-5} M)

JAMES W. LARRICK, ANDREW A. RAUBITSCHEK, AND GEORGE SENYK • Cetus Immune Research Laboratories, Palo Alto, California 94303. *Present address for* A. A. R.: Radiation Oncology Branch, National Cancer Institute, National Institutes of Health, Bethesda, Maryland 20205.

Methods

1. Forty milligrams of agarose into 5 ml dH_2O to make a 10× agarose solution. This solution is autoclaved and stored at room temperature.
2. Conditioned medium is added to melted agarose to prepare the supporting bed for soft agar cloning. Four milliliters of the 0.4% melted agarose is added to each 60-mm culture dish. They are cooled for 7 min at 4°C, then placed in a 37°C CO_2 incubator until needed.
3. Cells (usually 500–2000/dish) are mixed in 1 ml of agarose adjusted to the proper concentration (usually 0.31–0.36%) and placed over the supporting base of agar. The agarose is cooled for 7 min in a 4°C cooler.

Reference

Civin, C. I., and Banqueriga, M. L., 1983, Rapid, efficient cloning of murine hybridoma cells in low gelation temperature agarose, *J. Immunol. Meth.* **61**:1–8.

17
Cloning by Limiting Dilution

STEVEN K. H. FOUNG AND SUSAN PERKINS

Media

Cells should be cloned in the medium in which they are currently growing, with or without a feeder layer (e.g., irradiated mouse spleen cells, human embryonic lung fibroblasts, human red cells, or human mononuclear cells).

Methods

1. Count cells to be cloned. Two sequential dilutions are usually needed to achieve a low cell concentration for cloning. The number of cells per well to be plated depends on the growth characteristics of the cell. Ideally, one should clone at a concentration of 0.5 cells/well in 100 lambda of medium to maximize the likelihood of achieving mono-clonality. Plate cells in multiple 96-well, flat-bottom trays (Linbro) using the 60 inner wells only and with medium in the outer wells to maintain humidity.
2. The cells should be fed on day 5 and subsequently every 3–5 days.

STEVEN K. H. FOUNG AND SUSAN PERKINS • Department of Pathology, Stanford University School of Medicine, Stanford University Medical Center, Stanford, California 94305.

18
Reverse Plaque Assay

JAMES W. LARRICK, ANDREW A. RAUBITSCHEK,
AND GEORGE SENYK

The purpose of this technique is to determine the frequency of immunoglobulin-producing lymphocytes.

Materials

1. Staph protein A (Zymed):
   Five mg/10 ml in sodium chloride should be filtered, aliquoted, and
   stored ($-70°C$).
2. SRBCs:
   Washed 4–5 times with normal saline.
3. $CrCl_3$ molecular weight: 158)
   Used 4 mg/ml in water and prepared new each day.
4. Tissue culture medium
   Iscove's DMEM (IDMEM) or RPMI 1640
5. Lymphoytes or cell lines to be plaqued are washed once in Iscove's
   prior to use
6. Antiserum
   Rabbit antiserum (DAKO, affinity-purified) against human heavy
   and/or light chains is diluted in saline or Iscove's
7. Complement
   Guinea pig complement is absorbed with SRBCs at 4°C and diluted in
   saline or Iscove's

JAMES W. LARRICK, ANDREW A. RAUBITSCHEK, AND GEORGE SENYK • Cetus Immune Research
Laboratories, Palo Alto, California 94303. *Present address for* A. A. R.: Radiation Oncology Branch,
National Cancer Institute, National Institutes of Health, Bethesda, Maryland 20205.

Method

All reagents should be sterile filtered:

1. To 1 ml of packed SRBCs add 1 ml protein A with gentle mixing. This is followed by addition of 10 ml chromic chloride diluted 1:100 (with sodium chloride) just prior to the procedure. This mixture is rotated at 37°C for 45 min and washed four times with normal saline. A 10% solution in saline or in 10% IDMEM is prepared for use or in Alsever's solution for storage. Cells can be used for 1 month.
2. To 2 ml of lymphocyte suspension (10^4/ml) add 100 µl of 10% protein A–SRBC. Mix and dispense 100 µl/microtiter well.
3. Centrifuge microtiter plate 50 × g for 20 min, then at 200 × g for 5 min.
4. Incubate at 37°C for 1 hr.
5. Add 10 µl of 1:20 dilution of the appropriate anti-human serum.
6. Incubate for 1 hr at 37°C.
7. Add 10 µl of guinea pig complement, diluted 1:4.
8. Incubate 1 hr at 37°C.
9. Count plaques. If plaques are incomplete, continue incubation for 1–2 hr at 37°C and if necessary overnight at 4°C.

References

Gronowicz, E., Coutinho, A., and Melchers, F., 1976, A plaque assay for all cells secreting Ig of a given type or class, *Eur. J. Immunol.* **6:**588–594.

Pang, G. T. M., Gatman, M., Drummond, J. M., and Booth, R. J., 1981, A sensitive micromethod for measuring human reverse plaque hemolytic PFCs, *J. Immunol. Meth.* **40:**253–260.

Shimizu, K., Hirano, A., and Kunii, A., 1980, A plaque assay to enumerate circulating immunoglobulin secreting cells of each type of the different immunoglobulin classes, *Blood* **56:**199–202.

19
Assay of Interleukin 1 (IL-1)

James W. Larrick

Standard Thymocyte Assay

Principle

C3H/HEJ (low-LPS-responder) murine thymocytes will proliferate in the presence of submitogenic concentrations of PHA if IL-1 is present (Oppenheim *et al.*, 1980).

Materials

1. 6-Thioguanine-resistant LBRM cells
2. IL-2-dependent HT-2 cells
3. Ninety-six-well Costar flat-bottom plates
4. Iscove's medium supplemented with 10% fetal calf serum, 2 mM glutamine (Iscove's complete)
5. Phytohemagglutinin (PHA-P) (Burroughs Wellcome)
6. Hypoxanthine (Sigma) $100\times = 40$ mM
7. Azaserine (Sigma) $100\times = 500$ µg/ml
8. [^{3}H]Thymidine (NEN, 50 µCi/ml)
9. Scintillation vials, scintillation fluid, and beta-emitter counter

Method

1. Four- to six-week-old C3H/HEJ mice are sacrificed by CO_2 asphyxiation.

James W. Larrick • Cetus Immune Research Laboratories, Palo Alto, California 94303.

2. Thymus' are removed and thymocytes are teased free of connective tissue.
3. Cells are washed two times in warm Iscove's DMEM supplemented with 10% FCS, 2 mM glutamine, and 5×10^{-5} M 2-mercaptoethanol, and resuspended at 5×10^6/ml.
4. One hundred microliters of cells is placed in flat-bottom microtiter plates.
5. Burroughs Wellcome PHA-P is added at a final concentration determined to be one dilution below that which produces [³H]thymidine incorporation. This is usually 0.5–2.0 μg/ml final concentration.
6. One hundred microliters of unknowns and positive and negative control supernatants is added to the thymocytes.
7. The cells are pulsed for 4–6 hr with 0.5–1.0 μCi of [³H]thymidine on day 3.
8. Cells are harvested on glass fiber filter paper and processed as described for the IL-2 assay (Chapter 20).

The number of IL-1 units in an unknown is derived from the reciprocal of the dilution giving 50% of the maximum thymocyte [³H]thymidine incorporation.

One-Day Cell Line Assay

Principle

Interleukin 1 and suboptimal concentrations of PHA cause LBRM cells to secrete interleukin 2 (Conlon, 1983). Mitogenesis of IL-2-dependent HT-2 cells is measured. Because both types of cell are present in the same medium and the baseline growth rate of LBRM cells is high, the LBRM cells must be killed before HT-2 growth can be measured. This is accomplished by using a 6-thioguanine-resistant LBRM cell line (Larrick *et al.*, 1985).

Method

1. Fifty thousand LBRM cells and PHA-P (at optimal concentration) are added to flat-bottom, 96-well tissue culture plates in 100 μl of Iscove's medium.
2. One hundred microliters of unknowns and standards is added to the wells.
3. Cells are cultured 4–8 hr prior to the addition of 10^4 HT-2 cells in 50 μl of Iscove's medium.

4. On the following morning the cultures are fed with $100 \times$ hypoxanthine and azaserine.

5. In the afternoon, the cells are pulsed with [^{3}H]thymidine for 4 hr and harvested and counted as described above.

References

Conlan, P. J., 1983, A rapid biologic assay for the detection of interleukin 1, *J. Immunol.* **131:** 1280–1282.

Larrick, J. W., Brindley, L., Doyle, M. U., 1985, An improved assay for the detection of interleukin 1. *J. Immunol. Methods* In press.

Oppenheim, J. J., Togawa, A., Chedid, L., and Mizel, S., 1980, Components of mycobacteria and muramyl dipeptide with adjuvant activity induce lymphocyte activating, *Cell. Immunol.* **50:**71–81.

20
Assay of Interleukin 2 (IL-2)

JAMES W. LARRICK

Principle

An IL-2-addicted mouse T-cell line is cultured overnight in the presence of unknown or IL-2-containing medium (Gillis and Smith, 1977; Gillis et al., 1978). Thymidine incorporation is measured.

Method

Cell line HT-2 or CTLL (Gillis and Smith, 1977) is cultured in 5–10 U/ml of IL-2. Typically cells are washed and resuspended at 5×10^4 cells/ml in Iscove's DMEM supplemented with IL-2, 10% fetal calf serum, 2 mM glutamine, and 5×10^{-5} M 2-mercaptoethanol (freshly prepared every 3–4 days). Prior to assay, cells are washed two times in warm medium and resuspended at 10^5 cells/ml. One hundred microliters of cells is aliquoted into flat-bottom microtiter plates (COSTAR), and 100 μl of IL-2-containing medium, control medium, or unknown is added for 24 hr. During the final 5–6 hr of culture 0.5–1 μCi [³H]thymidine is added. Wells are harvested onto glass fiber filter paper using a Skatron or Cambridge Technology microtiter cell harvester.

Dried filter paper discs are placed in scintillation vials (Wheaton Scientific) with scintillation fluid (Scintiverse; Fisher Scientific Co.) and counted on a β-emitter counter.

Standardized units of IL-2 are just becoming available as recombinant IL-2 is purified. Conceptually, the number of units of IL-2 in an unknown is

JAMES W. LARRICK • Cetus Immune Research Laboratories, Palo Alto, California 94303.

the reciprocal of the dilution giving 50% of the maximum thymidine incorporation. Alternately, recombinant IL-2 has $(3-5) \times 10^6$ U/mg of protein.

References

Gillis, S., and Smith, K. A., 1977, Long-term culture of tumor-specific cytotoxic T cells, *Nature* **168**:154–155.
Gillis, S., Ferm, M., Ou, W., and Smith, K., 1978, T cell growth factor: Parameters of production and a quantitative microassay for activity, *J. Immunol.* **120**:2027–2031.

21

Assay of B-Cell Growth and Differentiation Factors

JAMES W. LARRICK AND ANDREW A. RAUBITSCHEK

Principle

Highly purified B cells are stimulated by anti-immunoglobulin to proliferate (B-cell growth factor; BCGF) or differentiate into immunoglobulin-secreting cells (PFCs) (B-cell differentiation factor; BCDF).

Materials

1. Ficoll–Hypaque-purified peripheral mononuclear cells (see Appendix, Chapter 5)
2. AET-treated sheep red blood cells (see Methods appendix, Chapter 6)
3. Plastic tissue culture flasks coated with human AB serum (e.g., 10 ml/150-cm² flask for 30 min at 37°C
4. Anti-μ antibody: the F(ab′)$_2$ fragment of goat anti-human heavy-chain-specific IgM (Cappel Laboratories)
5. Tritiated thymidine (New England Nuclear)
6. Cell harvester
7. *Staphylococcus aureus* (Bethesda Research Labs) washed and treated with 2-mercaptoethanol as described in supplier's literature.

JAMES W. LARRICK AND ANDREW A. RAUBITSCHEK • Cetus Immune Research Laboratories, Palo Alto, California 94303. *Present address for* A. A. R.: Radiation Oncology Branch, National Cancer Institute, National Institutes of Health, Bethesda, Maryland 20205.

Method

Purification of B Cells

1. Ficoll–Hypaque-purified peripheral blood mononuclear cells (see Appendix, Chapter 5) are twice rosetted with AET-treated sheep red blood cells (see Appendix, Chapter 6).
2. Monocytes are depleted by adhering 100×10^6 T-cell depleted-cells to human AB serum-coated tissue flasks for 1 hr at 37°C.

B-Cell Growth Factor Assay

1. Purified B cells are cultured in 200 μl of Iscove's DMEM with 10% FCS, 5×10^{-5} M 2-mercaptoethanol, 2 mM glutamine in flat-bottom, 96-well microtiter plates. Standard cell density is 1×10^5 cells/well.
2. Anti-μ antibody is added at a concentration of 10–20 μg/ml; the concentration of antibody giving the best signal must be determined for each lot of antibody.
3. Various concentrations of B-cell growth factors are added to the anti-μ-stimulated B cells.
4. B cells are cultured for 72 hr at 37°C in a CO_2 incubator.
5. During the final 4–6 hr of culture, cells are pulsed with 0.5–1.0 μCi of [^{3}H]thymidine.
6. Cells are harvested on a standard cell harvester on glass fiber filter paper. Paper discs are added to scintillation vials with scintillation fluid and counted in a liquid scintillation counter.

B-Cell Differentiation Assay

1. B cells are purified as described above.
2. Cells are cultured for 48–72 hr with 0.02% *Staphylococcus aureus* Cowan I bacteria in the culture medium described above.
3. For the final 72 hr of culture, various concentrations of B-cell differentiation factors are added.
4. On day 5 or 6 of culture, cells are washed and prepared for reverse plaque assay as described in Appendix, Chapter 18.

References

Hirano, T., Teranishi, T., and Onoue, K., 1984, Human helper T cell factor(s): III. Characterization of B cell differentiation factor I (BCDFI), *J. Immunol.* **132**:229–234.

Muraguchi, A., and Fauci, A. S., 1982, Proliferative responses of normal human B lymphocytes. Development of an assay system for human B cell growth factor (BCGF), *J. Immunol.* **129:**1104–1108.

Muraguchi, A., Buter, J. L., Kehrl, J. H., and Fauci, A. S., 1983, Differential sensitivity of human B cell subsets to activation signals delivered by anti-u antibody and proliferative signals delivered by a monoclonal B cell growth factor, *J. Exp. Med.* **157:**530–546.

22
Indirect Immunoglobulin ELISA Protocol

James W. Larrick and Andrew A. Raubitschek

Purpose

To detect human IgG, IgM, and κ and λ light chains by specific ELISA inhibition assay.

Materials

1. 50 mM NaHCO$_3$, pH 9.5
2. Wash buffer
   PBS with Ca^{2+} and Mg^{2+}, 0.1% Tween 20, pH 7.2. Do not add sodium azide preservative.
3. Dilution buffer
   Wash buffer with 1% BSA.
4. Substrate buffer
   a. 0.650 g/liter sodium phosphate, monobasic, monohydrate
   b. 0.736 g/liter sodium phosphate, dibasic, anhydrous
   c. 0.036 g/liter disodium EDTA, dihydrate; add water to 1000 ml, pH 5.95
5. Ninety-six-well Immulon I or II plates (Dynatech)

___

James W. Larrick and Andrew A. Raubitschek • Cetus Immune Research Laboratories, Palo Alto, California 94303. *Present address for* A. A. R.: Radiation Oncology Branch, National Cancer Institute, National Institutes of Health, Bethesda, Maryland 20205.

Method

1. Coat plates with 5 μg/ml human IgG(κ,λ) or 5 μg/ml human IgM in 50 mM $NaHCO_3$, pH 9.5, at 50 μl/well, 37°C, 1 hr, or overnight at 4°C.
2. Wash 1: Wash buffer.
3. Block plates with dilution buffer, 200 μl/well, 37°C, 1 hr.
4. Wash 2: Wash buffer.
5. Inhibition:
   a. One hundred microliters of supernatant or control.
   b. One hundred microliters of HRPase-conjugated anti-human reagent.

   Note: Remember that the addition of b constitutes a twofold dilution of these reagents. Peroxidase reagents must be added *after* supernatants are put in wells, 37°C, 1 hr.
6. Wash 3: Wash buffer.
7. Substrates:
   a. 5-Amino salicylic acid, 1 mg/ml in substrate buffer. H_2O_2,50 μl/100 ml substrate buffer.
   b. ABTS: 2,2-azino-di(3-ethylbenzthiazoline sulfonic acid).
8. Read: After plate has developed a good contrast of light and dark wells, on Titertek Multiscan, 450-nm filter.

Reference

Smart, I. J., and Koh, L. Y., 1983, Competitive inhibition enzyme immunoassays for the measurement of human IgG, IgA, and IgM, *J. Immunol. Meth.* **60:**329–339.

23

Purification of Human Immunoglobulins

James W. Larrick, Brian M. Fendly, and Janet Wang

We have used all of the protocols described below for the purification of mouse, rat, and human monoclonal antibodies. However, all of the protocols do not necessarily work for a given monoclonal antibody; therefore, investigators need to tailor the protocol to each monoclonal antibody.

Ammonium Sulfate Precipitation

Immunoglobulins precipitate in 40% saturated ammonium sulfate. Most monoclonals can be partially purified from culture medium or ascites by this technique. Antibodies can also be stored in this form at 4°C without loss of activity.

Materials

1. The solubility of ammonium sulfate is 103.4 g/100 g water at 100°C and 70.6 g/100 g water at 0°C
2. Ammonium hydroxide is used to adjust pH

James W. Larrick, Brian M. Fendly and Janet Wang • Cetus Immune Research Laboratories, Palo Alto, California 94303.

Method

1. Prepare a saturated solution of ammonium sulfate (SAS) by adding crystals.
2. Adjust the pH to 7.4 using ammonium hydroxide.
3. To precipitate antibodies, simply stir the SAS solution into the ascites or culture fluid until 40% saturation is reached. Precipitate will form after overnight storage at 0°C.
4. The precipitate can be stored free from bacterial growth in the 40% SAS at refrigerator temperatures.
5. To reconstitute the precipitated antibodies, the 40% SAS slurry is pelleted in a microfuge ($10,000 \times g$ for 5 min) and the precipitate is dissolved with a small amount of water. The antibodies are then exhaustively dialyzed against an appropriate buffer to remove any remaining ammonium ions and to prepare for further purification or use.
6. If the volume of fluid from which one wants to precipitate the antibodies is large, one can calculate the quantity of ammonium sulfate required to give 40% saturation. Crystals are gradually added to the antibody solution with gentle stirring at room temperature with appropriate adjustment of the pH to 7.4 with ammonium hydroxide.

Euglobulin Precipitation of IgM Monoclonal Antibodies

1. Human IgM antibodies precipitate at low ionic strength. Although many retain their activity if they are precipitated by dialysis vs. water, others require a higher ionic strength to be recovered in active form. Therefore, a series' buffers of gradually increasing ionic strengths should be tried to see which gives the best recovery of antibody activity.
2. The solution containing the IgM monoclonal is dialyzed in the cold vs. water or an appropriate low-ionic-strength buffer.
3. The precipitate is pelleted in a microfuge ($10,000 \times g$ for 5 min) and resuspended in phosphate-buffered saline, pH 7.4.

Gel Filtration Chromatography, DEAE Chromatography, Concanavalin A Chromatography, Protein A Affinity Chromatography

We have found the technical literature provided by Pharmacia (Piscataway, New Jersey 08854) to be a very useful source of information for column chromatography techniques. We have used Con A affinity chromatography and gel filtration chromatography to partially purify human IgM monoclonal antibodies and have found DEAE and protein A affinity chromatography to be useful for human IgG monoclonals.

Hydroxylapatite Chromatography

Reagents

1. 500 mM Monobasic sodium phosphate.
2. 500 mM Dibasic sodium phosphate.
3. Phosphate solutions: Titrate reagent 2 with reagent 1 to desired pH and make dilutions to desired concentration.
4. 200 mM phosphate pH 6.8 for washing.
5. Hydroxylapatite HTP from Bio-Rad.

Procedure:

1. Measure the volume of culture supernatant to be purified and determine the amount of HTP needed. A ratio of 300 ml supernatant to a gram of HTP is a good starting point.
2. Wash HTP with 100 mM phosphate twice according to manufacturer's instruction except letting the HTP settle for 5 min before removing the fine particles.
3. Add solid Dibasic phosphate to the culture supernatant to a concentration of 49 mM and Monobasic to 51 mM. pH should be between 6.7 and 7.0.
4. In batch operation: mix the buffered supernatant and washed HTP and incubate at 37° with gentle shaking for an hour or more. Let HTP settle overnight at 4°C. Remove the supernatant.
5. In column operation: pack the washed HTP into a column so that the ratio of height/diameter is within 2 to maintain a good flow property. Wash the column with 20 volumes of binding buffer before loading buffered supernatant.
6. Wash the bound HTP with 200 mM phosphate until no more protein is detected in the wash buffer.
7. Elute antibody with the phosphate of appropriate concentration and pH.

8. Dialyze the eluate or load it onto a desalting column to remove the excess salt.

Remarks:

1. For each human Mab a preliminary test should be carried out to determine the optimal eluting phosphate concentration and pH by running a small HTP column and eluting with a phosphate gradient.
2. The human Mab purified through one step elution is approximately 60 to 80% pure in our laboratory. IgG's elute at lower phosphate concentration than IgM; therefore, a lower concentration of phosphate buffer (<100 mM) should be used to wash off the contaminating proteins.

References

Stanker, L. H., Vanderlaau, M., and Juarez-Salinas, H., 1985, One-step purification of mouse monoclonal antibodies from ascites fluid by hydroxylapatite chromatography, *J. Immunol. Meth.* **76:**157–169.

Juarez-Salinas, H., Engelhorn, S. C., Bigbee, W. L., Lowry, M. A., and Stanker, L. H., 1984, Ultrapurification of monoclonal antibodies by high-performance hydroxylapatite (HPHT) chromatography, *Biotechniques* **May/June:**164–169.

Sampson, I. A., Hodgen, A. N., and Arthur, I. H., 1984, The separation of immunoglobulin M from human serum by fast protein liquid chromatography, *J. Immunol. Meth.* **69:**9–15.

24

A Nitrocellulose Strip Method for Isotyping Monoclonal Antibodies

DAVID B. RING, ROSY SHENG-DONG, AND TONY CHAN

Introduction

The immunoglobulin subclass of monoclonal antibodies is often determined by Ouchterlony diffusion or by microtiter plate EIA methods. The first method is slow and requires concentrated antibody, while the second method is also somewhat slow and typically requires that plates be precoated with specific antigen. We have found that nitrocellulose strips spotted with isotype-specific sera allow a convenient solid-phase assay for isotype determination. No specific antigen is required, less than 1 ml of hybridoma supernatant is needed, and the procedure requires about 2 hr if prespotted nitrocellulose strips are used.

Materials

1. Nitrocellulose sheets
   Schleicher and Schuell or BioRad: batches vary in their ability to be wet by applied droplets of antisera, and a batch that gives rapid, even absorption should be chosen.

DAVID B. RING, ROSY SHENG-DONG, AND TONY CHAN • Cetus Immune Research Laboratories, Palo Alto, California 94303.

2. Subclass-specific polyclonal antisera to immunoglobulin light and heavy chains
   We have used Litton Bionetics rabbit antisera to mouse κ, λ, α, γ1, γ2a, γ2b, γ3, and μ chains. DAKO has anti-human isotype-specific mouse monoclonal antibodies.
3. Phosphate-buffered saline containing 1% (w/v) bovine serum albumin (PBS/BSA)
4. Rabbit and anti-mouse–horseradish peroxidase conjugate (Zymed) diluted 1:200 in PBS–BSA
5. Fifty mM Tris–HCl, pH 7.6 (Tris buffer)
6. Tris buffer containing 0.03% diaminobenzidine and 0.05% hydrogen peroxide

Method

1. A grid of 5-mm squares is lightly drawn in pencil on the nitrocellulose sheet and 1-ml droplets of antiisotype sera are applied so that each row of squares receives one spot of each heavy and light chain reagent. The sheet is incubated 1 hr at room temperature in a moist chamber, rinsed quickly in PBS–BSA, and left overnight in PBS–BSA at 4°C. Strips are cut apart with a scissors and may be stored at 4°C in PBS–BSA containing 0.02% sodium azide. Alternatively, strips may be air-dried and stored desiccated at 4°C.
2. A series of small tubes is prepared containing 3 ml hybridoma culture supernatant or supernatant diluted with PBS–BSA. We find that 1:10 dilutions are generally successful and that some supernatants can be diluted as much as 1:200. A nitrocellulose strip is incubated in each tube for 1 hr at room temperature.
3. The strips are rinsed three times in PBS–BSA.
4. The strips are incubated for 1 hr at room temperature in diluted rabbit anti-mouse–horseradish peroxidase.
5. The strips are rinsed twice in PBS–BSA and twice in Tris buffer.
6. The strips are placed in Tris buffer containing diaminobenzidine and hydrogen peroxide until sufficient color develops on the anti-isotype spots (usually 3–4 min).

When this method was compared with a commercial EIA isotyping kit on 21 mouse monoclonal antibodies, the methods agreed on heavy chain type for 19 of 21 cases, and on light chain type for all cases. The two conflicts were resolved in favor of the strip method based on electrophoretic mobility of labeled antibody heavy chains (μ and α, both of which had typed as γ1 by EIA). With some antibodies, staining of more than one heavy chain spot is observed. We have attributed this to inadequate subclass specificity of the polyclonal sera spotted on the strips, or in one case to contamination of an antiisotype serum with a specific antigen recognized by certain monoclonal antibodies that were tested. Selection of the darkest staining heavy chain spot has generally yielded the right isotype (as confirmed by EIA and gel electrophoresis), but this will depend on the quality of anti-isotype sera.

Reference

McDougal, J. S., Browning, S. W., Kennedy, S., and Moore, D. D., 1983, Immunodot assay for determining the isotype and light chain type of murine monoclonal antibodies in unconcentrated hybridoma culture supernates, *J. Immunol. Meth.* **63:**281–290.

25

Immunoprecipitation of Antigens Using Polystyrene Balls

David B. Ring and Jeffrey A. Kassel

Introduction

Antigens recognized by monoclonal antibodies are often identified by immunoprecipitation procedures using fixed *Staphylococcus aureus* cells as an immunoadsorbent. While such methods work well in many cases, centrifugation and resuspension of the staphylococcal cells is tedious and time-consuming. If a monoclonal antibody does not bind staphylococcal protein A, a second polyclonal antibody must be employed to aid immunoprecipitation, and both the staphylococcal cells and second antibody tend to adsorb labeled proteins nonspecifically, leading to background in the final autoradiogram. If purified monoclonal antibody is available, an alternate immunoprecipitation method can be based on large polystyrene beads covalently coated with antibody. This method offers handling convenience and the advantage that several monoclonal antibodies can be simultaneously exposed to the total amount of labeled antigens in a target cell extract.

Materials

1. Eight-millimeter-diameter polystyrene balls (Precision Plastic Ball Co.)

David B. Ring and Jeffrey A. Kassel • Cetus Immune Research Laboratories, Palo Alto, California 94303.

2. Nitric Acid
3. Glacial acetic acid
4. Sodium dithionite
5. Sodium hydroxide
6. Suberic acid
7. Dimethylformamide
8. 1-Ethyl-3-(3-dimethylaminopropyl) carbodiimide· HCl (EDAC; Pierce)
9. Two-tenths molar 2[N-1morpholino] ethanesulfonic acid, pH 6.0 (MES buffer)
10. One percent (v/v) Triton X-100, 150 mM NaCl, 5 mM EDTA, 25 mM Tris–HCl, pH 7.5 (solubilization buffer)
11. Solubilization buffer containing 50 mg/ml bovine serum albumin (BSA)
12. Phosphate-buffered saline (PBS), pH 7.2
13. Laemmli SDS gel sample buffer

Method

Preparation of Modified Polystyrene Balls

1. Cover balls with 10% fuming nitric acid in glacial acetic acid. Incubate 3 hr in 50°C water bath.
2. Rinse three times with distilled water.
3. Cover with 1% sodium dithionite in 0.1 M NaOH. Incubate 3 hr in 50°C water bath.
4. Rinse three times with distilled water.
5. Cover with 0.1% EDAC, 0.2% suberic acid (suberic acid dissolved in dimethylformamide). Incubate overnight at room temperature.
6. Rinse three times with distilled water. Store in distilled water at 4°C until needed.

Covalent Linkage of Antibodies to Balls

7. Dilute purified monoclonal antibodies to 0.2 mg/ml in MES buffer.
8. Mark modified balls with a diamond scribe to distinguish balls bearing different antibodies.
9. Place balls in individual tubes and cover with 450 μl diluted antibody. Add 50 μl fresh 1% EDAC to each tube and cap. Incubate 24 hr at room temperature.

10. Rinse balls twice with PBS. May be stored several days at 4°C before use.

Immunoprecipitation

11. Prepare freshly labeled target cell extract. We have used several human breast cancer cell lines labeled with ^{125}I by the lactoperoxidase method or with ^{35}S by growth in [^{35}S]methionine. The solubilization buffer listed can probably be varied considerably.
12. In a small flask or 50-ml tube mix four parts labeled extract with one part solubilization buffer–BSA to give a final concentration of 10 mg/ml BSA. Add balls coated with monoclonal antibodies and incubate 4 hr on ice, shaking.
13. Pipette labeled antigen from vessel and rinse balls four times with solubilization buffer.
14. Place balls in individual tubes with 100 μl SDS gel sample buffer. Incubate 3 min in boiling water bath. Remove balls and run samples on gel.
15. Stain and dry gel, and autoradiograph as desired.

One advantage of this method is that ten or more monoclonal antibodies on separate marked balls can be exposed simultaneously to a preparation of labeled antigen. If the antibodies recognize different antigens, each will have access to several times more antigen than if the labeled preparation were divided into a number of aliquots for immunoprecipitation using staphylococcal cells. On the other hand, if many antibodies are expected to recognize the same antigen and the quantity of antigen is limiting, the method may be unfairly biased toward antibodies with higher affinity. We have found that the ball method gives very clean backgrounds, except for a complex of three polypeptides in the 50,000- to 60,000-dalton range. These proteins bind to balls coated with some, but not all, antibodies (and not to control beads uncoated with antibody). The 10 mg/ml BSA included in the immunoprecipitation is partly effective in blocking the nonspecific binding.

26

Immunostaining Using Monoclonal Antibodies

FRANK TRINGALE, SYLVIA T. HSIEH-MA, AND AUDREY M. EATON

Monoclonal antibodies are often evaluated for binding to normal tissues or tumors using immunoperoxidase or immunofluorescence techniques on frozen or paraffin sections. The use of frozen sections avoids exposure of antigens to the high temperatures and prolonged fixation used in paraffin tissue processing. Depending on the antigen in question, this exposure may decrease or eliminate its reactivity. On the other hand, paraffin sections generally have better cellular preservation than frozen sections. In addition, paraffin blocks are easily stored and may be retrieved from files for retrospective studies.

Immunohistochemical staining of mouse monoclonal antibodies against human tissue is performed by a two-stage indirect method. Mouse monoclonal antibodies to human antigens are added first, followed by peroxidase-conjugated goat anti-mouse Ig, which is then reacted with diaminobenzidine or followed by FITC-conjugated goat anti-mouse immunoglobulin. When evaluating human monoclonals against human tissue, the developing antibodies will obviously create high background staining by binding to endogenous human immunoglobulin in the tissue section. To avoid this problem, the monoclonal antibody is labeled directly with biotin, horseradish peroxidase, FITC, DNP, etc. (Hsu, 1981; Wilchek, 1984).

To avoid direct labeling of monoclonal antibodies it is possible to block human immunoglobulin by treating the sections with hetero-anti-human Ig prior to staining. The section is then stained indirectly by first adding anti-

---

FRANK TRINGALE, SYLVIA T. HSIEH-MA, AND AUDREY M. EATON • Cetus Immune Research Laboratories, Palo Alto, California 94303.

human monoclonal antibody, followed by FITC-labeled goat anti-human Ig or peroxidase-conjugated goat anti-human Ig and diaminobenzidine.

Because endogenous biotin may be present in normal tissues (Wood, 1981), it may be necessary to block it prior to immunohistochemical staining. The tissue is pretreated with avidin, followed by biotin to block the remaining binding sites on the avidin.

Materials

1. Microscopic slides
2. Albumin fixative (Fisher Scientific)
3. OCT compound (Lab Tek)
4. Cryomolds, 25 × 20 × 5 mm (Lab Tek)
5. Brass object holders (Lab Tek)
6. Microtome/cryostat
7. Acetone
8. Humidity control chamber
9. Normal goat or horse serum
10. Avidin D–horseradish peroxidase (Vector Laboratories)
11. Avidin D–FITC (Vector)
12. 3,3'-Diaminobenzidine (DAB) (Sigma)
13. PBS
14. Hydrogen peroxide 30%
15. Tris buffer, pH 7.0
16. Cover glass, 24 × 40 mm
17. Gills hematoxylin # 1 (Fisher Scientific)
18. Pro-texx mounting medium (Scientific Products)
19. Aqua-mount (Scientific Products)
20. Negative control medium RPMI 1640 with 10% fetal bovine serum with 0.1% sodium azide
21. Saran Wrap
22. Zip-loc bags

Methods

Tissue Sectioning. Frozen Sections

1. Cut fresh tissue into pieces that fit into cryomolds.
2. Fill cryomolds with OCT compound and orient tissue to the bottom of the cryomold.

Cells can be used unfixed or fixed with acetone, formaldehyde, paraformaldehyde, methanol, etc., before staining. For acetone fixation, fix cells with cold acetone for 60 sec in chamber before staining and omit formaldehyde fixation, step 9.

Biotin-conjugated monoclonal antibodies can also be evaluated in either an indirect immunofluorescent or an immunoperoxidase procedure. These methods can be used only on cell lines that do not have endogenous biotin. In the indirect immunofluorescent assay, avidin–FITC will be used as the second step antibody. In the immunoperoxidase method, avidin–peroxidase will be the second step reagent and diaminobenzadine is used as the substrate.

Eight-chamber slides provide increased ease of handling and the convenience of staining up to eight monoclonal antibodies on one chamber slide without cross-contamination. After staining, the plastic gasket can be easily removed and the slide mounted for microscopic observation. We have found that coating the chamber slide with laminin improves the adhesion of cells from 10 to 90% for human breast carcinoma cell lines MDA-MB-231, MDA-MB-157, and ALAB. We have found that coating with fibronectin greatly enhances the attachment of human fibroblast cell lines CC-95 (fetal foreskin) and WI-38 (fetal lung) and normal human breast cell lines HBL-100. Fibronectin also enhances the attachment of human breast carcinoma cell lines BT-549 and ALAB. Optimal concentrations of laminin or fibronectin may vary for different cell lines. Background staining due to the laminin or fibronectin coating is negligible.

References

Carlsson, R., Engvall, E., Freeman, A., and Ruoslahti, E., 1981, Laminin and fibronectin in cell adhesion: Enhanced adhesion of cells from regenerating liver to laminin, *Proc. Natl. Acad. Sci. USA* **78**:2403–2406.

Darmon, M., 1982, Laminin provides a better substrate than fibronectin for attachment, growth and differentiation of embryonal carcinoma cells, *In Vitro* **18**:997–1003.

Hsu, S., Raine, L., and Fanger, H., 1981, Use of avidin–biotin–peroxidase complex (ABC) in immunoperoxidase techniques, *J. Histochem. Cytochem.* **29**:577–580.

Johansson, S., Kjellen, L., Hook, M., and Timpl, R., 1981, Substrate adhesion of rat hepatocytes: A comparison of laminin and fibronectin as attachment proteins, *J. Cell Biol.* **90**:260–264.

Kawamura, Jr., A. (ed.), 1977, *Fluorescent Antibody Techniques and Their Applications*, University Park Press, Baltimore.

Kleinman, H. K., McGoodwin, E. B., Rennard, S. I., and Martin, G. R., 1979, Preparation of collagen substrates for cell attachment: Effect of collagen concentration and phosphate buffer, *Anal. Biochem.* **94**:308–312.

Marty, J., Kjeldsberg, C. R., and Groo, S., 1982, Improved immunoperoxidase stain on frozen sections: An avidin biotin peroxidase complex (ABC) technique, *J. Histotech.* **5**:61–64.

Sternberger, L. A., 1979, *Immunocytochemistry*, Wiley, New York.

Terranova, V. P., Rohrback, D. H., and Martin, G. R., 1980, Role of laminin in the attachment of PAM212 (epithelial) cells to basement membrane collagen, *Cell* **22**:719–726.

Wilchek, M., and Bayer, E. A., 1984, The avidin–biotin complex in immunology, *Immunol. Today* **5:**39–43.

Wood, G. S., and Warnke, R., 1981, Suppression of endogenous avidin–binding activity in tissues and its relevance to biotin–avidin detection systems, *J. Histochem. Cytochem.* **29:**1196–1204.

Yamada, K. M., and Olden, K.. 1978, Fibronectins—Adhesive glycoproteins of cell surface and blood, *Nature* **275:**179–184.

27
Immunoblotting

JANET WANG AND JAMES W. LARRICK

Introduction

The development of techniques for transblotting DNA to nitrocellulose paper by Southern (1975) led other investigators to transfer RNA and proteins to an immobilizing matrix. Towbin *et al.* (1979) reported a procedure for electrotransferring *E. coli* ribosomal proteins from polyacrylamide gel to nitrocellulose sheets followed by the immunologic detection of these proteins by specific antibody. In the past 5 years, the technique has been widely used for the detection of specific antigens in complex cellular lysates. By using radioactive protein A or a second "developer" antibody, Burnette (1981) and Howe and Hershey (1981) reported improved sensitivity in detecting antigens in cellular lysates. Gershoni and Palade (1983) have recently reviewed protein blotting and have gathered an extensive list of references. The following procedure of immunoblotting is used routinely in our laboratory.

Materials

1. Slab gel electrophoresis unit
    We have units from BioRad, Hoefer, and LKB. The designs of these units are basically the same.
2. Power supply
    All the above three suppliers carry power supplies for electrophoresis. A power supply with regulated ranges of 0–2000 V

JANET WANG AND JAMES W. LARRICK • Cetus Immune Research Laboratories, Palo Alto, California 94303.

and 0–300 mA can be used for both electrophoresis and
transblotting.
3. Cooling bath
   This is optional. An overnight electrophoresis at lower current is
   satisfactory. However, electrophoresis operated at refrigerated
   temperature (5–15°C) and elevated current (30–60 mA per slab
   gel) may be completed within 1.5–2.5 hr.
4. Electroblotting unit
   We use the unit from BioRad. It consists of a buffer chamber, gel
   holder, sponge pads, and/or Scotch Brite pads and cooling coil.
5. Staining boxes
   Plastic food containers from most stores can be used for either
   staining or developing blots.
6. Sample buffer
   A 5× reducing sample buffer consists of 50 mM Tris–HCl, pH
   8.3, 5 mM EDTA, 5% SDS, 25% mercaptoethanol, 50% glycerol,
   and 5% of 0.5% pyronin Y as tracing dye. Omit mercaptoethanol
   for nonreducing sample buffer.
7. Polyacrylamide gels
   Use only electrophoresis-grade chemicals for the gels. Stock solutions of 4× gel buffers and 30:0.8% acrylamide:Bisacrylamide are
   made in 500-ml batches and stored at 4°C. Ten percent ammonium persulfate solution is made fresh weekly and stored at
   4°C.
   a. 4× Separating buffer: 1.5 M Tris–HCl, pH 8.8
   b. 4× Stacking buffer: 0.5 Tris–HCl, pH 6.8
   c. Separating gel: 15 ml per 0.75 mm
   Ten percent slab gel mixture consists of 3.75 ml 4× separation
   buffer, 4.88 ml acrylamide: Bis, 35 μl ammonium persulfate, and 5
   μl TEMED as polymerization catalyst. Double the amount of
   acrylamide:Bis and reduce ammonium persulfate to 10 μl for 20%
   gel.
   d. Stacking gel: A 4.5% stacking gel consists of 1.5 ml
      acrylamide:Bis, 2.5 ml 4× stacking buffer, 100 μl ammonium
      persulfate, 50 μl of 10% SDS, and 10 μl TEMED
   A 10-ml stacking gel is adequate for two 0.75–mm slab gels.
8. Gel electrophoresis buffer
   Six grams Tris base, 28.8 g glycine, and 2 g of SDS per liter. The
   pH should be about 8.3 without adjustment. Make 10 liters at a
   time.
9. Nitrocellulose paper
   BA83, 0.20-mm paper from Schleicher and Schull.
10. Transblotting buffer
    Twenty percent (v/v) methanol, 25 mM Tris, and 192 mM glycine,
    pH 8.3. A 10× Tris–glycine stock solution is prepared and the 1×
    buffer is usually made fresh before each use.

11. Blotting filter paper

    #470 Schleicher and Schull 8 × 12 in. is cut into halves and used to increase the close contact of the gel and nitrocellulose paper.

12. PBS–phosphate buffer saline

    Eight grams/liter NaCl, 0.2 g/liter KCl, 0.275 g/liter KH_2PO_4, 1.15 g/liter Na_2HPO_4.

13. BSA–PBS

    One percent BSA in PBS.

14. Antibody

    Culture supernatant containing the antibody of interest is often used without dilution. Ascites can be diluted in BSA–PBS up to 1000 times. For purified antibody a 10 μg/ml concentration is used.

15. Developer–conjugate

    Peroxidase conjugated to rabbit anti-human immunoglobulin (Zymed) is routinely used in dilutions of 1:500–1:1000 in BSA–PBS.

16. Substrate for developer

    Five one-hundredths percent 3,3′-diaminobenzidine–4HCl in 50 mM Tris–HCl, pH 7.0, and 20 μl H_2O_2 (30%) per 100 ml.

Method

Gel Electrophoresis

1. Prepare 0.75–1.5 mm slab gel and stacking gel.
2. Dissolve 5–10 μg of antigen in either reducing or nonreducing sample buffer, and boil the contents in a water bath for 5 min.
3. Set power supply at 30 mA per slab gel and run the gel at 10°C until the dye front reaches ~2–3 cm from the edge of the gel. It takes 1.5–2.5 hr for completion under these conditions.

Transblotting

4. Prewet nitrocellulose sheets cut to the size of the gel in transblotting buffer.
5. Soak the electrophoresed gel in transblotting buffer while prewetting pads and filter papers with the same buffer.
6. Sandwich the gel and one or two sheets of prewetted nitrocellulose paper between a sheet of filter paper and a Scotch-Brite pad or a

sponge pad on each side within the gel holder. Care must be taken to remove air bubbles between the gel and nitrocellulose.

7. Insert the gel holder, with the nitrocellulose side facing the cathode, into the slot in the transblotting chamber filled with buffer.
8. Perform transblotting at 40 V overnight with 15°C cooling water circulating through the cooling coil.

Immunodevelopping the Blots

9. Remove the blot from the gel holder and block it with 100 ml BSA–PBS at room temperature for 1 hr. Stain the transblotted gel if desired.
10. Wash the blot once with PBS and repeat with two 5-min washings.
11. Incubate the blot with 50 ml of culture supernatant containing antibody of interest or with 50 ml of purified antibody in BSA–PBS. The time needed for incubation varies with the affinity of the antibody for its specific antigen. One hour at room temperature is sufficient for high-affinity antibodies. However, overnight or longer incubation in the cold room may be necessary for low-affinity binders or low antibody concentrations.
12. Wash the blot with PBS as in step 10.
13. Add 50 ml of developer–conjugate and incubate at room temperature for 1 hr.
14. Wash with PBS as before.
15. Add 100 ml substrate to the blot with gentle shaking until a slight increase in the background of the blot appears.
16. Discard the substrate and wash the blot twice with H_2O. Dry the developed blots between paper towels and let dry at room temperature.
17. The Coomassie blue staining technique of Laemmli (1970) (for gels) and of Burnette (1981) (for blots) is used to visualize antigen patterns on the electrophoresed gel or undeveloped blot.

References

Burnette, W. N., 1981, Western blotting: Electrophoretic transfer of proteins from sodium dodecyl sulfate–polyacrylamide gels to unmodified nitrocellulose and radiographic detection with antibody and radioiodinated protein A, *Anal. Biochem.* **112:**195–203.
Gershoni, J. M., and Palade, G. E., 1983, Protein blotting: Principles and applications, *Anal. Biochem.* **131:**1–15.
Howe, J. G., and Hershey, J. W. B., 1981, A sensitive immunoblotting method for measuring protein synthesis initiation factor levels in lysates of *Escherichia coli, J. Biol. Chem.* **256:**12836–12839.

Laemmli, U. K., 1970, Cleavage of structural proteins during assembly of the head of bacterio-
    phage T4, *Nature* **227**:680–685.
Southern, E. M., 1975, Detection of specific sequences among DNA fragments separated by gel
    electrophoresis, *J. Mol. Biol.* **99**:503–517.
Towbin, H., Staehelin, T., and Gordon, J., 1979, Electrophoretic transfer of proteins from
    polyacrylamide gels to nitrocellulose sheets: Procedure and some applications, *Proc. Natl.
    Acad. Sci. USA* **76**:4350–4354.

Manufacturers and Distributors

A useful general reference is *Linscott's Directory of Immunological and Biological Reagents* (40 Glen Drive, Mill Valley, California 94941).

Accurate Chemical & Scientific Corporation, 300 Shames Drive, Westbury, New York 11590; 516-433-4900, 800-645-7227

Aldrich Chemical Company, 940 W. St. Paul Avenue, Milwaukee, Wisconsin 53201; 414-273-3850

Amersham Corporation, 2636 S. Clearbrook Drive, Arlington Heights, Illinois 60005; 312-593-6300, 800-323-9750

Amicon Corporation, Scientific Systems Division, 25 Hartwell Avenue, Lexington, Massachusetts 02173; 617-861-9600

Astra Pharmaceutical Products, 50 Otis Street, Westboro, Massachusetts 01581; 617-852-6351

J. T. Baker Chemical Company, 222 Red School Lane, Phillipsburg, New Jersey 08865; 201-859-2151

BBL, Division of Becton–Dickenson and Company, Cockeysville, Maryland 21030; 301-666-0100

Beckman Instruments, Clinical Instruments Division, 2400–2500 Harbor Boulevard, Fullerton, California 92634; 714-871-4848

Beckman Instruments, Scientific Instruments Division, Campus Drive and Jamboree Boulevard, Irvine, California 92713; 714-833-0751

Becton-Dickinson FACs Systems, 506 Clyde Avenue, Mountain View, California 94043; 415-968-7744

Becton-Dickinson Immunodiagnostics, (formerly Schwartz/Mann), Mountain View Avenue, Orangeburg, New York 10962; 914-359-2700, 800-431-1237

Behring Diagnostics, P.O. Box 12087, San Diego, California 92112; 800-854-9256

Index

517